# RESPONDING TO THE HOMELESS
## Policy and Practice

# TOPICS IN SOCIAL PSYCHIATRY

Series Editor: Ellen L. Bassuk, M.D.

*The Better Homes Foundation*
*Newton Centre, Massachusetts*
*and Harvard Medical School*
*Boston, Massachusetts*

---

---

A Continuation Order Plan is available for this series. A continuation order will bring delivery of each new volume immediately upon publication. Volumes are billed only upon actual shipment. For further information please contact the publisher.

# RESPONDING TO THE HOMELESS
## Policy and Practice

## Russell K. Schutt, Ph.D.
*University of Massachusetts at Boston*
*and Harvard Medical School*
*Boston, Massachusetts*

and

## Gerald R. Garrett, Ph.D.
*University of Massachusetts at Boston*
*Boston, Massachusetts*

*With contributions by*

**Barbara A. Blakeney, R.N.**
*Boston City Hospital*
*Boston, Massachusetts*

**Stephen M. Goldfinger, M.D.**
*Massachusetts Mental Health Center*
*Harvard Medical School*
*Boston, Massachusetts*

**Elise Kline, Ed.D.**
*Long Island Shelter*
*Boston, Massachusetts*

**Ezra Susser, M.D.**
*Nathan Kline Institute*
*Orangeburg, New York*

**Friedner D. Wittman, Ph.D.**
*CLEW Associates*
*Berkeley, California*

PLENUM PRESS  •  NEW YORK AND LONDON

Library of Congress Cataloging-in-Publication Data

Schutt, Russell K.
    Responding to the homeless : policy and practice / Russell K.
Schutt and Gerald R. Garrett ; with contributions by Barbara A.
Blakeney ... [et al.].
        p.   cm. -- (Topics in social psychiatry)
    Includes bibliographical references and index.
    ISBN 0-306-44076-8
    1. Homeless persons--Services for--United States.  2. Homeless
persons--Government policy--United States.  3. Homeless persons-
-Medical care--United States.  4. Homeless persons--Mental health
services--United States.  5. Social work with the homeless--United
States.   I. Garrett, Gerald R.   II. Blakeney, Barabara A.
III. Title.  IV. Series.
    [DNLM: 1. Health Policy--United States.  2. Health Services-
-United States.  3. Homeless Persons--United States.  4. Social
Problems--United States.   WA 300 S396r]
HV4505.S38   1992
362.5'8'0973--dc20
DNLM/DLC
for Library of Congress                                    92-3455
                                                              CIP

ISBN 0-306-44076-8

©1992 Plenum Press, New York
A Division of Plenum Publishing Corporation
233 Spring Street, New York, N.Y. 10013

Printed in the United States of America

*To Ruth Eisaman Schutt and Pearl Odessa Garrett*

# Foreword

*Responding to the Homeless: Policy and Practice* is largely a product of a unique collaboration between Russell K. Schutt and Gerald R. Garrett and their Boston community. As such, it offers a rich perspective on the problem of homelessness that is derived from the authors' shared experience with researchers, academics, students, providers, policymakers, and homeless persons themselves.

Schutt and Garrett take the reader into the shelters and acquaint him or her with the philosophical and practical dilemmas facing line workers as well as policymakers. They also take the reader into the community to better understand the housing market and the dysfunctional continuities among shelter, housing, treatment, and social supports. There are sensitive discussions of the salient health problems that too commonly touch the lives of homeless individuals, such as substance abuse and AIDS. The volume also includes clear descriptions of the sometimes elusive processes of counseling and case management for homeless individuals. The sidebars of "what to do" and "what not to do" contain useful information that will both inform and empower individuals who are working on the front lines, and inspire and prepare future caregivers.

While the eminently readable organization and style of the book are suggestive of a highly practical handbook on the basics of homelessness, the authors and their contributors have also produced a scholarly volume that is replete with current research findings, programs descriptions, case studies, and vignettes. The authors draw upon history, experiences, and empirical data to produce a reference work that will be useful for a wide audience of readers over time.

The book appropriately underscores the complexity of the daunting social problem that homelessness is. It describes the diversity of the homeless population, the multineed nature of homeless persons, and the multiple causes and pathways leading to homelessness for any given individual. The authors devote substantial discussion and detail to each of these topics and utilize their own varied perspectives to acquaint readers with a range of relevant issues. The chapters focused on homelessness when complicated by severe mental illness and substance abuse are excellent.

*Responding to the Homeless* is likely to be a source of insight for all those who simply wish to better understand the realities of homelessness in the United States. This volume accurately portrays the complicated interaction between homeless individuals, their helpers, and the social context—and, in so doing, compels action.

IRENE S. LEVINE, Ph.D.
*Director, Office of Programs for the*
*Homeless Mentally Ill*
*National Institute of Mental Health\**
*Washington, D.C.*

---

*The opinions expressed in this Foreword are those of the author and do not necessarily reflect the official policies or positions of NIMH.

# Preface

The number of Americans who were bereft of lodging and sustenance became too large to escape recognition in the early 1980s. Coming after 30 years of postwar prosperity and a decade of urban revitalization, the tragic circumstances of homeless persons captured the attention of reporters and commentators across the nation. Abject poverty cast long shadows across a prosperous landscape.

Although most cities offered a few missions, emergency shelters, or short-term benefits for homeless persons, the growing number of such persons soon overwhelmed the capacity of existing resources. Cities began to expand their emergency shelters, sometimes only after lawsuits, and private charities and churches began to focus their attention and resources on the needs of homeless persons. Citizen advocacy groups and coordinating committees were formed across the nation, adding a new voice to those who were redefining and responding to the problem of homelessness. The federal government began to complement state and local efforts with special programs to aid homeless persons.

Working in an atmosphere of crisis, often imbued with missionary zeal, those individuals who sought initially to help homeless persons created a wide array of emergency shelters, soup kitchens, and drop-in centers. Many of these individuals pressured governments and charities to increase housing opportunities, to expand emergency bed capacity, and to mobilize a wide array of resources to eliminate homelessness entirely.

But homelessness did not diminish; rather, tragically, it seemed to increase through much of the 1980s. Many emergency shelters found that they were serving the same homeless persons for months, and then for years. As a result, these shelters began to reexamine their goals: How should care be provided for those who were ill or infirm? What should be done to help shelter users who were addicted to alcohol or drugs? What about serious mental illness? Could shelters themselves develop sites for permanent housing?

These questions were answered in different ways by different shelters, stimulated in part by variations in preference between local and state governments, and by changing federal programs. But service options for homeless persons increased, contacts with service agencies multiplied, and the service delivery role of shelters expanded. Professional training and service experience began to complement motivation and a willingness to work irregular hours as qualifications for shelter staff.

Early surveys of homeless persons revealed diverse backgrounds and needs. Now, research findings required translation into programmatic initiatives to alleviate suffering resulting from physical and mental illness, substance abuse, and family disruption. Many shelters began to assess their guests' needs, to connect guests to service agencies, and to train their staff members, all the while continuing to meet emergency survival and health needs.

The origins of this book are to be found in this same process of change in the mission of shelters. In 1984, Dr. Schutt responded to a request by Boston's Long Island Shelter for assistance with computerizing their case records in order to describe more adequately the service needs of their guests. Graduate students in a computer applications course adopted this request as a class project and began the process of coding, analyzing, and refining intake data collected by the shelter's case managers.

This class project led to more ambitious plans. Based on Dr. Schutt's work with the computer class, Dr. Schutt and Dr. Garrett, who was building on his research with Howard Bahr on homeless persons a decade earlier, collaborated on a grant proposal to secure more funding for the intake record study. For 2 years, funds from the National Institutes of Health Biomedical Research Support Grant program administered by the University of Massachusetts at Boston permitted the hiring of regular research assistants to continue the work. An extensive report to the shelter and a revised intake form were the result.

After the grant expired, graduate assistants and interns in our graduate program in Applied Sociology continued to process intake forms and interview new shelter guests. This work resulted in several more reports to the shelter on the needs of shelter users, numerous publications, and several master's theses. Undergraduate interns from the university's Alcohol and Substance Abuse Studies Program also participated in service activities at the shelter.

We also secured a University of Massachusetts grant with which to organize a conference on homelessness. We then collaborated with Dr. Ellen Bassuk of the Harvard Medical School and Nancy Kaufman of the Massachusetts Executive Office of Human Services on a joint national conference. Papers we presented at this conference served as preliminary drafts of two chapters in this book.

After the conference, we were awarded two Public Service Grants from the University of Massachusetts to produce a videotape-based training program for shelter staff. Entitled *Working with the Homeless*, the videotape and manual have since been adopted by shelters and service agencies throughout the country.

Other collaborative efforts ensued. As consultants to the Massachusetts Department of Public Health's Stabilization Services for Homeless Substance Abusers Project, one of nine research demonstration projects funded by the National Institute for Alcohol Abuse and Alcoholism, we helped to train case managers and other service staff. We conducted other workshops in collaboration with staff from shelters and other agencies. Some components of these training programs are integrated into the chapters in this book.

Through these various projects, the boundaries between academic and applied work were crossed. Students became involved in local shelters as interns, assistants, and researchers; the University of Massachusetts at Boston became a source for policy insights and practical advice about homelessness; and professors and service personnel became joint participants in the evaluation of service policies.

We have used our experiences in this university–community collaboration to develop an evaluation of and response to homelessness that is described in this book. Our goals are to present to service personnel the findings and insights of academic research, as well as to make available for classroom use the experience and practical wisdoms of service delivery personnel.

*Responding to the Homeless: Policy and Practice* is applied sociology, then, in a very practical sense. It integrates the findings of social scientific research about the problem of homelessness with the background developed by those persons who work directly with homeless persons, and it does so in a format intended to make the book useful to practitioners on the job as well as to students in the classroom. Each group, we believe, can learn from the other, just as our involvement with service delivery personnel and homeless persons themselves has enriched immeasurably our academic understanding of homelessness.

If this book helps students in social work, nursing, and other service-oriented professions learn how to help homeless persons, if it makes the work of shelter staff more effective, if it leads to improved public and private agency policies about homelessness, it will have served its purpose. But, in addition, we hope that the book helps our academic colleagues make homelessness more real to their students in substantive courses and internships alike, and generates more insightful academic research.

Of course, there are many points of contention about homelessness that will not be resolved by a shared base of information (Schutt, 1989), but these debates can be recast so as to focus more explicitly on policy preferences, rather than on misunderstandings about the phenomenon subject to debate.

The organization of the book reflects our applied perspective in two ways. First, each chapter combines historical and research information on homelessness with a description of different aspects of the problem encountered in the field and a review of methods of responding to the problem. Second, the book is consciously interdisciplinary, spanning the fields of sociology, psychiatry, and psychology; nursing and social work; and economics, public administration, and politics. The practical solutions demanded by practitioners cannot be constrained by the tenacious boundaries of academic disciplines.

*Responding to the Homeless* begins with a historical overview of homelessness in America, an analysis of the policies that shaped the size and composition of the homeless population in the 1980s and 1990s, and a description of the types of people who are homeless and the forms in which they experience homelessness. The second chapter reviews the range of responses to homelessness: the different types of shelters and their operations, the role of shelter staff, and the programs that extend beyond shelters. Chapter 3 first reviews research on the value of services for homeless persons and then focuses on service work within shelters. General principles and alternate models of case management are discussed, and the generic skills required by case managers and counselors are identified: how to assess clients, how to refer clients, how to respond to interpersonal conflicts, and how to cope with stress and burnout.

Chapters 4, 5, 6, and 7 focus on the major health care problems found among homeless persons: mental illness, alcohol abuse, drug abuse, and physical illness and injury. Each of these chapters provides background information on the health problem and its prevalence among the homeless, describes specific types of disorders, and reviews methods of assessing and treating these disorders.

Housing is the focus of Chapter 8. A description of types of housing available to the poor is followed by a historical review of their development and/or demise; in addition, the efforts that shelters and other organizations can make to improve housing options are reviewed. The book concludes with an overview of options for responding to homelessness and a discussion of the directions needed for future research and theory about homelessness.

We have included distinctive panels throughout the book to highlight case studies, policy dilemmas, treatment approaches, and research results. Most of the chapters include sections containing practical advice for practitioners in the format of "What to Do" and "What Not to Do."

But in spite of our effort to be comprehensive, the book has important limitations. We have not treated in any detail the specific problems and needs of homeless families—that is, parents, usually single mothers, who are homeless with their dependent children— or of homeless youth—usually adolescents who are runaways or "throwaways." Although much of the book can be applied directly to the plight of these very large segments of the homeless population, there are more specific wisdoms pertaining to families and youth that are not included in this book.

We also caution our readers that the book is not a medical text, nor are its directives in any way a substitute for treatment by trained medical personnel. Medical personnel should be consulted about all health care problems. However, this book should help medical personnel not only to understand the nature of the shelters but also the homeless persons with whom they work. It should also help staff without medical training to respond to emergency medical needs and to make appropriate referrals for medical care.

So this book is not a substitute for the advice and services of trained medical personnel; it also is not a prescription for ending the problem of homelessness in America. What follows is a tool to increase the effectiveness of those who work with the homeless, a resource for those who develop policy about homelessness, and a text for those who seek to understand homelessness.

# Acknowledgments

We have incurred a great many debts in the course of writing this book—first and foremost, to the book's other contributors: Barbara A. Blakeney, R.N. (Chapter 7), Stephen M. Goldfinger, M.D. (Chapter 4), Elise Kline, Ed.D. (Chapter 4), Ezra Susser, M.D. (Chapter 4), and Friedner D. Wittman, Ph.D. (Chapter 8). They have demonstrated the superior knowledge that results from years of practical experience combined with very fine analytic abilities. We are indebted particularly to Barbara Blakeney, whose practitioner-oriented "What to Do" format in the health care chapter served as a guide for the other chapters. In fact, Ms. Blakeney's guidelines for responding to emergency alcohol and drug problems were incorporated directly into the two chapters on these topics. Between ourselves, Dr. Schutt was primarily responsible for the preface, the first three chapters, the final writing of Chapter 4, the final editing, and the final chapter; Dr. Garrett wrote Chapters 5 and 6 and portions of Chapter 7, and made numerous other contributions throughout the book.

We thank Ellen Bassuk, M.D., series editor, for her interest in this project, for her frequent encouragement and editorial advice, and for the example she has set of how to bring members of the academic community into service to the larger community. We also thank Robert A. Dentler, Ph.D., and Irene S. Levine, Ph.D., for their thoughtful editorial comments on the book.

Boston's Long Island Shelter has for years exemplified the spirit of collaboration between service providers and academic institutions, and we are honored to have been able to work with them on so many occasions. Debbie Chausse initiated our relationship and Richard Weintraub, Director of the Long Island Shelter, has helped to maintain the relationship over many years. William Dillon and Barbara Blakeney, Long Island's Director of Health Care, also have played critical roles.

Important resource materials for the book were made available through the generosity of Irene S. Levine, Director of the Office of Programs for the Homeless Mentally Ill, National Institute of Mental Health; Barbara Lubran, former Chief, and Robert Huebner, Chief of Homeless Demonstration Projects at the National Institute on Alcohol Abuse and Alcoholism; Dennis McCarty, Director of the Massachusetts Division of Substance Abuse Services; Milton Argeriou, Director, Stabilization Services Project in Boston; Pamela J. Fischer, Johns Hopkins University; and Deborah L. Dennis of the National Resource Center on Homelessness and Mental Illness. We thank them all, and the other experts whose material is incorporated in panels throughout the book.

A variety of service providers in eastern Massachusetts participated in interviews that helped to lay the foundation for Chapter 2 and, to a lesser extent, Chapter 8. We thank Paul McGerigle, Elyse Jacob, Randy Bailey, Susan Do, Dominic O'Donnell and Lindya Udori, Ira Greiff, Carol Johnson, Nancy Mahan, Karen McCarthy, Bob Richards and Susan Fazio, Sally Rizzo and Irene Lee, and Paul Robinson.

We also are indebted to the University of Massachusetts at Boston for its many efforts to facilitate faculty involvement in community affairs and for its support of our research and service efforts, both directly through grants and indirectly through its support of the graduate program in Applied Sociology. Dr. Fuad Safwat, Dean of Graduate Studies and Research, has provided needed resources at many critical points and has facilitated the development of the innovative graduate programs that make work such as ours possible. And without the assistance of many fine students in the graduate program, the research and service activities which this book reflects would not have occurred—we thank each of these students and apologize (although with some pride) that their names are too numerous to mention here. A special expression of gratitude goes to our outstanding secretary, Anne Foxx.

Most important, we thank the many other service providers and homeless people whom we have tapped for insights. We would never have been able to write this book without their willingness to collaborate on service and research projects and to share with us their experiences, techniques, and concerns.

R.K.S.
G.R.G.

# Contents

# List of Panels

## Chapter 1

## Chapter 2

## Chapter 3

## Chapter 4

## Chapter 5

## Chapter 6

## Chapter 7

## Chapter 8

## Chapter 9

# The Problem of Homelessness

## INTRODUCTION

Huddled in doorways and on heating grates, standing in lines at soup kitchens and shelters, homeless persons have become an all-too-familiar part of urban American life. Each winter, newspapers report the tragic deaths of these people: freezing on the streets, burning in makeshift shelters, wasting away from a host of illnesses. And throughout the year, homeless persons are vulnerable and victimized: beaten, raped, stabbed, strangled. Securing the basic necessities of life—food, clothing, human companionship—becomes a daunting, sometimes life-threatening, task.

Confronted with the myriad problems of homeless persons, some people react with disbelief and avoidance, others with compassion and concern. A few reach into their pockets, reorient their schedules, or change their careers to work with the homeless. For these volunteers, employees, and advocates, the homeless are no longer part of the "other America"; they come into focus as unique families and individuals, each with his or her own history, outlook, and needs.

This chapter provides a comprehensive and historical framework for understanding the particulars of homelessness to which most citizens and all service providers are exposed—the tragic stories on the streets as well as the moments of sharing in the shelters. We begin by describing the nature of homelessness and then review its history and the policies about homelessness in the United States. Next, we review recent research and develop a description of the homeless population. Finally, we describe the various meanings of "homelessness" according to how long the experience of homelessness lasts.

## THE NATURE OF HOMELESSNESS

Homelessness can be defined simply as the inability to secure regular housing when such housing is desired. Homelessness is symptomatic of extreme poverty, but it is a condition of more extreme deprivation—the absence of a place to call one's own. Spending a night in a bus station does not qualify as homelessness if it occurs while a person is in transit to a vacation destination; it is homelessness when it is the sequel to eviction from regular housing or to a futile housing search. Living for several months with friends or family is not homelessness for adults if the arrangement is preferred to other regular housing alternatives; it becomes home-lessness when there are no other alternatives.

In this book, we focus our attention on those persons who live routinely on the streets or in emergency shelters—a focus that excludes some who are literally homeless and includes a few who are not literally homeless. But it is on the streets and in shelters where most homeless persons are found and where most efforts to help them occur. And the techniques we discuss for helping homeless persons, like the knowledge we review about homelessness, can easily be generalized to other settings.

Homelessness is, after all, not a problem that is limited to particular settings or to certain kinds of people; nor can it be understood from the perspective of one discipline or one point in time. We find the problem of homelessness across a wide array of institutions, touching the lives of vast numbers of Americans. We find the antecedents of homelessness in urban poverty and in family dislocation, in state psychiatric hospitals, and in the corner tavern (Erickson and Wilhelm, 1986). We will fail to grasp the nature of the homelessness problem or respond effectively to it if our vision extends no further than the outstretched hand at the entrance to a public building.

Even the definition of homelessness requires making a categorical distinction in what really is a long continuum. Many persons who, at best, are marginally housed are often termed the "hidden homeless." Although we do not focus directly on their problems in this book, the situation of the hidden homeless underscores the similarity of the problems of extreme poverty and homelessness.

Many extremely poor persons live on the verge of homelessness (Robbins, 1986). The numbers of families living with others as subfamilies has doubled between 1978 and 1983 (Hopper and Hamberg, 1984). In 1983, 2.6 million house-holds were overcrowded, with 1.01 or more persons per room; 700,000 were extremely overcrowded (1.51 or more persons per room) (Hartman, 1986). In New York City, 17,000 of 150,000 public housing units were doubled up in 1983 (Robbins, 1986), and a total of 103,000 families were doubled up citywide (*New York Times*, September 21, 1986:44). In the summer of 1982, 27 percent of the individuals in food lines in Phoenix, Arizona, were not homeless but were trying to extend their limited resources in order to avoid becoming homeless (Phoenix South Commu-nity Mental Health Center, 1983). About one third of Florida's indigent population who were not receiving welfare or social security benefits were living free of charge with relatives or friends (Statewide Task Force on the Homeless, 1985).

In any state, within any city, there is room for, even need of, a variety of different responses to homelessness, informed by diverse visions and alternative definitions. Some parts of the problem can best be resolved with a focus on alcoholism, others with a focus on poverty and unemployment. Some parts of the problem defy such simple categorization: When does a drinking problem begin to "explain" ineffective efforts to cope with repeated bouts of unemployment? Can an abused spouse be helped just by getting a room of her own after spending months living in fear of assaults on the street?

In the final analysis, social policies and programs that seek to lessen the problem of homelessness must be informed by a larger vision that rejects simplistic solutions and constraining definitions. The roots of homelessness are as numerous as modern society is complex, and the problems faced by homeless persons are as multifaceted as the range of human experience. Without recognition of these larger dimensions of the homelessness problem, proposed solutions can be expected to fail.

## HISTORY OF HOMELESSNESS

In the United States, homelessness has occurred since colonial times, but the numbers and types of persons who are homeless and the popular interpretations of their plight have varied markedly. Almost 100 years of research reveal four basic influences on this variation: the number of poor persons, the supply of affordable housing, the level of personal disability, and the supply of social services and supports.

Homelessness occurs when individuals are too poor to secure permanent housing at either market or subsidized rates; this poverty in turn can reflect a level of personal disability that exceeds the capacity of available service or social supports. The "homelessness equation" identifies the basic interrelations among these factors:

$$homelessness = f(poverty/housing, disability/supports)$$

The homelessness equation indicates that the higher the level of poverty in relation to the supply of housing, and the higher the level of disabilities relative to available social and service supports, the higher the level of homelessness (Schutt, 1990).

When the poverty rate increases and the supply of affordable housing remains constant or declines, the likelihood of persons' becoming homeless and of remaining homeless increases. If the supply of social or medical supports decreases when the level of substance abuse, mental or physical illness does not, or increases, homelessness increases and personal disabilities are more in evidence. But if the supply of housing increases, homelessness will decrease.

Poverty was the primary focus of the earliest social scientific attempts to explain homelessness, although the influence of other factors was acknowledged. McCook's "tramp census" in 1893 and other early sources highlighted economic marginality—unemployment, sporadic work histories, and residential transience (Anderson, 1923; McCook, 1893). Several studies (Anderson, 1934, 1940; Rice, 1918; Sutherland and Locke, 1936) identified many homeless persons as "ordinary unskilled working men" who were unable to find employment in a changing labor market.

But disabilities and "moral inferiority" were also common themes in this early literature: researchers estimated that physical disabilities and alcoholism com-

Panel 1–1

## A Tragic Ending

After a long and sometimes bitter struggle, a group of tenants of a rooming house won concessions from their new landlord who had wanted to evict them in order to develop the property. As part of the process, the landlord agreed to pay the tenants' lawyer to hire a housing search worker to assist in the tenants' relocation . . . and to provide them with a sizeable "moving bonus" if they relocated by a certain date.

The housing search worker met with the tenants on a regular basis to develop a plan with each and assist them in the relocation process. . . . The relocation program appeared to be going smoothly except in one case: tenant Roy M., a 54-year-old single man who had a history of alcohol and drug abuse and psychiatric problems. Roy had been living in the rooming house for several years except for occasional hospital admissions for depression and alcohol detoxification.

In their meetings together, Roy was either surly or noncommunicative with the worker. He usually had an objection to any housing opportunity the worker presented; either it was in a "bad" neighborhood, it was too expensive, or it was inconvenient to get to public transportation. If he did finally agree to see an apartment, he apparently sabotaged the effort by missing his appointment or showing up intoxicated.

. . . As the deadline approached, the worker met with Roy to inform him that time was running out. If he did not take action soon, a golden opportunity would be lost. She reminded him that the landlord had the right to relocate the tenants and that the reconstruction was going to take place as planned. If he did not take advantage of the offer, he would end up losing the moving benefits ["sweetened" by the landlord with additional incentives] and, given the housing market and his own limited resources, he could very well end up living in a shelter or on the streets.

To her amazement, Roy was very cooperative and agreed to accompany her the next day to see an apartment. He even expressed his gratitude to her for her caring and hard work; and he gave her a gift as a token of appreciation—a locket his mother had left to him. The worker thanked Roy and encouraged him in his new found cooperative attitude. They agreed to meet the following morning to visit the new apartment.

That night Roy bought a bottle of scotch, went to his room, consumed all of the bottle, and then plunged to his death from the building's roof.

Prepared by Debbie Chausse, Long Island Shelter, Boston, Massachusetts.

pounded the problems of about one third of homeless persons (Anderson, 1923). Mental illness did not seem much in evidence, although measurement methods were crude: Solenberger (1911) identified 0.5 percent of Chicago's homeless men as insane and 0.2 percent as having been inmates of "insane asylums" (Cook, 1910; Laubach, 1916; Solenberger, 1911).

Early in the twentieth century, provisions for the homeless reflected an image of homelessness as a voluntary and transitory condition—labor colonies and detention camps were common responses (Bahr, 1973:198–201). Alcoholism was considered a crime, and public inebriates were often jailed (Stark, 1987:8); the insane were often sent to institutions.

The population of homeless persons swelled during the Great Depression of the 1930s. Although little systematic research was conducted, several surveys suggest a migrant homeless population of unemployed young men, often found in transient camps, and a local homeless population of unemployed older men who relied on municipal shelters and religious missions. The relative incidence of alcoholism seems to have declined, perhaps to 1 in 10, as poverty exerted proportionately greater influence (Culver, 1933; Rossi, 1989; Stark, 1987; cf. Sutherland and Locke, 1936).

During World War II, the homeless population faded in the midst of a feverish war effort and remained small in the prosperous postwar decades. In the 1950s and 1960s, flophouses and missions in the skid row districts provided shelter largely to single, unattached, middle-aged, or older men. At least one third were identified as chronic alcoholics, and research often focused on alcoholics' unique problems and survival strategies (Bahr and Caplow, 1968; Bogue, 1963). Several studies reported that about 11 percent of the skid row homeless were mentally ill, but estimates (and measurement procedures) varied widely (Bahr and Garrett, 1976; Blumberg, Shipley, and Shandler, 1973; Bogue, 1963).

Agencies providing services to the homeless in this period were oriented primarily to alcoholics. Jailing for public drunkenness was still a primary response. Missions run by religious groups provided shelter and necessities for perhaps 10 percent of the homeless, and longer-term social services for those willing to work in the mission and participate in religious services (Bahr, 1973). Mission accommodations were often sparse:

> I am in this mission. This is a big room. I lie up here and listen to the snores of a thousand men. . . . Here is a stiff who has lived his life, and now he is dying under these lousy blankets in a mission. Who is there to care whether he lives or dies. (Tom Kramer, as quoted in Bahr, 1973:14)

Public shelters, typically large and impersonal, were maintained in a few cities.

> Late at night they flop on the concrete floor of the big room. . . . During the day they get two meals served up with only a tablespoon to make sure no one gets killed—at least on the premises. Most of the time they just wait in line. . . . There are lines for patients. Lines for men who have gripes. . . . (Bahr, 1973: 131–132)

The most common skid row lodging was the SRO—the single-room occupancy hotel (Bahr, 1973:54–63; Wiseman, 1970). Although their cleanliness and atmosphere varied, most SROs provided few amenities: for sleeping, five-by-seven-foot cubicles topped by wire mesh; for daytime recreation, lobbies filled with chairs and listless men.

Indigent chronic mentally ill persons were more likely to be found in hospitals than on the streets:

Feeble-minded or seriously psychotic men . . . usually are picked up rather promptly by the police, and the screening process in the courts causes them to be institutionalized. (Bogue, 1963:49)

Skid row districts were not pleasant places, but these districts and their lodging houses provided settings for homeless persons to conduct their affairs largely away from the public eye. In the 1960s and 1970s, public policy changes expanded the numbers of homeless persons while they chipped away at the size of skid row districts. The result has been a far more visible presence of homeless persons and a wider array of disabilities among them.

## POLICY BACKGROUND

Shrinking low-income housing opportunities, deinstitutionalization of the chronically mentally ill, and reduced income supports were the most important policy changes to affect the size of the single adult homeless population in the 1960s, 1970s and 1980s. New approaches to treating alcoholism and to administering public welfare services have also shaped the crisis of homelessness in America.

### The Housing Market

Throughout the 1970s and 1980s, the core of national urban policy was the redevelopment of city centers. This trend was motivated in part by the economic and social benefits of eliminating dangerous and decaying districts. It was stimulated by growing interest in urban living by the burgeoning population of young singles and childless couples (Carliner, 1987). But, at the same time, redevelopment conflicted with the housing needs of the very poor. Lacking financial resources and political influence, skid row residents offered little resistance to displacement.

The impact of redevelopment was dramatic: one million single-room units, almost one half of the total supply, were lost in the 1970s (Mapes, 1985, citing the 1984 GAO report). In New York City, over 30,000 single-room units were lost between 1975 and 1981, while the SRO vacancy rate fell from 26 percent to less than 1 percent (Bahr, 1973; Kasinitz, 1984; Mair, 1986). In Chicago, SRO capacity declined by almost one fourth from 1980 to 1983 (Rossi and Wright, 1987; see also Chapter 8).

Increasing housing prices and decreasing public housing subsidies exacerbated the trends spawned by redevelopment. Rents increased at double the rate of tenant incomes during the 1970s—30 percent fewer rental units were available at 30 percent of a $3,000 income. By 1980, the median rent-income ratio for renters with under $3,000 annual income was more than 60 percent— a huge burden for a meager income (Dolbeare, 1983; Hartman, 1986; Hope and Young, 1986). But federal housing policy did not respond: funds for subsidized housing fell by 60 percent from 1981 to 1985 (Mapes, 1985). Rental subsidy programs that supplement prospective tenants' incomes (primarily HUD's Section 8 Certificates) have helped many poor persons, but often certificate holders still cannot find housing they can afford (Carliner, 1987).

The overall consequences of these changes in housing policy have been dramatic: each year about 2.5 million Americans are displaced from their housing; each year half a million low-rent units are lost through conversion, abandonment, inflation, arson, and demolition (Hartman, 1986; Hopper and Hamberg, 1984).

## Income and Income Supports

In the early 1980s, a sharp rise in unemployment exacerbated the financial strains created by changes in the housing market. Unemployment was 10.7 percent in November, 1982, the highest level since the 1930s (Bassuk, 1984; Sebastian, 1985). The demand for cheap, temporary, manual labor, the primary income source for many homeless men, continued to decline. After a decade of stability, the number of poor persons (measured in terms of both cash income and the value of in-kind transfers) rose by 49 percent between 1978 and 1983 (Danziger and Gottschalk, 1985; Statewide Task Force on the Homeless, 1985); focusing just on the extremely poor, Rossi (1989) found an increase of 224 percent between 1970 and 1989.

Some of those unable to support themselves, whether primarily because of personal disability or inadequate earnings, could avoid homelessness through government transfer payments. However, sharp declines in the early 1980s, in both the level and availability of such benefits, placed many more individuals at risk of homelessness. Eligibility for the federal government's program of Supplemental Security Income (SSI) was restricted in 1981, and many disabled persons were removed from the rolls (although many were restored to SSI in 1984, after legal action); many states severely reduced the scope of general assistance, often the only welfare benefit available to single adults; and many poor working families were dropped from the AFDC (Aid to Families with Dependent Children) rolls, even as subsidies for single mothers did not keep pace with inflation. The value in constant dollars of both general assistance and AFDC benefits fell by about one third (Hopper and Hamberg, 1984; Solomon, 1985; Wolch, Dear, and Akita, 1984).

The combined effect of these changes in the housing market and in incomes was to increase the rent-to-income ratio. The supply of low-cost housing units fell, and the number of poor households rose. Between 1975 and 1983, for example, the number of rental units available for under $250 per month declined from 10.8 to 8.8 million, but the number of households with incomes of less than $10,000 per year (in constant dollars) increased from 8.9 to 11.9 million (Carliner, 1987).

## Mental Health Services

The Supreme Court's decision in *Shelton* v. *Tucker* (1960) affirmed the right of the mentally ill to treatment with the "least restrictive alternative." The decision itself was an early indicator of growing concern with patients' rights and recognition of the nontherapeutic, often unsafe and nonhygienic conditions in state psychiatric hospitals. States began to change their involuntary commitment laws to require proof of a person's dangerousness. The ability of the new psychotropic drugs to control some of the most troublesome symptoms of psychosis and the availability of Medicaid to nonhospitalized patients also stimulated increased interest in deinstitutionalizing psychiatric care.

Given congressional sanction by the Community Mental Health Centers Act of 1963, increasing numbers of psychiatric patients in state and in Veterans Administration (VA) hospitals were released (Hope and Young, 1984; Hopper and Hamberg, 1984). Between 1959 and 1980, the number of persons in state mental hospitals fell by 73 percent (Mapes, 1985), while the Veterans Administration reduced its psychiatric beds from 59,000 to 28,500 between 1963 and 1981 (Hope and Young, 1984).

The closing of state hospital beds was not accompanied by the equally rapid growth of alternative care facilities (Peele, Gross, Arons, and Jafri, 1984). Of an intended 2,000 community mental health centers that were to provide outpatient care, only 789 were built (Mapes, 1985). In California, the number of state hospital beds fell from 37,000 to 5,000 between 1960 and 1983, while the total state population grew by 150 percent (Wolch, Dear, and Akita, 1984).

The community mental health centers (CMHC) that were built tended to provide less than comprehensive care, and they were not funded to serve the poor—Medicaid and Medicare provided funding primarily for nursing home and inpatient care (Bassuk and Gerson, 1978). Most of the CMHCs turned their attention to the more treatable, and better endowed, "worried well" (Torrey, 1988). The end result was fewer opportunities for stable psychiatric care, and even for food and shelter, for the poor and indigent.

Many discharged patients returned to their families; many others were placed in nursing homes; some managed to survive in SROs and other cheap lodgings with their Social Security Income checks (Hope and Young, 1986). But as cheap lodging disappeared from urban areas, as already impoverished families were unable to maintain mentally ill members, residential alternatives disappeared for former and prospective patients. In California, one third of those no longer in the hospitals were also not in residential programs; perhaps one third of these were homeless and without treatment (Wolch, Dear, and Akita, 1984).

## Detoxification

In the early 1970s, decriminalization of public drunkenness also reduced the use of jails as overnight shelter for homeless alcoholics. Stimulated in part by landmark court decisions in the 1960s and in part by growing acceptance of a disease model of alcoholism, Congress passed the Uniform Alcoholism and Intoxication Treatment Act to decriminalize public inebriation (Neuner and Schultz, 1986; Peele et al., 1984). The act defined a continuum of medical treatment as an alternative to jailing alcoholic derelicts, although the impetus for adopting this model did not come until federal funding was appropriated through the Comprehensive Alcohol Abuse and Alcoholism Prevention, Treatment and Rehabilitation Act Amendments (Garrett, 1989).

A vast network of detoxification centers and sobering stations developed, but these facilities provided only temporary respite for persons living on the streets. In fact, Fagan and Mauss (1978) suggested that the network of "detox" centers promoted a new revolving-door recidivism that paralleled the street-to-jail-to-street cycle of homeless men in earlier decades.

## Social Services

The administration of public welfare was transformed in the 1970s. Since the modern welfare system began in the 1930s, clients had been assigned to case-workers who, at least in theory, determined clients' continuing eligibility for welfare and maintained an ongoing personal service relationship with their clients. The Social Security Act of 1969 changed all this: income maintenance work was assigned to different employees than social service provision. In addition, many states adopted in the early 1970s a "flat grant" system of welfare payments that simplified eligibility determination. As a result of these changes, welfare clients had fewer and less significant contacts with caseworkers (see Schutt, 1986, for a more thorough discussion).

For many welfare recipients, the decline in caseworker contact was a welcome reduction in intrusiveness; but for others, less flexibility and human contact were additional assaults on already fragile support systems (Preston, 1984). The ability of these welfare recipients to manage in the face of evictions or other setbacks was impaired.

## Summary

By the early 1980s, a decline in the supply of low-cost housing, an increase in the level of poverty, and changes in social service policies had increased the risk of homelessness for many Americans. The effect of these trends was exacerbated by the increased prevalence of single-parent families, drug abuse, and AIDS. At both the institutional and the personal levels, the threads which bind together the social fabric and help to maintain the stability of impoverished persons had frayed; a larger and more diverse homeless population was one result.

## THE HOMELESS POPULATION

The policy changes of the 1960s and 1970s produced a different and more heterogeneous homeless population in the 1980s. The average age of guests in adult shelters was younger—about 34—but as many as 15 percent were between 17 and 25; about one in five were 46 or more years old. Many more guests were women—about one in five—and families. About one third were veterans (comparable to the proportion of veterans in the male population), and a disproportionate number were members of minority ethnic groups (Wright, 1989).

In the 1980s, most single adult homeless persons had completed high school; one in five had had some education beyond high school. Few were working at the time they were homeless (about one in ten), but most had worked at some time in the past. Two thirds received no financial benefits, such as welfare or social security.

> Tom Smith, 32, faces his work day just like many other riders on the T: Some
> days, he can think of better things to do. On paydays, he is glad for all the times
> he has dragged himself out of bed. . . . What makes Smith different from his
> fellow riders is where he lives: the Pine Street Inn, a shelter for the homeless.
> (*Boston Globe*, March 30, 1986:1)

A substantial proportion of the 1980s homeless population was comprised of families, usually women with two or three young children, frequently preschoolers, About 2,300 homeless families received shelter in New York City in 1984; 90 percent were single, female-headed households. Younger and less educated than other adult homeless persons, the mothers often have had a long history of economic and residential instability and severe stress (Phillips, Kronenfeld, and Jeter, 1986). One third of homeless mothers interviewed in a Massachusetts study had been abused as children; two thirds reported a major family disruption; two thirds had minimal or no supportive relationships (Bassuk, 1986). Many homeless children suffered from academic, physical, and behavioral problems (Bassuk, 1986; Phillips et al., 1986).

Teenage runaways and "throwaways" comprise another portion of the homeless population, with estimates ranging from one quarter to two million persons (Brickner and Scanlan, 1990). Family disruption following death, divorce, separation, and desertion is often the precursor of running away, but chaotic family life involving substance abuse, physical abuse, and neglect also is likely (Saltonstall, 1984). Many homeless youths have been in foster or institutional care.

## Poverty

Homeless persons have very limited economic resources to use in coping with their health problems or in improving their residential circumstances. Few of the homeless are employed at any given time; welfare benefits are a more common source of income, but large numbers of the homeless simply have no discernible economic resources. Just 5 percent of the homeless in inner-city Los Angeles reported current paid employment. Although two thirds had engaged in some paid work during the previous year, half had worked no more than 1 month. The annual income of almost half was less than $1,000; for three quarters, it was less than $5,000 (Farr, Koegel, and Burnam, 1986).

In Chicago, one third of the homeless had worked for pay in the preceding month, but only one tenth reported steady work and it had been an average of 4 years since the last steady job (Rossi, Fisher, and Willis, 1986). The median monthly income from all sources was just $100 (Rossi and Wright, 1987). Among Boston's homeless, 12 percent reported current employment; half had not worked for at least 18 weeks and almost half had never worked for more than 5 months in one job (Schutt and Garrett, 1985).

There are a range of benefits possibly available to homeless persons: (1) Medicare, a federally administered health insurance program for the elderly, is open to anyone eligible for Social Security benefits; (2) Medicaid, a joint federal-state program for the indigent, is open to those on AFDC, but with other eligibility criteria varying between the states (often only those on AFDC or SSI are eligible); (3) Supplemental Security Income and Social Security Disability Insurance (open only to those former workers with disabilities that prevent them from working), have eligibility rules that vary by state; (4) Old Age and Survivors Insurance; and (5) welfare programs such as AFDC and General Assistance (Wright, Weber-Burdin, Knight, and Lam, 1987).

Few of the homeless receive benefits from any of these sources. Among the homeless in Los Angeles, only 8 percent reported current receipt of some kind of disability payments; less than one quarter had received disability benefits at any point in their lives (often for work-related injuries). Few (9 percent) received General Relief ($228 per month) or some other form of welfare, although 59 percent had received such benefits at some time in their lives. Many had lost their General Relief benefits within the preceding year; some never tried to procure them again, whereas others cycled on and off the relief rolls in relation to their success in establishing entitlement and the gravity of their need (Farr et al., 1986).

In Chicago, less than half of the homeless received any income maintenance benefits. Their average total cash income was less than $6 per day; their median daily income was $3.50. In monthly terms, the corresponding figures are $168 and $100. One in five received the General Assistance payment of $144 per month; another one in five received AFDC or other income maintenance benefits. Only 36 percent of those who qualified for General Assistance were receiving benefits at the time of the survey, although refusal rates were fairly low (24% for General Assistance) (Rossi et al., 1986). Only one third of Boston's homeless who came to the Long Island Shelter received any financial benefits. The most common benefits were food stamps (44% of those receiving any benefits), General Relief (33%), and SSI (29%) (Schutt and Garrett, 1985).

The availability of financial benefits is lessened by various restrictive eligibility rules and complex application procedures (relaxed in recent years to make benefits more accessible to the homeless population) (Crystal, 1985). General Relief (GR) requirements in Los Angeles indicate one type of barrier to entry into the welfare system. Employable GR recipients are required to work on county projects for 70 hours each month and to procure signatures from 20 prospective employers from whom they have sought work. Individuals who fail to meet these criteria are cut off from GR for 60 days; at the end of this period, they can reapply (Farr et al., 1986). In addition, those who reside in shelters are ineligible for food stamps; it is difficult for the mentally ill to manage SSI; singles are ineligible for AFDC (Mapes, 1985).

Delays in receipt of benefits are a major problem for those who become homeless. In Florida, for example, an expedited procedure for eligibility of home-less applicants for SSI benefits only leads to receipt of a check within 19 days of application, under "ideal" circumstances. Homeless families who apply for AFDC in Florida do not receive their first benefit checks for 30 to 45 days. Eligibility for Food Stamps may be easiest to establish, and a fixed residence may not be required, but benefits generally are very low—a maximum of $79 per month for single individuals in Florida; a maximum of $264 for a family of four (Statewide Task Force on the Homeless, 1985). Flynn (1985) reported the case of a woman who was evicted after being laid-off from a low-income job. Although she applied for

---

*Panel 1–2*

**Financial Benefits**

For the chronically mentally ill, as well as for other disabled groups, Social Security payments are the main source of income support. The Supplemental Security Income Program (SSI) provides payments to the aged, blind, and disabled; the Social Security Disability Insurance Program (SSDI) provides benefits to those unable "to engage in any substantial gainful activity by reason of any medically determinable physical or mental impairment which can be expected to result in death or which has lasted or can be expected to last for a continuous period of no less than twelve months" (42 U.S.C. 423(d)(1)(A), 1382c(a)(3)(A)].

The Social Security Act was amended [section 1611(e)(i)] to allow individuals residing in public emergency shelters for at least 1 month to receive up to 3 months of SSI benefits in any 12-month period (residents of private shelters have always been eligible) (Statewide Task Force on the Homeless, 1985). In 1984, the Social Security Disability Reform Act established new criteria for evaluating mental disorders and automatic re-review of those terminated from benefits (Health and Welfare Council of Central Maryland, 1985). Nonetheless, the minimum social security benefit in 1984 was just $314 per month. Other benefits potentially useful to a wider range of the poor have also been reduced.

In some states, General Assistance is not available, and in most it provides only limited funds. In Massachusetts, for example, General Relief pays $268.90 per month (Flynn, 1986). In many states, General Assistance has been severely reduced in scope. In 1983, for example, the restructuring of Pennsylvania's General Assistance Program cut back the eligibility period of nearly 30,000 individuals in Philadelphia from the entire year to only 90 days per year (Crystal, 1985; Hopper and Hamberg, 1984; Philadelphia Health Management Corporation, 1985). Overall, the real value of GA benefits declined by 32 percent during the 1970s (Hopper and Hamberg, 1984).

---

welfare benefits, she did not receive them before the storage company with which she had left her possessions auctioned them all off.

The consequences of failure to receive financial benefits may not be just financial. Those persons in Chicago who succeeded in obtaining General Assistance benefits were significantly less depressed than those who had been denied benefits; a similar pattern occurred for women with dependent children who were denied AFDC benefits (Rossi et al., 1986).

## Social Ties

Social ties are often the means by which the very poor manage to maintain a stable residence. For example, half of all General Assistance recipients in Chicago were living with relatives or friends; another one third received financial assistance from relatives or friends (Rossi and Wright, 1987).

Most studies of the homeless have found lower levels of social integration

---

*Panel 1–2*   (Continued)

AFDC is a primary, but often inadequate, source of income support for poor families. From 1970 to 1985, median AFDC benefits, in constant dollars, declined nationwide by about one third, and benefit levels are now well below the poverty line in many states (Solomon, 1985). In Florida, for example, cash benefit levels were $284 per month in 1984 for a family of four (Statewide Task Force on the Homeless, 1985). In 40 states, a working mother of three is ineligible for benefits when her monthly income exceeds $479. New regulations enacted in 1981 caused half of the 500,000 working families who were receiving AFDC to lose their benefits and 40 percent to have their benefits reduced (Hopper and Hamberg, 1984).

Food Stamp benefits are the most accessible for many of the very poor, but the average monthly benefit per person in 1983 was just $43, after being cut by 14 percent since 1981. In 1984, Food Stamp benefits provided the equivalent of just 47 cents per meal (Hope and Young, 1986; Hopper and Hamberg, 1984).

Medicaid is the federal government's principal means-tested health care benefit for the indigent, paying for the full cost of covered services and not restricting the patient's choice of physician. Medicare provides partial payment (about 45 percent) of recipients' medical expenses, primarily those who receive Social Security retirement benefits.

Medicaid or Medicare benefits are available to several classes of individuals. Some elderly homeless persons with little income may qualify for Old Age benefits in the SSI program. This program does not require a disability test and entitles the recipient to Medicaid as well as Medicare benefits. Homeless families with children may be eligible for Aid to Families with Dependent Children, and because of this eligibility, for Medicaid. However, Medicaid and Medicare benefits pay only for medical services, not for rehabilitation expenses or maintenance of social support services.

---

(Bahr, 1973). About half have never married, about half do not have any children; many have no relative or friend nearby. Few of Chicago's homeless had ever married and most of those who had were separated or divorced. One third were not in contact with any relatives, spouse, or children; about 60 percent were not in contact with someone they considered to be a good friend. Just 24 percent reported they were not in contact with any family and that they had no friends, although among women who were 40 years of age or over such social isolation was as high as 41 percent; it declined to a low of 6 percent among women under 40 and ranged in men from 21 percent of those under 40 years to 27 percent of those 40 years and over (Rossi et al., 1986).

In Baltimore's shelters, 45 percent of homeless men had no friends, compared to just 7 percent of housed men in the same community (Breakey, 1987; Fischer, Breakey, Shapiro, and Kramer, 1986). Less than 20 percent of Boston's homeless at the Long Island Shelter had relatives in the Boston area; less than 15 percent had any friends in the area (Schutt and Garrett, 1986b).

A study of the homeless in inner-city Los Angeles yielded more indications of meaningful social ties. Two thirds reported feeling attached to their families; almost three quarters had had contact with at least one relative within the past year—for 64 percent of these, the contact was at least once a month. About one quarter were estranged from their families; half had had a break with at least one family member. Seventy-one percent reported contact with friends within the last year; such contact had occurred within the past month for 60 percent, and almost one third reported seeing friends every day. However, interviewers sensed that the actual level of support available from friends and family was negligible (Farr et al., 1986).

Prior social relationships often were troubled:

> An aspiring lawyer who lived for months on the streets of New York . . . 38-year-old Ivy League graduate . . . became despondent after he twice failed the Florida bar and was rejected by his girlfriend, had been on the streets since last spring. (*Boston Globe*, January 1, 1986:63).

> My step-father just punched me out whenever he felt like it and my Mother didn't try to make him stop. The last time the neighbors took me to the hospital all bloody. I won't go back. (Saltonstall, 1984:6).

Street friendships may form for survival purposes, for pooling resources to buy drinks, and for companionship. But often these relationships are poor substitutes for stable social ties:

> A "street friend" . . . is: "Someone you can live with them [sic], spend time with them, think they'll do anything for you but they rip you off and take your money and they don't even need it sometimes when they take it. They take it just to show you that they can and how good they are at it. Even when you need it yourself and they know you need it. So I don't have any friends—street friends. Like I see the same people at the Greyhound all the time, then I go away or they go away and I don't wonder about them or what's happened to them. They'd be mean to me if they wanted to be or could be. That's what street friends are. They are all mean." (Saltonstall, 1984:11)

## Mental Illness

Although insufficient economic and social resources are a problem for almost all homeless persons, major health problems also limit the opportunities of many. When housing costs are high, unemployment, low wages, or meager levels of welfare or social security benefits are enough to make some individuals and families homeless. When limited economic and social resources are coupled with physical illness, psychiatric problems, or substance abuse, the risk of homelessness increases sharply.

Most studies estimate that between 25 percent and 50 percent of single homeless adults suffer from serious and chronic mental illness—many have been ill for a long time, although living on the streets exacerbates and, at times, initiates mental illness. About one third of the single adult homeless have been hospitalized for psychiatric problems at some time in the past, although younger mentally ill homeless persons may never have experienced long-term hospitalization. Almost two thirds in a Birmingham sample were clinically depressed (LaGory, Ritchey, and Mullis, 1990). Rates of chronic mental illness are much lower among adults in family shelters (Arce, Tadlock, Vergare, and Shapiro, 1983; Bachrach, 1986; Bassuk, 1984; Farr et al., 1986; Lamb, 1984; Levine, 1984; Schutt and Garrett, 1986b).

> Shouting, "I'm possessed by the devil," a homeless man yesterday stormed to the altar of St. Pius V Church in East Lynn, pressed a knife against his chest and threatened to kill himself before being subdued by police, authorities said. (*Boston Globe*, June 6, 1986:25)

> I wonder if suicide is my destiny. I feel lonely all the time and I feel depressed; maybe I've set up a pattern for myself I can never get out of. If I believed I'd be in a better space I'd kill myself in a minute. (Saltonstall, 1984:11)

## Alcoholism

Alcoholism among the homeless is a major problem: as many as half of individual adult homeless persons in some cities appeared to suffer the symptoms of alcohol abuse and about one third were chronic alcoholics. Two distinct groups are apparent: one is composed of older white men, often with failed marriages— the traditional skid row population. The other group of homeless alcoholics is composed of younger persons, many of whom are members of minority groups and some of whom are women; they often also suffer from mental illness and are more likely to have legal problems (Farr et al., 1986).

Social relations can become destructive among homeless alcoholics. "The road into the respectable community is cold and lonely, while Skid Row provides instant warmth and friendliness for some" (Blumberg, Shipley, and Shandler, 1973:78). Binge drinking among homeless alcoholics is common, as the drinker seeks to maintain the positive feelings that wear off an hour or two after a drink. However, the alcoholic's behavior when not intoxicated becomes comparatively normal, unless there is psychiatric impairment (Fischer and Breakey, 1987; Lipton et al., 1983; Ropers and Boyer, 1987a, b; Wiseman, 1970).

> The homeless panhandler who died Sunday in a South End doorway had turned his back on a comfortable middle-class life on Cape Cod. He had been married, had served in the Army and had had the trappings of a comfortable life—a wife, a job in a Taunton manufacturing plant, a beautiful house with a swimming pool in Carver—when he "dropped out of sight." Just three months before he left, he had lost two-thirds of his stomach in an operation brought on by serious stomach ulcers. "He was very ashamed of his alcoholism and the effects it had on his body, mind and spirit." (*Boston Globe*, February 19, 1986:13)

For some homeless persons, the problems of mental illness and substance abuse are confounded. In a study of homeless adult individuals in Los Angeles, 12 percent had dual diagnoses of chronic substance abuse and major mental illness. Of the homeless people entering Bellevue Hospital's psychiatric emergency service, 41 percent used alcohol, drugs, or both. About one quarter of adult users of Boston's Long Island Shelter had indications of both alcohol abuse and mental illness.

The distinction between "pure" and dually diagnosed alcoholics parallels in many respects the distinction between the "old" and "new" groups of homeless alcoholics. Dual diagnosis alcoholics tend to be younger, are more often women, and are less likely to have been married or to have children than alcoholics without other diagnoses. They tend to have been on the streets longer and to have more legal problems than other groups. Whether they turn to substance abuse programs or the mental health system for help, those having both mental health and substance abuse problems may encounter staff who are unable or unwilling to respond effectively to their "other" problem (Farr et al., 1986; Schutt and Garrett, 1986b, 1987).

## Physical Illness

Physical illness can precipitate homelessness. Illnesses, too, are often caused by the extreme rigors of the homeless lifestyle: regular exposure to the elements, constant mobility, exacerbation of chronic illnesses, inadequate resolution of acute health problems, infectious diseases, and physical danger. Between half and two thirds may experience physical illness within 1 year.

Common illnesses among the homeless include infestations (scabies and lice), trauma (from accidents), peripheral vascular diseases (from not lying down at night), cellulitis, thermoregulatory disorders, leg ulcers, and tuberculosis. Chronic diseases are of particular concern. These disorders require continuous intervention and monitoring by the patient and by health care workers. Some of the common chronic ailments among the homeless, such as hypertension, arteriosclerotic cardiovascular disease, chronic obstructive pulmonary disease, and diabetes mellitus, present symptoms only after significant damage has occurred; infrequent medical contact compounds difficulties in detecting and treating these diseases (see Chapter 7) (Brickner et al., 1984; Filardo, 1985; Sebastian, 1985).

## Victimization

Residential instability and poverty, particularly when coupled with mental illness or substance abuse, often result in high rates of legal problems—particularly criminal victimization. Rates of victimization are much higher among the homeless than in the general population: over half of those using a Detroit family shelter reported victimization within the previous 6 months (Solarz, 1986); homeless persons in inner-city Los Angeles reported a similar rate of victimization (Farr et al., 1986).

Victimization is more likely for those with a history of mental illness, perhaps because of the attention their behavior may attract or to poor skills in avoiding danger. Women are more at risk of assault, while men are more likely to be robbed; overall, homeless women are particularly at risk for victimization (Stoner, 1983). About 10 percent may have become homeless as a direct result of abuse within the family or because of the depletion of economic resources by associated legal problems (Solarz, 1986).

## Criminal Involvement

Current and past criminal involvement is also common, acknowledged by over 60 percent of the homeless in one study. Such criminal activity as trespassing, break-ins, and shoplifting may supplement meager economic resources. For some, criminal activity is more chronic and perhaps 5 percent become homeless upon release from prison (Solarz, 1985). About one third of the inner-city homeless in Los Angeles had been picked up by the police within the last year; a comparable percentage had spent time in jail during this period (Farr et al., 1986). Among Chicago's homeless, almost one in five had been in federal or state prisons, two in five had been in jail, and one quarter had been sentenced and placed on probation (Rossi et al., 1986). About one in five persons at two large Boston shelters were on probation or parole; those with indications of psychiatric problems, and particularly those who also abused alcohol, were much more likely to have such legal problems (Schutt, unpublished data).

## DURATION OF HOMELESSNESS

The homeless population is not composed of a homogeneous or constant group of individuals, nor is it easily distinguished from other social groups. Migrant farmworkers also lack a fixed residence; many chronic mental patients periodically experience periods of homelessness, and some persons "sheltered" in jails and prisons would otherwise lack a regular residence (Bachrach, 1984b).

Among those persons usually considered homeless, some are homeless for a short time, some for many years; others cycle into and out of the state of homelessness. While some persons first become homeless after losing a stable residence, others avoid homelessness by living with family or friends until strained budgets or interpersonal conflicts make the streets or public shelters more feasible alternatives. Homelessness represents a variety of situations that share, at some point, the loss of a residence by a person.

## Chronic Homelessness

Chronic homelessness occurs among those persons who are unable to maintain any social or financial supports. Among the homeless in Los Angeles (Farr et al., 1986), 15 percent had been homeless for longer than a year, without any periods of residential stability. From 1985 to 1986, one quarter of Chicago's homeless had been homeless for 2 or more years (Rossi and Wright, 1987). In Charleston, West Virginia, nearly 40 percent of the men and 25 percent of the women used a shelter an average of more than 1 week per month and more than 3 months per year (Carter, 1985).

Boland (1986:13) presented the case of a chronically homeless alcoholic:

John was once a first-class carpenter, but for the past ten years, alcohol has ruled his life. He is no longer employable in his trade. Now 45 years old, John has spent most of the past seven years living at an emergency shelter for alcoholics. He receives no benefits from income support programs. When he is sober, he earns a little money at odd jobs. . . . John never married and has little contact with his family. His alcoholism is so severe that he has experienced brain damage.

Among the mentally ill, chronic homelessness occurs when social supports and financial resources are very limited. Current practices result in the return of patients to community settings after their behavior has been stabilized in a hospital. Discontinuation of medication, and sometimes rejection of further treatment, may follow. Negative attitudes toward service delivery personnel often develop in this situation; in turn, these attitudes decrease the likelihood of effective care (Levy and Henley, 1985).

Terry's (1986:52–53) notes described a 53-year-old schizophrenic woman who was chronically homeless:

She [consistently] had inappropriate behavior, i.e., urinating in sinks, defecating in showers, showering with all her clothes on, screaming and talking to herself, and assaulting other guests for no reason . . . filthy, lice infested . . . inappropriate clothes for the weather . . . bounced around from agency to agency. The shelter . . . did not want to put her out on the street. . . . They tried to get her pink papered [institutionalized] several times, but no one would take her: she was "in touch with reality" . . . she did not want treatment and refused medicine.

## Episodic Homelessness

Episodic homelessness stems from crises and problems that are less continuous than those involved in the chronic condition. Two thirds of the homeless in inner-city Los Angeles were episodically homeless, experiencing periods of stability, living on their own or with friends or family, since they first became homeless (Farr et al., 1986).

Baxter and Hopper (1981:35–36) described the case of an episodically homeless man:

Joseph is a 92-year-old man currently living on the streets. . . . He gets SSI, but his money ran out earlier than expected this month. . . . He had been staying at an "old men's home" . . . after briefly being hospitalized owing to a fall on a subway train. . . . He left the home because of the way he was treated there. . . . He then moved to the Salvation Army House on the Bowery, but soon left because the meals cost too much. Now stays in a hotel when he can, on the streets otherwise. Survives on his monthly check, handouts, and loans from friends.

## Temporary Homelessness

Many individuals and families become homeless temporarily because of natural disasters or other calamities. Children and women may become homeless temporarily after an episode of abuse within the family. The psychiatrically impaired who are normally cared for within their family may also become homeless temporarily when the family system becomes too taxed by their demands or behavior. Temporary homelessness often is resolved by reintegration into the system of social supports that is still accessible to the temporarily homeless person (Levy and Henley, 1985). When a support system no longer exists or has become inaccessible, the temporarily homeless may become episodically or chronically homeless.

Boland (1986:14) provided an illustrative case of a family that may only be temporarily homeless:

> Tammy and Lucas and their two children . . . lived in a rented house. Tammy worked part-time in a local variety store. Luke worked as a skilled laborer in an Auburn shoe factory . . . the shoe factory closed. Luke was laid off. Luke received unemployment compensation until the first week of August. It was not enough. In May they missed their first car payment. In June they fell behind on the rent. In August the car was repossessed, making job hunting more difficult. In September they were evicted. They set up a tent on a friend's property. In November the weather turned cold. They went to the town office to apply for assistance. They are staying in a motel as they look for an apartment.

---

*Panel 1–3*

### Changing Forms of Homelessness

There is no sharp dividing line between the chronically homeless and those homeless for shorter periods. Chronic homelessness is itself usually the end point of a long period of increasingly unstable residential arrangements. Several comparative studies indicate how the downward slide into chronic homelessness can occur.

In Chicago, Rossi (1988) found that General Assistance clients remained housed by living with others, usually their parents, or by receiving some subsidy from relatives. However, these extremely poor households were not able to support unproductive and behaviorally difficult household members for many years, leading, in the long run, to the homelessness of these members. In fact, mental illness and alcoholism were ten times more common among the homeless than among the housed General Assistance clients. Several other studies confirm that homeless persons have higher levels of disabilities and lower levels of social and financial supports than the domiciled poor (Farr et al., 1986; Fischer, Shapiro, Breakey, Anthony, and Kramer, 1986; Sosin, Colson, and Grossman, 1988).

The comparison by Bassuk and Rosenberg (1988) of homeless mothers with housed AFDC recipients reached similar conclusions: the homeless mothers had fewer social supports (the housed welfare mothers often had close ties with an extended family), had more often been abused, and showed higher levels of substance abuse and serious psychiatric problems.

Individuals come to a shelter in quite different circumstances. The chronically homeless are more likely to have frayed social ties, serious illnesses, and a fatalistic attitude about their homelessness. Those temporarily, and to a lesser extent episodically, homeless are more likely to have access to social and financial resources that can be used to reconnect to the settled society. Temporarily homeless persons are likely to experience high levels of anxiety about their insecure residential status.

## CONCLUSIONS

The problem of homelessness in the United States today has been shaped by a century of social and economic changes and social policy efforts. Far from being a clearly distinct group in the larger population, homeless persons experience the same personal problems and suffer from the same weaknesses as many others. In the homeless population, however, these problems become magnified. For the homeless, the social service system has failed, family stability has ruptured, and alternative resources are inadequate.

Understanding the situation of persons who are homeless requires stitching together the various threads of their past experiences with housing and work, friends and family, health and social services. Responding effectively to an individual's evident problems ultimately requires comprehending much of the fabric of his or her life. So too with the problem of homelessness itself: the short-term solutions, whether building another shelter or holding another charity ball, have to be followed by long-term strategies that tap the resources of many social institutions.

# Shelters and Services

## INTRODUCTION

An emergency is created when any individual or family becomes homeless. Lack of a home means inadequate food, poor health, diminished social supports, and continual stress—an absence of the most basic moorings of individual identity and well-being. The primary goal of most of the 5,400 shelters in the United States is to meet these emergency needs, preventing them from progressing quickly to even more complete misery and death (U.S. Department of Housing and Urban Development [HUD], 1989).

Beyond the common commitment to helping homeless persons survive, shelters differ in many ways. In appearance, some shelters could be mistaken for bus station waiting rooms, while others appear to be like military barracks; some shelters provide cozy bedrooms in renovated church basements or in rehabilitated apartment buildings. For their funding, shelters draw on diverse sources: private charities, public grants, church tithes. Shelter services may include support for the mentally ill or substance abusers, religious programs, transitional work opportunities, and group therapy. The skills and temperament required in a person to work with shelter users vary accordingly.

In brief, the physical characteristics of shelters, their funding sources, service programs, and staff skills and orientations vary almost as much as homeless persons and the numerous local communities in which they appear. "Working with the homeless" means different activities in different shelters and at different times.

This chapter provides background information on shelters and the services available through them. The major influences on shelters' impact on homeless persons and on the experience of shelter work are each discussed: shelter philosophy, type, staffing and management, as well as the larger service network. Several key debates about shelters are summarized: Should shelters provide an array of services? Are professionals necessary?

## SHELTER PHILOSOPHY

The particular features of a shelter reflect the answers given by its founders and operators to a few basic questions: What should the shelter seek to accomplish? Who should finance the shelter? Who should work in the shelter? When should the shelter call on other service providers for assistance? From these answers, a shelter philosophy emerges.

### Shelter-Based Services

First and foremost, shelters vary in their goals—in what they seek to accomplish with their guests. Although many shelters focus on meeting only the emergency survival needs of their guests, others provide a range of services for less immediate needs—physical and mental health, substance abuse, family counseling, job assistance, literacy training.

Boston's historic Pine Street Inn focuses on emergency needs: "We hammered out a philosophy of the place. . . . We said we wanted to provide food, shelter, and lodging to people who are homeless. That's it. We kept it simple" (Hirsch, 1989:108); "providing the 'basics' to the homeless in an atmosphere of care and respect" (Pine Street Inn, 1985:1).

The Catholic Charities Parish Shelter program in Chicago goes beyond emergency concerns:

> The program emphasizes casework planning and follow-up. . . . caseworkers help . . . occupants to develop immediate as well as long-term goals for regaining permanent independence. . . . Each resident enters into a contractual agreement with the shelter, taking personal responsibility for his or her stabilization process. In addition, residents undertake a number of tasks designed to facilitate self-sufficiency. (Redburn and Buss, 1986:119–120)

The survey by the U.S. Department of Housing and Urban Development (1989) of shelters in population areas of 25,000 or more indicated the prevalence of a service orientation. Between 80 percent and 95 percent of shelters provided food and/or showers/baths, laundry facilities and/or television, and clothing, but many went beyond these basic services. More than three quarters referred guests for some form of psychiatric counseling or provided counseling themselves, although often on an informal basis. Almost two thirds of the shelters made referrals for housing and jobs; some had employment and training services, and 70 percent required guests to do chores. One in five shelters required participation in religious activities.

A simple count of programs offered does not begin to indicate the diversity of services provided by shelters nor the operational complexity that a diverse program mix can produce. Increased administrative work and efforts to coordinate efforts between programs inevitably are one result.

### Funding Sources

As with other organizations, those who fund shelters influence shelter philosophy, although they may turn shelter operations over to others. Shelters funded by

---

*Panel 2–1*

## Services in Shelters?

The merits of a focus on emergency needs or service provision has been a subject of heated debate. Baxter and Hopper (1984) argued that shelters should remain oriented toward emergency needs—homelessness is not fundamentally a social service or mental health problem; shelters should focus on ensuring immediate survival. Even shelter directors and staff often express the fear that by developing a comprehensive range of services, shelters are taking an undesirable step toward institutionalization—becoming long-term inferior solutions to meeting the housing and service needs of the very poor.

Others, often mental health professionals, criticize shelters that function only as temporary respites, unable to assess or treat their clients' biopsychosocial needs (Drake and Adler, 1984; Goldfinger and Chafetz, 1984; Lipton and Sabatini, 1984). A shelter without access to or provision of mental health care, Goldfinger and Chafetz (1984:105) assert, "can serve only as a temporary respite but is without ameliorative value." In the words of one shelter employee in Boston, the question is simply, "Are we a program or are we a shelter?"

---

*Panel 2–2*

## The Shattuck Shelter: Program Activities

*Daytime*

| | |
|---|---|
| Saturday, Sunday | Work Crew Projects |
| Monday | Religious Visitors |
| Tuesday | Expressive Therapy (Field Trip Every Other Week) |
| Wednesday | Social Services Team Meeting |
| Monday–Friday | Medical Respite Rounds with Physician or Nurse Practitioner |

*Evenings*

| | |
|---|---|
| Saturday, Sunday | Alcoholics Anonymous (AA) Group, Medical Clinic |
| Monday | Podiatry Clinic (biweekly), AA, Health Care Clinic |
| Tuesday | Dental Clinic, Women's Group, AA, Health Care Clinic |
| Wednesday | Medical Clinic, AA |
| Thursday | Expressive Therapy, Health Care Clinic—M.D., AA |
| Friday | Medical Clinic, AA |
| Monday–Friday | Social Services and Department of Mental Health Case Management |

hospitals or other health care agencies are most likely to emphasize intensive services. Traditional missions, not including those operated by the Salvation Army, often receive funds solely from church contributors and emphasize emergency and spiritual needs rather than intensive services. Shelters begun by social activist groups and sustained by their volunteer efforts often also eschew an emphasis on intensive services (Hope and Young, 1986:40–41).

The government, at all levels, is a major source of shelter funds. In 1984, 80 percent of city and county governments provided some services for homeless persons (HUD, 1984): 60 percent subsidized private shelter operators; 37 percent funded rehabilitation and other services; 20 percent operated shelters (rarely more than two shelters). In addition, almost half of the local governments provided vouchers for temporary housing in hotels, motels, or apartments and one fifth rehabilitated and/or leased shelter buildings, at minimal charge, to nonprofit groups.

---

*Panel 2–3*

**Minimum Requirements for Emergency Shelters**

(Cincinnati, Ohio)

Minimum Requirements for Shelters Requesting City Operating and Capital Improvement Funds

An emergency shelter provides crisis relief for the homeless on a daily basis with no fee or religious participation required. It provides the basic needs of a place to sleep, humane care, reasonable security, safety, and referrals to other agencies.

The following requirements are categorized as Essential (E) or Desirable (D). A shelter is expected to comply 100% with the essential requirements and 70% with the desirable requirements. In order to receive city funds, shelters will be asked to answer *Yes* or *No* to the following statements, and to sign their responses.

A. *Administration*

(E) 1. Our shelter is a legal entity according to the provisions of Chapter 1702 of the Revised Code (that is, we are a nonprofit corporation).                    Yes   No
(E) 2. Our shelter shall have a policy statement which includes our shelter's purpose(s), population served, program(s) description, shelter criteria and a nondiscrimination policy. Our shelter does not require religious participation, and does not discriminate on the basis of race, religion, or national origin.                                                                 Yes   No
(D) 3. Our shelter has an organization chart delineating the administrative responsibilities of all persons working in the shelter.                          Yes   No
(D) 4. Our shelter has space designated for securing all documents in order to insure client confidentiality.                                                    Yes   No

B. *Personnel*

(E) 1. Our shelter has enough adequately trained on-site staff persons (paid or volunteer) to meet the needs of residents and insure the safety of the facility during all hours the facility is open to residents. (A recommended ratio during awake hours should be 1 staff to 50 residents for an adults-only facility, and 1 staff to 25 residents for a facility housing children.)     Yes  No

(D) 2. Our shelter has a written position description for each type of position, which includes at least job responsibilities, qualifications, and salary range.     Yes  No

(D) 3. Our shelter has written personnel policies in effect which include at least a code of ethics for all our personnel.     Yes  No

(D) 4. Our shelter's staff has been trained in emergency evacuation, first aid procedures, and CPR procedures, and has received on-going inservice training in counseling skills, handling tensions in a nonviolent manner, emergency assistance skills, etc.     Yes  No

(D) 5. Our shelter has an organized method of selecting and training all volunteers. In addition, volunteers have job descriptions and identifiable lines of authority.     Yes  No

C. *Fiscal Management*

(E) 1. Our shelter carries out fiscal activities which are consistent with sound financial practices based upon a budget approved by our board.     Yes  No

(D) 2. Our shelter has records of accountability for any client's funds or valuables we are holding or managing.     Yes  No

(D) 3. Our shelter has received an independent audit and will make available all financial records as may be required by the city.     Yes  No

D. *Procedures*

(E) 1. Our shelter has written policies for intake procedures and criteria for admitting people to our shelter.     Yes  No

(E) 2. Our shelter reads to all residents our house rules, regulations, and disciplinary procedures; asks residents to sign a copy, and/or posts a copy in a conspicuous place.     Yes  No

(E) 3. Our shelter keeps a daily office log which documents the activities of each shift, and any unusual or special situations and instructions regarding special clients (such as children, medicine, illness, etc.). Our shelter requires the staff person in charge of each shift to sign the log for that shift.     Yes  No

(D) 4. Our shelter maintains an attendance list which includes, at least, name, age, and sex of all persons residing in our shelter.     Yes  No

(D) 5. Our shelter refers people to the appropriate shelter or agency if we cannot provide shelter.     Yes  No

(D) 6. Our shelter provides all residents with a one-page handout which summarizes our program, or posts a copy in a conspicuous place.     Yes  No

*(Continued)*

*Panel 2–3*   (Continued)

E. *Medical*

(E) 1. Our shelter has available at all times first aid equipment and supplies in case of a medical emergency.   Yes   No

(D) 2. Our on duty shelter staff has available a life squad phone number. Our shelter's staff rely on life squad personnel or a physician to determine medical status.   Yes   No

(D) 3. Our shelter has at least one staff person on duty who is trained in emergency first aid procedures.   Yes   No

(D) 4. Our shelter has a written policy regarding the possession and use of controlled substances, prescription medicine, and over-the-counter medication.   Yes   No

F. *Food Service*

(E) 1. (For shelters which provide food service): Our shelter has made adequate provisions for sanitary storage and preparation for food.   Yes   No

(E) 2. (For shelters which serve infants, young children, or pregnant women): Our shelter has made provisions to meet their nutritional requirements.   Yes   No

(D) 3.(For shelters which do *not* provide food services): Our shelter has a nearby food system available for our residents.   Yes   No

G. *Safety*

(E) 1. Our shelter has a fire safety plan, including a fire detection system.   Yes   No

(E) 2. Our shelter has an emergency evacuation plan posted.   Yes   No

(E) 3. Our shelter has an office phone to contact fire or emergency squad or police.   Yes   No

H. *Equipment and Environment*

(E) 1. Our shelter has a housekeeping and maintenance plan.   Yes   No

(E) 2. Our shelter provides each person with at least a crib or bed with linen, or a mat.   Yes   No

(D) 3. Our shelter has an adequate ventilation and heating system.   Yes   No

(D) 4. Our shelter is clean and in good repair.   Yes   No

(E) 5. Our shelter has reasonable access to public transportation.   Yes   No

(D) 6. Our shelter has adequate and separate toilets, wash basins, and shower facilities for men and women.   Yes   No

(D) 7. Our shelter can provide space in which to meet with individual residents.   Yes   No

(D) 8. Our shelter has laundry facilities available to residents, or access to laundry facilities nearby.   Yes   No

(D) 9. Our shelter has secure storage for checking in/out residents' personal belongings.   Yes   No

Shelter Director                                   Chairperson, Board of Trustees

_____        _____

Date: _____        Date: _____

The role of local governments in funding shelters in turn obscures the state and federal roles: homeless services were usually paid from state and federal sources; only 20 percent of local governments used locally generated revenues. Across different states, the total state financial contribution for homeless persons is highly variable; a study of six states in Fiscal Year 1987–1988 found a range of state spending on homeless programs from lows of 12 cents per capita (based on the total population) in New Mexico, 15 cents in Georgia, 23 cents in Wisconsin, and 54 cents in Ohio, up to $2.27 in California and $13.83 in Connecticut (Burt and Cohen, 1988).

Several national funding programs have played a decisive role in developing shelter-based services throughout the country. The most prominent effort has been the Health Care for the Homeless Program funded in 1985 by the Robert Wood Johnson Foundation and the Pew Memorial Trust, in conjunction with the United States Conference of Mayors (Wright and Weber, 1987:19–20). Each of the 19 local projects funded was required to draw on a coalition of organizations to provide community-based care with interdisciplinary health care teams (see Chapter 7).

The Stewart B. McKinney Homeless Assistance Act of 1988 funded numerous new programs. The National Institute of Mental Health used "McKinney money" to fund demonstration projects oriented to chronically mentally ill homeless persons. The projects sought to develop a comprehensive system of training, case management, outreach, day program, mental health treatment and/or networking activities in particular cities. Several case management projects relied on para-professionals, but in general the projects encouraged shelter professionalization.

In 1988, the National Institute on Alcohol Abuse and Alcoholism funded nine McKinney research demonstration grants (NIAAA, 1988). Each project involved

---

*Panel 2–4*

**The Stewart B. McKinney Homeless Assistance Act**

The McKinney Act was signed into law on July 22, 1987. It created numerous pro-grams to protect and improve the lives and safety of the homeless, including physical and mental health care programs, education and job training, emergency food and shel-ter services, income assistance, transitional and long-term housing, and substance abuse programs. The McKinney Act also established the Interagency Council for the Homeless and mandated that the Council review all federal activities and programs to assist homeless individuals; reduce du-plication among federal agency programs; monitor, evaluate, and recommend im-provements in programs conducted by fed-eral agencies, state and local governments, as well as private voluntary organizations; provide technical assistance to eligible agencies and programs; collect and dis-seminate information about homelessness, including publication of a bimonthly bulle-tin; and report to Congress and the Presi-dent on the nature and extent of homeless-ness and evaluate the federal response.

Source: Garrett and Schutt, 1990:41

delivery of community-based alcohol and/or drug abuse treatment and rehabilitation services; in addition, each included some innovative component—outreach programs in the streets and shelters, intensive case management, and supportive housing arrangements. Again, most of the projects encouraged professionalization within shelters.

The federal government has also sponsored one major funding program for shelters that encouraged delivery only of emergency services. The Emergency Food and Shelter Program of the Federal Emergency Management Agency (FEMA), established in 1983, provided funds only for food and other consumable supplies in shelters (Cooper, 1987; GAO, 1987). By 1984, states had distributed $140 million of these FEMA emergency funds. The Department of Housing and Urban Development (HUD) also began an Emergency Shelter Grants Program in 1986 to fund rehabilitation and conversion costs for shelters, in addition to their operating costs.

Both the FEMA and HUD programs were expanded with the addition of funds generated by the Stewart B. McKinney Homeless Assistance Act of 1987. In many states, McKinney funds quickly became the primary source of federal support for homeless programs and exceeded substantially the provision of state dollars. Specific McKinney funding programs that required state matching dollars garnered less state participation (Burt and Cohen, 1988).

In spite of the importance of public funds, shelters have primarily been operated by the private sector: in 1984, secular groups operated 54 percent, while religious groups operated 40 percent. City and county governments operated only 6 percent.

## SHELTER TYPES

The various possible combinations of shelter service approaches, funding sources, and staffing requirements result in several basic shelter types. Each plays an important role in meeting the needs of some homeless persons.

### Emergency Municipal Shelters

In earlier decades, municipal shelters typically provided barracks-style accommodations without "frills." New York's "Muni" was the most renowned:

> Late at night they flop on the concrete floor of the big room. . . . During the day they get two meals served up with only a tablespoon to make sure no one gets killed—at least on the premises. Most of the time they just wait in line. . . . There are lines for patients. Lines for men who have gripes. Lines to get meal tickets from clerks protected behind metal screening. . . . Lines stretch endlessly through the brick limbo and lead back to oblivion. . . . Only the staccato commands of the shelter employees puncture the stillness. "Hey, you, get over there," the guards shout as they herd the men into the elevators. "Move, Mac. On your feet, fella. Hurry up, Pops." The contempt echoes off the dirty green wall and produces flashes of resentment in the faces on the line. (Bahr, 1973:131–132)

Within the public sector, the traditional "muni" approach is still common. For example, the Keener Building on Ward's Island (outside of New York City) is "a paragon of institutional thrift: a skeletal staff, rudimentary bedding (light mattresses on metal frames), and walls innocent of any ornament but graffiti. The one concession to relief of tedium is a new mess-hall, open only during mealtimes." TVs in the common rooms seldom work, newspapers are out-of-date. Many of the guests, too incapacitated to do otherwise, "languish in nearly unbroken torpor, confined to the building throughout the day but for an occasional, supervised walk." Violence is common; the temptation of acquiring a dollar or two by assaulting an alcoholic is too much for some to resist (Baxter and Hopper, 1981:54–58).

The municipal women's shelter in Manhattan is more oriented to services—personal hygiene supplies, clothing, a locker, and services are each available—but the "no frills" approach is still in evidence: bedtime is at 10:00 P.M.; housekeeping duties must be performed when requested by an attendant; medication, funds, and personal belongings must be turned over to staff; phone calls and cigarette distribution are announced with a loudspeaker; guests must make their beds army-style (Baxter and Hopper, 1981:63–67).

Boston's Pine Street Inn is the most prominent example of a privately run municipal-style shelter. Pine Street focuses on emergency services, but in a specially designed building that facilitates cleanliness, basic comforts, and the management of over 300 guests.

Pine Street's philosophy is to allow anyone to use the shelter with no questions asked and to avoid forcing people into treatment. The only intake procedure is a quick frisking, and there are just two rules: no violence and no drinking. All except the elderly, sick, or uncontrollable must line up nightly to receive a bed pass and are deloused and given sleepwear before retiring. The rudimentary services

---

*Panel 2–5*

### Difficulties with an Open Door Policy

Shelters that welcome all homeless persons but do not provide support services face a dilemma: Some of the persons most likely to be attracted to a "hands off" shelter are very troubled. "The staff has never considered Pine Street to be a suitable place for someone with serious mental illness. These men and women are in need of more than 'the basics' which characterize Pine Street. Still, with no other alternative, we have not refused to take anyone in. But these Guests of ours need more professional services. They are the most vulnerable of men and women relegated to a life on the streets. Some will not eat, others do not wash, still others refuse warm clothing in the dead of winter. All are easy prey for streetwise hoods. Some wander to the Inn on their own, others are often brought by the Boston Police . . . now the numbers are straining Pine Street's ability to offer shelter to these homeless men and women."

*Source*: Pine Street Inn: *Newsletter*, Fall 1985, 23:1.

provided include regular van trips to detoxification centers and hospitals, a highly regarded nursing clinic, and some referrals—to lodging opportunities, social security offices, detoxification centers, and the like.

## Missions

Religious missions, common sights in the skid row districts of earlier years, continue to shelter homeless persons in some cities. Mission philosophies range from viewing homeless persons as sinners in need of salvation to providing treatment for needy souls. Salvation Army missions offer a range of therapeutic opportunities; some mandatory, others voluntary. Spiritual therapy at Salvation Army missions has included attendance at services and "self-denial" contributions of earnings to the mission; "companionship" therapy involving enforced group living; and low-wage salvage work termed "work therapy." Formal therapy may be available, although few participate; vocational counseling therapy and structured milieu therapy, involving curfews and deportment regulations, have been more popular (Bahr, 1973; Wiseman, 1970).

## Private Nonprofit Emergency Shelters

The role of the nonprofit sector in providing emergency shelter expanded in the 1980s. Mainline churches began to establish or sponsor shelters that often were quite different from the old missions—small in size, committed to the dignity of homeless individuals, and, for the most part, not concerned with religious conversion. Some other secular nonprofit organizations have developed service-oriented shelters for special groups, while some advocacy groups have taken up sheltering the homeless as a political act.

Smaller shelters usually provide an environment quite unlike a barracks— more homelike and caring; their roots are often in a church or other concerned community. These shelters tend to survive through donations and voluntary labor. Volunteers work together with the homeless to prepare food, celebrate holidays and birthdays, and maintain lunch programs for other needy persons. Guests are not required to divulge personal information, to accept social services, or to participate in religious activities, although staff members seek to aid guests in their efforts to secure assistance from other agencies. When length-of-stay limits are not maintained, many guests become, in effect, long-term shelter residents; vacancies are rare (Baxter and Hopper, 1981:69–73).

Some combination of strict behavioral rules, preclusive admission policies, or frequent barring are used by many private shelters to keep order and to maintain the safety of guests and staff. An alternative approach is to provide more intensive services to help guests cope with the stress of being homeless and a range of personal troubles.

## Service-Oriented Shelters

In the 1980s, service-oriented shelters ranged from dormitory-style accommodations with some ancillary services to long-term shelters providing quasi-

*Panel 2–6*

## Behavioral Rules

Shelters can manage the most difficult problems associated with substance abusing or mentally ill guests by making clear rules against disruptive behavior and penalizing the violators with expulsion.

*Action, Inc. Emergency Shelter Rules*

1. The Shelter opens at 8:00 P.M. and closes at 7:00 A.M. each day of the week including Saturday and Sunday.
2. No area, space, or chair is reserved. It is first come–first chair basis.
3. Absolutely no visitors are allowed on the premises.
4. Wake up time is 6:00 A.M.
5. Area must be picked up prior to leaving.
6. Everyone except staff must be out of the shelter and off the property by 7:05 A.M.
7. No one is allowed to "hang out" on the property before 7:55 P.M. and after 7:05 A.M.
8. Blankets and sleeping bags must be rolled up after use.
9. No violence, threat of violence, or rowdy behavior will be tolerated.
10. No type of weapons including "knives" are permitted on the guests during their overnight stay.
11. Smoking is allowed only in a designated smoking area.
12. No alcohol and/or drugs are allowed on the property in the shelter or on the grounds around the area.
13. All guests must clean up after themselves before they leave.
14. At the discretion of the shelter supervisors, a half-hour clean-up period will be conducted. All guests are asked to participate.
15. Lights will be turned on or lowered by the direction of the staff.
16. Everyone is expected to participate in making out a guest intake form.
17. After 11:00 P.M. is quiet time. No loud socializing, singing, yelling, partying, etc., etc., will be tolerated. Be considerate of your neighbor.
18. Residents must clean up after themselves.
19. If you are asked to leave for not following these instructions, you must LEAVE IMMEDIATELY.
20. You will be given another chance the following night if the staff tells you that you have another chance.
21. Once in, guests cannot leave. If guests leave for any reason, they cannot be allowed in again.
22. Remember, the STAFF has the final say while you are in the shelter.

therapeutic environments. Boston's Long Island Shelter assigns beds on a nightly basis to 350 guests. The beds which are in large dormitories are separated into small groups by dividers. In addition, case managers conduct a detailed intake interview with new guests and routinely make referrals to service agencies. The shelter also provides a transitional employment program, a literacy program, a stabilization program for alcoholics, a full-time nursing clinic, and a psychiatric

---

*Panel 2–7*

**Preclusive Admission Policies**

Smaller shelters, particularly those that rely on volunteer staff, often limit admissions to those who seem appropriate to the shelter's mission and programs.

GUIDELINES FOR REFERRAL

*Introduction*

The philosophy of the Somewhere Shelter is to recognize each person's right to be respected with dignity and to be provided with the basic human needs of food, clothing, and shelter. We are a temporary shelter which specifically addresses the needs of the people who are in a temporary crisis situation but have the coping skills necessary to be reintegrated into a more normal living situation and/or work force. We are not an emergency, walk-in shelter. Guests will have been referred to us by an agency and gone through a screening process before being accepted.

*Guidelines*

1. Our shelter can accommodate 6 adult men and women, 18 years and over.
2. We cannot accommodate families or children.
3. Persons should be ambulatory for fire safety reasons.
4. Persons not suitable for our Shelter are:
   a. Active alcohol or drug users
   b. Persons showing signs of disruptive behavior or serious mental illness.
5. Before referring a homeless person to us, please ask a few basic questions.
6. If a person seems appropriate for our Shelter, you can call us and give the card information to the staff person answering the phone who will inform you if we have an available bed and if we can accept the person.
7. If the person is accepted [he or she] will be expected to be at [a transit public stop] at 6:00 P.M. to be escorted to the Shelter.

NOTE: If a person is not appropriate, please see the attached list for possible referrals.

---

nurse. Shelter guests in these programs are assigned regular beds and make a commitment to maintain their program standing by signing a contract.

Among services offered by other shelters are vocational rehabilitation and job placements through local businesses (Heckler, 1984), a savings program that requires employed guests to bank a portion of their earnings as a future rental deposit, and art therapists who engage interested guests (Schutt, 1986).

Some specialized shelters provide more intensive services to a specific group. The Massachusetts Department of Mental Health's three shelters in Boston provide a more stable setting for severely mentally ill homeless persons. Staff evaluate guests clinically at intake and develop treatment plans in case conferences. Three programs seek to rehabilitate guests who are at particular levels of functioning: identification of and efforts to resolve personal problems; supervised rehabilitative

---

*Panel 2–8*

## A Day in the Life of Shattuck Shelter

In the winter, the Shelter is always filled. As each guest arrives, he or she is greeted at the door, then registered, and given a towel. New guests are taken aside by a Shelter Coordinator to complete a Registration Card, read the rules of the Shelter, and urged to have a medical screening at the Shelter Clinic. Telephones are constantly ringing. "No, we are all filled up. . . ."

The Shelter is crowded by 5:30 and there is the constant din of conversations, the clattering of chairs, and the blare of the TV. A long line of men and women has formed waiting for dinner to be served. Card games and dominoes have begun. Guests wander between the sea of beds, back and forth to the dining area. After dinner, the card games, conversation, and TV begin again. Some guests lie down, exhausted after a long day on the cold streets. Many of the guests who work late now begin to arrive from their jobs and pick up dinners that have been saved for them. At the Reception Counter, requests are constant: "Can I have a razor?" "Is the Social Worker in?" "Did I get any mail today?" "Do you have change for a dollar?"

At 5:45, a Police car pulls up outside the Shelter. Immediately, a staff member helps to bring in an inebriated man who has a small bleeding cut on his forehead. Medical Clinic staff clean and bandage the wound and return to their office where several guests are lined up waiting to be seen.

Meanwhile, at the back of the Shelter, another line forms as the clothing room is about to open. In the Staff Office, a mental health case manager and social worker are conferring with a Shelter Coordinator about a mentally ill guest. The Coordinator agrees to keep an eye on the guest and enters the information into the Shelter Log. In another office, women guests gather for their weekly arts and crafts group.

By 8:30, guests are preparing for bed. Hand washed clothes are draped over radiators. Late arrivals quickly wash up. At 9 o'clock, lights are out. A few guests mingle in the bathrooms.

*Source: The Shattuck Shelter News, Fall/Winter 1985, 1(1):3, 4.*

---

work followed by a community workshop; hygiene and recreation activities for those most severely ill. Guests also run a social club in which other homeless persons can participate.

The Women of Hope shelter in Philadelphia is a low-demand permanent residence administered by the Sisters of Mercy for 24 chronic mentally ill women (91 percent are schizophrenic) who have been homeless for a long period (Reyes, 1987). Shelter staff begin to build trust with potential guests on the street in an outreach program. A preliminary assessment of guests is done upon their entry to the shelter; however, the assessment is done informally and unobtrusively over 2 to 4 weeks. Case managers then develop a comprehensive treatment plan focusing on mental health, physical health, social service needs, residential services, and the activities of daily living. There is much individual attention, all activities are

---

*Panel 2–9*

**Struggling against Shelterization**

One of shelter providers' most commonly expressed fears is that their guests will become acclimated to shelter life and lose interest in regular housing. Several common policies reflect the fear of "shelterization": Guests may be allowed to remain for only brief contiguous periods, perhaps 3 or 4 days at a time; physical separation of a shelter's social worker in a separate building "so as not to give the wrong impression that we are a social service agency"; closing on weekends "to prevent settling in."

---

voluntary, and staff members emphasize the dignity and worth of each guest, participating actively with them in advocacy efforts.

Yet another concern often voiced about shelter-based service provision is that shelters may thereby become a poor, but accepted, substitute for regular service agencies that should be responsive to homeless persons themselves.

> At no point was it determined as a matter of policy that shelters were to be a substitute for other human service systems, such as those for mental health, education, foster care, and skilled nursing care. However, that is what seems to be happening in many parts of the country. (Institute of Medicine, 1988:36)

## Client-Run Shelters

Efforts by homeless persons themselves to develop shelter programs have been limited. In Philadelphia, the Committee for Dignity and Fairness for the Homeless was started by three homeless men but soon secured FEMA money for a shelter program. The shelter provides 40 cots in a church basement and two meals each day. Shelter staff deliver sandwiches to those on the streets with an outreach van and encourage the homeless to come to the shelter. At the shelter, a paid professional caseworker assesses client needs and develops a daily task schedule. Clients who seem not to be able to "accept responsibility" for themselves are referred to another provider.

In Los Angeles, the "Homeless Organizing Team" established a makeshift settlement called *Tent City* on state land during the 1984 Christmas season (Heskin, 1987:179–180). Although the homeless were soon removed from the site, the Los Angeles Labor Council built an alternative plywood shelter for 138 persons that was maintained for several months on a temporary basis. However, when 60 homeless persons occupied a former children's playground on skid row to establish a shantytown (termed *Justiceville*), they were arrested. Soon after, they formed a nonprofit group to work on homelessness.

These five shelter types seldom appear in a pure form—a shelter may have characteristics of more than one type, and many shelters change over time—often beginning with a strictly emergency orientation and then adding services over time. Nonetheless, the differences between shelter types can result in quite different work experiences. Both shelter management and individual staff should be aware of their own service philosophy and seek to prevent needless friction about services through appropriate selection, socialization, or change strategies.

## SHELTER STAFF

Working with homeless persons is not a fashionable career. The hours are long, the pay is low, and the conditions are, at times, trying. "I feel good if I'm able to go through the day and say hello to everyone [at the shelter] and have them say hello back. . . . Eliciting a smile from somebody here is a mighty big reward" (*Boston Globe*, July 27, 1987:15).

Since shelters range from large bureaucratic organizations to small quasi-therapeutic support groups, their staff run the gamut from career government employees and highly trained professionals to concerned volunteers and recovering alcoholics. Staff at large shelters usually include administrators, health care and social service professionals, and paraprofessionals who supervise beds and meals. Small shelters may employ only a director and one or two paid staff with relatively undifferentiated duties. Many shelters also use volunteers and guests in transitional work programs to provide some basic services.

Direct care staff, often termed *counselors* or *house managers*, provide the most essential shelter services. Direct care staff duties may include: daily upkeep to maintain the shelter's cleanliness and safety; ordering supplies; logging guests' entry to and exit from the shelter; assisting with referrals, intake, and transportation; providing limited, informal counseling; introducing new guests to the shelter; and supervising food service.

Newer shelters tend to use volunteers more than established shelters; in fact, publicly administered shelters may include no formal role for volunteers. More often, volunteers play some role in donating and/or preparing food. Volunteers may also be encouraged to meet with and provide social support to guests and to advocate with agencies for guests' needs.

St. Francis House in Boston, a day program with a psychosocial rehabilitation emphasis, uses volunteers extensively with 270 supplementing the work of 40 paid employees. Volunteers help in meal preparation, cleaning, and clothing distribution, talk with guests and engage them in recreation activities, provide clerical support, and help in fund raising (Reyes, 1987).

Nurses usually work in a clinic within a shelter, assisting guests with their medical problems and referring them to hospitals when necessary. Nurses may keep guests' prescription drugs and help them maintain a regular medication schedule. Psychiatric nurses are available in some shelters to help guests with mental health problems and/or to refer guests with mental health problems to other facilities.

Many shelters provide a "work experience program" (WEP) for guests with an interest in and capacity for maintenance work. Program participants receive a regular bed in a special area within the shelter, a small stipend, and the right to

---

*Panel 2–10*

### Quincy Interfaith Sheltering Coalition
### Job Description: Evening Counselors

The Evening Counselors are very important in the shelter's operation. They are the first personnel clients meet and they set the tone of the shelter. They must enjoy working with people yet be able to enforce rules and keep order. Their duties will include, but are not limited to the following:

- Conduct the Admissions Process, including the screening of clients.
- Supervise the evening meal and give assistance where needed.
- Supervise showers.
- Supervise evening activities, keeping order and enforcing all rules.
- Spend time with clients, being attentive to problems or concerns.
- Make referral to Case Managers as appropriate.
- Attend at least 75% of staff meetings and training sessions.
- Keep all required documentation and records.
- Responsible to make lunches as directed by the Food Service Coordinator.
- Will do assigned cleaning and laundry.
- Facilitate a positive atmosphere within the shelter for both the clients and employees.

---

remain at the shelter during the day and for an extended period. In exchange, WEPs perform maintenance and food service chores.

## Case Management

Case managers help to connect guests with needed services. Although there is no consensus on the appropriate backgrounds or duties for case managers, they can play a critical role by arranging appointments and referrals; arranging and monitoring service delivery; coordinating agency personnel, and advocating for patients (Bachrach, 1984b:43).

Case managers help to identify shelter guests' social service and income support needs and then work with guests to meet these needs. At Boston's Long Island Shelter, case managers interview all new guests with a 14-page instrument that reviews their residential, work and health history, and needs. The Shattuck Shelter records critical information on medications and personal identity during intake interviews; guests are then encouraged to meet with a case manager for a more formal assessment. In addition to evaluating guests' problems, case managers may develop plans for securing housing and social services, provide counseling, and participate in program development and case conferences.

An important part of case management duties is helping guests to secure needed services—legal aid, medical care, income supports, and social services. Larger shelters may actually have a separate position for an "advocate" or a "referral counselor" who calls other agencies on behalf of guests. Advocates may also help guests locate housing or services and then accompany guests to their appointments.

At the Westside Drop-In Center in New York, case managers are paraprofessionals, without advanced degrees. These caseworkers are responsible for almost all client needs: they develop case plans with the client, are held accountable for implementing the plan and following up as necessary, and are available to help clients in all areas of need. However, specialized services and formal counseling are provided by outsiders. Case aides also play a critical role in the Westside supported housing option, the Traveler's Hotel.

The Women of Hope shelter in Philadelphia (Reyes, 1987) uses mental health aides who were formerly homeless themselves. The aides help with housekeeping, assist clients with appointments, bathing, and in developing and implementing treatment plans. The aides also keep client information and provide an interested companion for conversation. They "know what it is like to be close to the edge of a mental breakdown while living on the street."

But not all programs find nonprofessional staff to be adequate. Marsha Martin, Director of New York's Midtown Outreach Program, explained why the program uses only staff with a Master's degree and experience:

> A successful encounter on the streets requires staff to immediately assess a situation and to make decisions quickly. This is why we need people with professional degrees. We tried less qualified people (BSW's, RN's, LPN's and volunteers) but they were not capable of doing the job. (Heckler, 1984:157)

Paraprofessionals at the Queens Mens' Shelter in New York, both the shelter guards and the "Institutional Aides," often shared clients' perspectives about their problems, but also tended to hold stereotyped, cynical, sometimes even hostile attitudes toward the clients (Morrissey, Dennis, Gounis, and Barrow, 1985).

Conflicts between paraprofessional and professional staff are not uncommon. At one shelter, case aides felt they were being treated as second-class citizens

---

*Panel 2–11*

### Case Aides in Action

Case aides staff the residence 24 hours a day, with back-up help available to the one person on duty. The case aide plays many functions—covering the front desk; providing security; monitoring the lounge and individual women; keeping a log; and engaging the women individually and in small groups in a range of formal and informal discussions and activities. This continuous monitoring provides information for formal casework provided by the agency and on-site by staff from another mental health/social service agency. This allied agency also provides group therapy and recreational activities as well as a consultant psychiatrist (Reyes, 1987).

---

### Panel 2–12

## Professionals or Paraprofessionals?

What social and educational backgrounds are preferable for shelter staff? Some mental health professionals argue that staff who lack clinical training are insensitive to psycho-pathology and unable to provide needed treatment (Segal and Baumohl, 1980). A director of a privately funded shelter in the Boston area recounted that he stopped relying on volunteers to provide regular staffing, because "the population is too diverse, needy; incredibly complicated cases."

Paraprofessional staff often stress the importance of experience: "Staff who have been homeless themselves can relate better to guests" (Schutt, 1987:47). And formerly homeless advocates point to the value of their experiences:

> I've had body lice and horrible skin infections from sleeping on the steam grates. I know what these people are going through. I've been as bad off as any of them, so I know it's possible for them to get better.

> Source: Joseph Rogers, president and founder of the Mental Health Association of Southeastern Pennsylvania, as quoted in the New York Times, October 4, 1987:51.

Politics can also shape the perceptions of the need for professional staff. In a battered women's shelter described by Pahl (1979), radical feminists focused on the oppression of women and "tended to stress the normality of the women who came to stay at the refuge, rather than their need for help," while other staff focused on the women's personal problems and emphasized their need for professional help.

---

because college-trained case managers expected the aides to perform routine chores but not to influence guest policies. In another shelter, "everyone felt responsible for everything" and professional social workers and paraprofessional coordinators found themselves responding to guests' requests in different and often contradictory ways (Schutt, 1987).

Shelters can reduce these problems by requiring case managers to work with case aides as a team, by dividing responsibilities between paraprofessionals and professionals more clearly, and by requiring professionals to consult with para-professional staff before setting policies.

## THE SERVICE SYSTEM

As the shelter population has multiplied, so too have efforts to coordinate shelter activities and their relations with service agencies. By 1988, all but three states had statewide coordination strategies: an interagency coordinating council, a designated state coordinator, or a special governor's task force. Half of the states had passed legislation or adopted policy initiatives explicitly concerning homeless-

---

*Panel 2–13*

**Conflict Over Professionalism in Cincinnati**

"These professionals wanted a nine-to-five therapeutic program, five days a week—in total opposition to what the community saw as a priority," says Buddy [a community activist who helped to found Cincinnati's Drop-Inn Shelter]. "We wanted a seven-night-a-week program that could keep our people alive. They said shelter and rehabilitation couldn't work together,

and community involvement threatened their control of the center. Eventually, Over-the-Rhine folks took control, and we got what we wanted—a community-based program that runs all week and has a staff that suits our needs—one that's racially balanced, has half men and half women, and uses recovering alcoholics.

*Source*: Hope and Young, 1986:112.

---

ness, and state funding for programs for the homeless grew by 80 percent in 1987–1988 alone (Toff, 1988).

In spite of these developments, research to date suggests many deficits in the service system for homeless persons. Service providers in six states reported that low-income and supportive housing were not available in sufficient numbers, that more case management was needed, and that health care, transportation and benefits, and jobs programs were inadequate (Burt and Cohen, 1988).

More systematic studies in Washington, D.C. (Dockett, 1986), St. Louis (Johnson, 1988), Chicago (Sosin et al., 1988), and California (Vernez, Burnam, McGlynn, Trude, and Mittman, 1988) found that the provision of emergency services—food and shelter—was relatively successful. Nonetheless, shelter staff often did not know who in the service network could provide particular services, mental health services often were lacking, housing options were never sufficient, and many persons did not receive benefits they were eligible for. Hospital admission policies and bureaucratic agency requirements often deflected homeless mentally ill persons (Turner and Shifren, 1979) and agencies often shunned the dually diagnosed (Farr et al., 1986).

## Outreach Programs

The effectiveness of shelters is shaped in part by factors over which shelters themselves have little direct control, such as the preference of some homeless persons to stay on the streets rather than in shelters. This avoidance may be due to negative experiences with shelters, general distrust of service agencies, or to the unconcern with personal well-being produced by alcohol abuse or the disordered thinking associated with psychosis. Efforts to engage this portion of the homeless population require outreach in the community.

Several communities have developed aggressive outreach programs. Street teams in New York's Midtown Outreach Program visit locations that homeless persons frequent, offering assistance, leaving a phone number, and encouraging guests to use available services. The program's focus is on the chronically mentally ill homeless; it often requires multiple contacts to gain the trust of some homeless person so that they are willing to use a shelter or accept other services (Martin, 1986:4–6, cited in Ridgway, 1986). Outreach workers find that it takes approximately 9 months to engage their clients in food, shelter, and health care programs; another 3 to 6 months to secure cooperation in obtaining benefits and medication oriented to the clients' longer term needs; and another 9 to 12 months to obtain permanent housing, with ongoing case management support (Reyes, 1987).

In 1982, New York City added Psychiatric Outreach Teams to its Midtown Outreach Program in order to deliver professional psychiatric care in shelters and drop-in centers in Manhattan. Each team included a psychiatrist, a psychiatric nurse practitioner, a physician's assistant, and a psychiatric aide. They administer medications, refer clients to agencies, and involuntarily transport for evaluation homeless persons who appear to be dangerous to themselves and others (Reyes, 1987:27–30).

Other cities have developed different outreach approaches. Santa Monica uses four outreach teams from four agencies. The coalition arrangement avoids duplication of services and encourages cooperation and joint planning. The Center City Project in Philadelphia uses a mobile outreach team to initiate case management efforts, a mobile emergency team to respond to acute crises, and a winter emergency service to bring homeless persons to shelters during dangerously cold spells (Reyes, 1987).

## Day Programs

Another problem confronted by shelters is the homeless person's need for daytime activities. Although 60 percent of shelters (HUD, 1984) are able to remain open during the day, the others require that their guests leave; often this means a day of wandering the streets or congregating in public libraries and other public places. In order to provide more rewarding daytime opportunities, some organizations have opened day programs.

A drop-in program or "community living room" can supplement the caring activities of a shelter during the day. Drop-in programs for psychiatric patients can provide a secure environment in which staff gradually gain clients' trust. Minimal rules—no screaming, cleanliness—facilitate the maintenance of order and development of friendships. Furniture is arranged to encourage social contact while telephones, tables, and newspapers encourage the performance of life tasks. Staff lead field trips, mediate with the police, nurses, and other authorities, and may make referrals for health care, day labor, and the like (Breton, 1984; Segal and Baumohl, 1985).

Saint Francis House in Boston provides a comprehensive day program to homeless men and women using a psychosocial rehabilitation model (Reyes, 1987). Four hundred homeless persons are served each day; about half are chronically mentally ill. St. Francis House seeks both to provide a "home" during the day and to engage homeless persons in supportive rehabilitation services. The program includes a health clinic, art therapy, counselors for alcohol abuse, housing and employment, case managers, as well as such group activities as discussions of health and benefit programs, movies, singing and prayer, outings, AA meetings, and women's and men's groups. A range of service agencies send representatives to St. Francis House to help guests obtain their services.

## The Service Network

A third external problem that shelters confront is the need to secure a range of services from other agencies to meet the many needs of their guests. In fact, describing service provision only within a shelter can be misleading, since some rely heavily on other agencies to provide services. Guests with psychiatric problems may be sent to a local mental health clinic; substance abusers to a detoxification center. Ultimately, shelter operations can only be understood within the context of related service agencies.

The human services network for homeless people has never been highly structured. In the 1960s, Wiseman described the service route for homeless alcoholics: a "loop" from municipal court to a city screening facility to missions, the streets, and jail; a path traversed in many directions and having no end (Wiseman, 1970). Stoner (1984:4) characterized the system of service provision for homeless people as "a loosely organized network of emergency shelters which have no defined system or consistent organizing element."

Recent observations are no more positive. In 1988, representatives of six states pointed out numerous service system problems: insufficient case managers, inadequate health care, lack of transportation, inadequate services for children and youth and the dually diagnosed, unaffordable housing, and gaps in benefits, education, and job training opportunities, minimum wage coverage, and services for the nearly homeless (Burt and Cohen, 1988). One service provider described the service system for homeless persons as

> a pinball machine, with homeless individuals as pinballs which bounce, almost randomly, from one community agency to another. (Koegel, 1987:63)

For shelter staff seeking to connect guests with health and social services, the absence of an effective interagency network severely hampers success.

> Although the separate elements of the continuum may be of high quality, well designed, and staffed with the best meaning of clinicians, the absence of an effective interagency network may render their work ineffective. (Goldfinger and Chafetz, 1984:100)

The difficulties encountered by the Residential Care Center for Adults (RCCA) illustrate the problem (Dennis, Gounis, Morrissey, and Holz, 1986). Although the initial plan for the RCCA assumed referral linkages to local agencies and service providers, no advance effort was made to develop such linkages. Service agencies frequently rejected clients referred by the RCCA staff as inappropriate for the agency. Ultimately, the RCCA had to focus on developing more programs itself.

---

### Panel 2–14

## Accessibility versus Comprehensiveness

The effort to provide many services within one comprehensive residential shelter program may solve many coordination problems, but it also tends to discourage from participation those who are more resistant to treatment, as New York's experience with the Residential Care Center for Adults revealed.

> The ideal of client movement along a continuum of coordinated services addressing different levels of need may be difficult to achieve outside of a relatively self-contained, quasi-institutional system. The trade-off here is that the effort to narrow the "gaps" or "cracks" can result in limiting services to a narrow segment within the homeless population—those who will be least resistant to moving from the relatively unrestrictive environment of the streets or shelters to a more institutional setting. (Morrissey, Gounis, Barrow, Struening, and Katz, 1986:104)

The Institute of Medicine's report, *Homelessness, Health, and Human Needs* (1988: 27–36, 94–96) identified another aspect of the accessibility/comprehensiveness trade-off in the delivery of health care services: shelters simply do not provide the service capacity required to respond effectively to many health problems.

Access barriers to those eligible for health and other benefits from regular service agencies included lacking the required documents, transportation problems, not having a watch, conflicts between shelter hours and appointment times. On the other hand, shelter-based clinics, which were more accessible to homeless persons, had other problems: limited hours, dependence on volunteers, limited access to less common medications and medical specialties, inability to screen systematically, difficulty in obtaining malpractice insurance.

Many shelters have referral counselors to help their guests secure services from other agencies, but the most effective efforts involve system-wide service coordination. In Philadelphia, the Center City Project for the homeless mentally ill is a relatively successful coordination effort. Developed by the city's Office of Mental Health and Mental Retardation, the project provides two programs: a highly structured crisis-oriented unit for the episodically or transitionally homeless—typically treatment-resistant young adult chronics; and a less structured program for the chronically homeless—typically older deinstitutionalized schizophrenics. The high structure program emphasizes crisis intervention, a mobile emergency team, specialized care, and community rehabilitation facilities. The less structured program links homeless persons with SRO units; it includes mobile outreach teams, day services, shelters, respite care, and a personal care center (Reyes, 1987).

Multiservice centers are another approach to coordinating service delivery. In Portland, Oregon, the Burnside Community Council sponsors Baloney Joe's, a multiservice center and job clinic that also provides emergency shelter during the winter and low-cost housing and ongoing emergency shelter for homeless women with children (Heckler, 1984). Burnside Projects also sponsors other services, including free warm jackets and sleeping bags, a Clean-Up Center, outpatient alcoholism treatment, and a pretrial release program. Finally, the Burnside Consortium (HIE, 1988; Korenbaum, 1984) renovates and operates SROs, providing multiple programs for both the homeless and other SRO residents.

Another approach to system coordination is to maintain a centralized intake unit from which homeless people are sent to shelters offering a variety of services. New York City's Human Resources Administration accepts homeless people for its 18 shelters primarily through two intake units. Shelter-based services include medical clinics in seven shelters and on-site mental health rehabilitation programs in three shelters.

St. Louis developed a Homelessness Services Network in response to a right-to-shelter suit (HIE, 1988). The network combines several features that enhance service coordination: it is overseen by a board including 50 public and private groups, and all services are delivered by a private vendor under contract to the city. A Reception Center provides a 24-hour walk-in central intake point; a day shelter is available for women with children; a comprehensive counseling and placement program provides skills training on such issues as parenting, budgeting, and tenant rights and responsibilities; transportation is available. Outreach services are provided by volunteers who visit sites where homeless people congregate.

In order to be effective, the service system must include a continuum of housing opportunities, outreach workers who make the initial connection to homeless persons, case managers available in shelters and day programs, and coordination among related agencies. The continuum of housing opportunities should have three elements: basic emergency shelter, with an open-door policy and survival services; transitional housing, in which residents are required to take some responsibility for their own welfare and staff provide longer-term social services; long-term residences, or homes with some services (Stoner, 1984:7).

## CONCLUSIONS

The emergency shelter system developed in response to a growing national crisis, without sufficient time for careful planning or resource acquisition. In its early years, this system reflected, in a sense, policy-making from the ground up, and it has been characterized as fragmented, loosely structured, and lacking any consistent organizing element.

Yet there are important lessons to be learned from the emergency shelter system for those who seek to make policy for and deliver services to the homeless population. Within this system are contained a wide array of innovative approaches to responding to the needs of homeless persons. The factors that have shaped the development of this system are a catalog of the opportunities and constraints that face those who seek to improve it.

Implementation of sophisticated service systems is not easy. Program managers complain about the lack of public sympathy with the mentally ill homeless; their lack of political lobbying clout; the dearth of research and conceptual models to guide new approaches; the tendency to label persons as a requirement for receipt of services; the lack of low-cost housing alternatives and income supports;

and the relative lack of interagency coordination (Ridgway, 1986:49–51; Rog, Andranovich, and Rosenblum, 1987:4). But when the political will to respond to the problem of homelessness strengthens, the shelter system contains within it the seeds for a successful assault.

Any service that is offered must begin where the potential clients are, so that the shelters and streets have to become acceptable sites for service outreach. Shelters also can serve as a base of operations for health care and other programs that are offered by other agencies. When traditional boundaries between shelters and traditional service agencies are spanned, shelters can be the starting point for a service continuum; and for some persons, shelter-based services may be all that is needed in order to regain a more stable lifestyle.

**3**

---

# Counseling and Case Managing

## INTRODUCTION

> I remember when I first hit the Row for good, and I was still alive enough to feel it. I remember patrol cars—and dark bottle-strewn alleys and nights. And my own flesh crawling with lice, and with half-forgotten shame. I remember the smell of warm port wine, and the sounds of groans, and men puking in doorways.
>
> I remember watching the old men, and waiting for my brain to be numbed like theirs. I remember the waiting—and only the small struggles against it—for that chronic disease of the Row, hopelessness, to take firm hold of the body, dull the senses, still the torment.
>
> The hopelessness—the sense of failure. That begins before you get to the Row, but it's like a slight infection then—if you could get over it while you're still out there. If there was anything—anyone—out there to stop you. . . . (Blumberg et al., 1973:35–36)

Working with homeless persons is more than just a job: it is reaching out to people in extreme crisis; it is creating a bond to restore stability; it is showing that society can respond to the needs of its most destitute members. Working with homeless people involves the most delicate interpersonal problems and the least tractable interorganizational conflicts—it involves being there after others have left.

Most shelter staff who work with homeless persons are employed as counselors, who supervise shelter guests directly, or case managers, who help shelter guests secure needed services. This chapter focuses on the basic skills needed by these counselors and case managers—skills that also are required by other shelter staff and by staff in related agencies. Five basic skills are discussed: how to establish relations with homeless persons; how to maintain rapport with homeless persons; how to help homeless persons connect to service agencies; how to manage interpersonal conflicts involving shelter guests; how to reduce feelings of burnout and stress among shelter staff.

We also attempt in this chapter to answer three controversial but related questions about service provision: Are homeless persons interested in services? Can services help homeless persons? What role should case managers play in service provision? Our answers to these questions help to connect our discussion of service delivery skills to recent research findings about homeless persons and to the variation in case managers' roles between shelters and over time.

## ARE HOMELESS PERSONS INTERESTED IN SERVICES?

Homeless persons are often thought to reject offers of assistance, particularly assistance with mental health or substance abuse problems. And it is clear that homeless persons are not all waiting for services, even for shelter, with arms outstretched. Some actively refuse offers of help, while others accept help grudgingly and soon lose interest; some use encounters with service providers as occasions for acting out their frustrations (Levine, 1984; Segal and Baumohl, 1980). The resistance to services resulting from these attitudes can be extreme:

> Wendy weeps. It is cold and lonely on the grate. From time to time, bundled in a rough gray army blanket, she glances down the street. She pulls blackened hands out of the sleeves of her plaid wool jacket and warms them over the current of hot air. There is nowhere for her to go unless she wants to sit on a chair at the intake until dawn, two hours away, which she doesn't. . . . How it's come to this again, she wishes someone could tell her. . . . She couldn't even take care of herself anymore, burning herself against radiators. . . . She hugs her bottle close to her. She's sick as a dog. But, she says, "Psshh! You can have it. I'm out here. I got my vodka." (Hirsch, 1989:393–394, 400)

There are several reasons for homeless persons' negative attitudes toward services. Concern with more immediate needs may decrease interest in social or health services. For example, dropout and recidivism rates are very high for both homeless alcoholics and chronically mentally ill persons receiving treatment without housing, but when housing is provided in conjunction with treatment, dropout rates plummet (Rosenheck, Gallup, Leda, Gorchov, and Errera, 1989; Sadd and Young, 1987). Some homeless people reject help because of prior negative service experiences, although they can be engaged by outreach workers after a prolonged period of trust-building and assistance with basic needs (Breakey, 1987).

In spite of these understandable reasons for rejecting services, research indicates that many homeless persons respond positively to offers of help that are made in an appropriate manner. None of the 50 formerly homeless psychiatric inpatients studied by Lipton, Nutt, and Sabatini (1988) refused a residential placement upon discharge; only 9 percent of the homeless mentally ill veterans studied by Rosenheck et al. (1989) refused help or only wanted basic services at the time they first entered an intensive service program; just 7 percent of the 123 homeless persons studied by Morse, Calsyn, Volker, Muether, and Harmann (1988) refused attempts at engagement and service linkage.

Surveys of homeless persons' service interests find substantially less interest in mental health services than the prevalence of serious mental illness would

---

*Panel 3–1*

**Philadelphia's Diagnostic and Rehabilitation Center**

In the 1960s, Philadelphia developed a special center to help homeless alcoholics stabilize their lives. Some of the difficulties experienced by counselors in this "Diagnostic and Rehabilitation Center" (DRC) were in clients' level of interest in services (Blumberg et al., 1973).

According to their initial assessment at the DRC, the homeless alcoholics were socially isolated, guilty, suspicious, and despondent; they lacked social maturity and integrity and had little self-control or self-esteem, all as compared to the general population.

In part, as a result of these personality traits, clients tended to give DRC counselors oversimplified descriptions of what the clients wanted. Clients seldom looked beyond their immediate needs or else could not express long-term needs.

In order to gain the trust of alcoholics who came to the DRC, the counselors had to prove themselves by helping with some concrete benefit, such as medical services. Crisis intervention when needed was effective particularly in strengthening relations with clients. Lunchroom conversations also helped.

But the best efforts did not always have the intended effect. It seemed that over four in every ten alcoholics were trying to "con" the case manager on a regular basis; conning in turn was an important predictor of failure in the program. Most agencies did not want skid row alcoholics, so DRC counselors had to prepare clients for punitive treatment, fully document the client's needs, provide support during the process, and follow through after rejection.

---

suggest, but interest in housing and benefits is high (Ball and Havassy, 1984; Mulkern and Bradley, 1986; Schutt, 1991). The key is to provide help with the most immediate needs first—sandwiches for those living on the streets, showers, clean facilities, a pleasant environment, and physical health care for those staying in shelters—before attempting to address problems in social relations, psychiatric difficulties, or substance abuse. Persistence and a gradual approach can pay off in the long run.

Clearly, client "interest in services" is a moving target, sometimes a hidden target, that cannot be described fully by a survey administered at one point in time. Clients' expressions of their service interests are likely to change as they develop a relationship with service staff and learn what services are available. Staff understandings of clients' service interests may change as their rapport with clients improves.

## DO SERVICES MAKE A DIFFERENCE?

Will the delivery of services make a difference in the health and subsequent residential stability of homeless persons? Four recent studies have investigated the value for homeless mentally ill persons of services and supported housing; each found some beneficial effects of a combination of services and housing, but they differed in their assessment of the effect of case management itself.

Lipton, Nutt, and Sabatini (1988) assigned homeless subjects randomly to a comprehensive residential program in New York. After 1 year, those in the residential program were more likely to be in permanent housing, spent fewer nights homeless outside of the hospital, and were more satisfied with their living arrangements, although they did not differ in the severity of their illness. One month after clients were assigned randomly to a comprehensive service program in St. Louis, they were significantly more satisfied with their services, had been housed for more days, had spent less time homeless, and were more stable socially than were other clients (Morse et al., 1988).

Two nonexperimental studies* found that health and subsequent residential stability improved for homeless persons in supported housing, but findings about the value of case management itself were inconsistent. Homeless veterans fared better when they were seen more frequently by a program clinician/case manager (Rosenheck et al., 1989), but case management had no independent effect for homeless persons in New York City (Barrow, Hellman, Lovell, Plapinger, and Struening, 1989). (In fact, most participants in the New York study who were not placed in housing dropped out of the service program.)

The comprehensive study by Blumberg et al. (1973) of services for homeless alcoholics in Philadelphia also indicated the possibility of different effects of different service approaches. Blumberg focused on the operation of the Philadelphia Diagnostic and Relocation [now Rehabilitation] Center experiment, in which some clients were connected to an "anchor counselor" who coordinated services for each client, maintained a consistent tie to each client, and provided sympathetic counseling, emergency cash, and easy access to other staff and information. Intensive counselors met clients at lunch, after work, and at AA meetings, visited them in detoxes and helped them to get out of jail, engaged them in weekly group therapy, and scheduled visits to social and cultural events. At a half-way house—the comparison condition—there was little counselor involvement with clients.

The success rate was highest with intensive counselors and lowest in the traditional halfway house. Apparently, the lack of counselor involvement and the halfway house's provision of "instant stability" (since all living needs were met) generated unrealistic expectations. Some clients rushed into jobs before they were able to forego drinking. Intensive counselors, on the other hand, were more likely

---

*In experimental research, subjects are assigned randomly to the treatment group (in this case, those receiving the special services) and the control group (those not receiving the services). Random assignment ensures that the groups are equivalent in all respects except for the treatment (with a certain margin of error). Nonexperimental studies do not use random assignment, so differences between treatment and control groups may be due to differences in the individual characteristics of persons in these groups. Statistical techniques can be used to control for any such individual differences that have been measured, but when subjects have decided for themselves whether to enter treatment or not, it is likely that subjects will differ on many characteristics related to treatment outcome; statistical controls are unlikely to be adequate.

to develop in-depth relations with clients and their families, and thus helped to create ongoing support structures for the critical postdetoxification period.

Sadd (1985) also indicated the importance of social supports for successful rehabilitation of homeless alcoholics, although in this research social support was not provided by case managers. Among patients in a detoxification program using a social support approach, 68 percent showed up for their appointments; among patients in a medical detoxification program, only 30 percent to 35 percent kept their treatment appointments. Eighty-two percent of those in the social detox program felt that the program's atmosphere made it easier to detox, compared to just 28 percent of those in the medical detox program.

In spite of significant differences in client reactions to these two different detoxification programs, there were few ultimate rehabilitation successes in either setting. Other studies indicate that the success rate is generally very low in public detoxification programs. In a wide range of studies, three quarters of the detox-ification patients left without a referral to aftercare; of those who received a referral, acceptance rates ranged from 30 percent to 100 percent. A large proportion of those referred never enrolled; the dropout rate for those entering outpatient treatment was very high (two thirds left after their second appointment); and the retention rate in residential programs also was low (Sadd and Young, 1987).

Overall, the research evidence suggests that case management combined with a residential program is very effective in improving several aspects of client status. When case management is delivered by itself, its effect is less certain, but probably often positive in the short run. Little is known about long-term success, but it clearly is difficult to achieve in the face of severe health problems.

## Differences Between Subgroups

One possible explanation for the mixed evidence of positive benefits of case management is that the particular groups that have been the object of different studies benefit to a differing extent from this service.

Young adults who are chronically mentally ill and homeless are often regarded as particularly treatment resistant (Appleby, Slagg, and Desai, 1982; Bachrach, 1982; Kellerman, Halper, Hopkins, and Nayowith, 1985; Lamb, 1982), but chron-ically mentally ill young adults in New York City were no less likely to obtain or remain in housing than others, nor to make successful psychiatric treatment linkages (Barrow et al., 1989).

Homeless persons with diagnoses of both mental illness and substance abuse generally have greater problems of health and welfare, but being dually diagnosed had no independent effect on homeless clients' success in securing housing or psychiatric treatment in New York City (Barrow et al., 1989; see also Wright and Weber, 1987).

Virtually all homeless persons are extremely poor, but variation in economic status even within this range still seems to matter. Homeless persons who are receiving economic benefits have shorter episodes of homelessness, better health status, and greater service satisfaction than those without any income source (Rossi, 1989; Sosin et al., 1988). Socioeconomic background was positively and independently associated with securing housing and psychiatric treatment among homeless mentally ill persons in New York City (Barrow et al., 1989), as was early referral to entitlement services.

The effects of situational factors on distress in the general population are mediated by psychological dispositions, particularly cognitive flexibility and powerlessness. Lack of cognitive flexibility and a sense of powerlessness—belief in an external locus of control—result in demoralization and ineffective coping. Social support may also act as a buffer against the negative effects of stressors (Kessler and McLeod, 1985); in fact, social support and a sense of control may be alternative psychosocial resources (Mirowsky and Ross, 1989).

Similar patterns appear in studies of homeless persons. Both personal mastery and social support reduced levels of depression among homeless persons in Birmingham independent of other characteristics, and both played a mediating role for other influences on depression (LaGory et al., 1990). Contact with family members was associated with shorter episodes of homelessness among Health Care for the Homeless Clinic clients—an association that accounted for lower rates of chronic homelessness among women (Wright and Weber, 1987).

These studies add an important dimension to understanding homeless persons' service needs and interests. Service providers need to be sensitive to the possibly complicating influences of youth, substance abuse, minimal economic resources, lack of a sense of mastery, and social support. An effort should be made to identify each client's status with respect to each of these characteristics and to plan services accordingly. However, the research evidence suggests that caution is warranted about the implications of these characteristics: providers must keep an open mind and avoid jumping to conclusions about the service interests or service responsiveness of particular types of homeless persons.

## THE PROCESS OF CASE MANAGEMENT

The specific functions of case managers vary from shelter to shelter, but case management is most often thought of as a process of working with clients to identify their service needs and then helping clients procure these services from other agencies. Case managers may also be responsible for outreach to potential clients, one-on-one counseling, and reassessment of service needs and opportunities. Less formally, a case manager can be a supportive friend; a guide to available services; an advocate for unmet needs; a bridge between the shelter and other agencies; and a means for reconstructing ties to the settled society.

### Case Management Alternatives

In spite of many similarities in what all case managers do, the specifics of the job differ between settings. Some case managers provide clinical help directly, others only refer clients to clinicians; many case managers are responsible for their own case loads, while others focus on particular client needs or a portion of the case management process as part of a team. Many case management skills are

*Panel 3–2*

## A Guest's Perspective on Case Management

Case managers try to develop effective service relations with their clients and attempt to help clients secure services from other agencies. The recollections of a formerly homeless alcoholic illustrate these two components of successful case management (Sullivan, 1986:14–15):

> I started to go to St. Francis House [a day program in Boston] for lunch . . . I was feeling lost, lonely and I felt that I was one of the bums of the world . . . had no self-esteem. After lunching at St. Francis House for a few weeks, I realized that the staff noticed me and appeared to be glad to see me. This was something very special for me, as nobody had been glad to see me for a long time. I had a long straggly white beard and long tangled hair full of lice.
>
> Everyone made me feel welcome at St. Francis House but two of the counselors were very friendly towards me. . . . I was very reluctant to talk or open up in any way, as my experience in the past was that people who kept quiet, kept out of trouble. I would not [go on Welfare]. After 9 months of Chris telling me how it was my right to accept welfare and that I was not taking anything that was not mine, I gave in. . . . She told me where to go for my birth certificate. . . . She then sent me for my Social Security Card. To go into any of these buildings was a great

> trauma for me at this stage. I tried to go where Chris had sent me but I got as far as the 2nd floor and turned back. Each time I went back to St. Francis House I expected Chris to be either annoyed with me or to give up on me. But she did neither. She just talked to me and seemed to understand my situation. Chris came with me next time. When the bureaucrat behind the desk tried to dismiss me, Chris stood up for me and we came away with my Social Security receipt. The next step was to go to the Welfare Office. . . . I would never have gotten past the door, if Chris had not been with me.

It required friendly overtures over a period of weeks until Mr. Sullivan responded to case managers, months of encouragement until he was interested in services, and repeated attempts until he secured these services. Case managers must be prepared to spend much of their time overcoming resistance both from clients and from service agencies, and to retain their patience and good cheer all the while. But the payoff for these efforts can be substantial. Mr. Sullivan, for example, finally secured pension funds from his former union and was then able to move into a low-income housing project.

generic—other shelter employees, from nurses to counselors, use some of them. Effective case management can be provided by staff in multiple agencies—for example, local mental health agency case managers may visit homeless persons in shelters or meet with them elsewhere and collaborate with shelter case managers.

### Service Broker or Service Provider

The supportive interpersonal relationship that case managers develop with clients must be complemented by effective interorganizational relations with service agencies. When clients experience a personal crisis, when they have fear of applying for social benefits, when social relations in the shelter deteriorate, case managers must be able to provide direct interpersonal support. Nonetheless, every shelter relies on other agencies for meeting some of the needs of at least some of its clients, and it is up to case managers to make the connections required.

The balance struck by case managers and shelters between managing interpersonal and interorganizational relations varies between individual case managers and between shelters. Case managers in some shelters are expected primarily to help clients meet their needs through service agencies; these case managers often are termed *service brokers*. Case managers in other shelters concentrate on developing supportive relations with clients and in providing more direct help; these case managers may be termed *intensive* or *clinical case managers*.

Although intensive case managers working with homeless persons are a far cry from traditional clinicians providing individual therapy in scheduled 50-minute periods, several features distinguish the intensive case management role from the service broker role (adapted from Rog, Andranovich, and Rosenblum, 1987):

- Intensive case managers (ICMs) have clinical training or at least close supervision by a clinician.
- ICMs are ready to provide at least quasitherapeutic services and seek to establish strong, supportive, interpersonal relations.
- ICMs have a small client-to-staff ratio.
- ICMs provide services to the same clients frequently and for extended periods of time, with ongoing follow-up and support.

The need for an intensive case management style varies with the type of clients served and with the goals of service delivery. The problems involved in mental illness and substance abuse require more intensive help and a deeper understanding of the client, as do the problems involved in caring for young children. Clients with multiple health problems requiring the services of several agencies may require a more intensive approach.

The more ambitious the goals that a shelter sets for its clients, the more likely that intensive case management will be required. Developing natural family or peer support systems and encouraging a shift from dependence on drugs or alcohol to reliance on these support systems require the persistence and depth of an intensive case management relationship. A service broker relationship is unlikely to provide an adequate basis for teaching independent living skills (Rog et al., 1987).

## Generalist or Specialist

Intensive case managers are likely to be viewed as generalists, and are responsible for aiding clients with most of their service needs. Case managers who function as service brokers, however, may serve either as generalists or specialists. Each approach has some advantages and disadvantages (Levine and Fleming, 1987:17–18).

The *generalist* model of case management provides each client with a single person to relate to. This approach is more likely to develop trust among participants and allows case managers to use a variety of skills and have greater autonomy in their work. But high staff turnover, burnout, and inadequate communication with other staff are common problems.

The *specialist* model of case management involves a group of case managers who work as a team; each team member is responsible for a limited component of the case management process, such as assessment, advocacy, or residential placement. The model provides greater continuity of care, results in better planning and a larger knowledge base about clients; also it is likely to reduce staff burnout by reducing the complexity of case managers' responsibilities, and allows for more flexibility in responding to clients. But this approach also requires much more frequent communication, through meetings and informal interaction, and smoother coordination with other staff. Another disadvantage is that clients may play off team members against each other.

Whichever specific case management model is adopted, case managers must build relationships with clients that reflect the reality of the client's past experiences, present situation, and future options (Rog et al., 1987). Needs and problems must be assessed honestly. Suggestions from the client should be encouraged and respected. Interest in longer term goals, such as education, family formation, and employment, even if abandoned long ago, should be encouraged. Support should be provided after the initial transition to a more settled residence. Reflected within the case management relationship should be the seeds of successful independent living.

## How to Approach and Assess Clients

The case manager's first goal is to build rapport with current and potential clients—to lay the foundation for a relationship that can endure inevitable setbacks and pressures. Building rapport is an individualized and continuous process: some will resist overtures, others will welcome any attention; progress can begin unexpectedly, as can regression of the relationship.

### Approaching Prospective Clients

Mental health workers must often make special efforts to develop rapport with individuals in need of psychiatric services. Even when mentally ill individuals feel that they are ill, prior negative experiences with psychiatric services and the fear of stigmatization by others result in reluctance to seek out or accept services. But these fears appear even among those who are not seriously mentally ill. Thus, Kathleen Owens's innovative approach to establishing rapport can serve as a model for many case managers (see Panel 3–4).

Such success stories are not easy to come by; progress in much smaller steps and at a slower pace is usually the most that can be expected, and even then the highly developed clinical expertise and the interpersonal empathy reflected in Kathleen Owens's story are prerequisites. Staff involved in such aggressive outreach must be prepared for unanticipated responses and the more difficult issues that may be unveiled. But Owens's open, aggressive, yet very empathic outreach approach is one to be emulated. And, like Owens, all shelter staff should spend

*Panel 3–3*

## A Brief History of Case Management

In the United States, different approaches to case management, and different names for it, have been popular at different times. Case management has its origins in the Charity Organization Societies of the late nineteenth century. Begun in 1877, in Buffalo, New York, local Charity Organization Societies attempted to provide poor relief in a more systematic way than previously had been the case, emphasizing the importance of understanding persons in their environment. Volunteers, called "friendly visitors" visited the homes of new welfare recipients in order to assess objectively the recipient's situation, to emphasize the value of working, and generally to encourage the poor to change their ways.

Unfortunately, few communities were able to recruit enough volunteers to visit their welfare clients, and friendly visitors' judgmental approach often failed to change clients' lives. By the early years of the twentieth century, many communities were relying on full-time staff for social services. In 1917, Mary Richmond, a leading social worker, proposed a new, more professional approach to poor relief.

Casework, Richmond (as quoted in Steiner, 1966:181) suggested, should involve "those processes which develop personality through adjustments consciously effected, individual by individual, between men and their social environment." In

other words, caseworkers would help individuals to adapt to their environments through one-on-one counseling and support. Caseworkers would need advanced training and the type of professional association that helped doctors and lawyers maintain their knowledge base and limit access to job opportunities to those who were properly trained.

Thanks in part to growing recognition of the work of Sigmund Freud and in part to increasing acceptance of the professional model of work in other occupations, Mary Richmond's casework model received wide acceptance. Both social work schools and professional social work associations grew. But the Great Depression stymied the efforts of professional social workers to lessen the problems of the poor on a case-by-case basis.

Public relief on a vastly enlarged scale required many new recruits to welfare jobs—many more than the number of professionally trained social workers. New welfare programs—the foundation for current programs—included social security insurance, assistance to the disabled, and welfare for dependent children. Government relief workers handled large caseloads and had little time for the field work and individual counseling recommended by Richmond.

The postwar years witnessed a decline

some time just "hanging out" with guests in the shelter in order to begin the process of trust-building.

As a client becomes willing to discuss her situation and needs with the case manager, increasing attention should be given to more comprehensive assessment. Assessment continues throughout the relationship and may be more or less formal, depending on shelter policies, client preferences, and the needs of agencies from which services will be sought. Finding out what the client wants, and not just what

---

in the resources and personnel necessary for relief efforts, and a return to the effort to professionalize relief workers. But the mid-1960s welfare explosion again sent welfare caseloads soaring and again brought large numbers of new recruits into the profession (Schutt, 1986).

Two federally mandated changes helped to lessen the increasing demands made on welfare workers. The provision of income maintenance was separated from the delivery of social services by the Social Security Act of 1969—the work of determining eligibility and distributing checks could then be handled by less skilled employees, while case workers could focus on social service needs that required more training. Second, a new flat grant system determined benefit amounts with a fixed and simplified formula, so that little training was required for eligibility workers.

Complementary changes occurred in mental health services in the postwar years. Widespread disenchantment with the squalid conditions and high costs of state mental hospitals, high expectations for the new psychotropic medications, and recognition of the value of less stigmatizing forms of community-based treatment stimulated the movement to deinstitutionalize the treatment of mental patients. The Community Mental Health Act of 1963 began a large-scale reduction in the population of state

mental hospitals that continued throughout the 1970s.

By the 1980s, the fabric of social services which was able to support the poor and disabled had been rearranged and, in some ways, weakened. Chronically mentally ill persons were less likely to be warehoused, but more likely to have to fend for themselves in the community. Welfare mothers were less subject to intrusive inquiries from social workers, but were also less able to receive individualized help with family problems and money management. Although many of the resulting problems disappeared from public view amid crowding, crime, and substance abuse in poor neighborhoods, the social service needs of homeless persons wandering downtown areas were inescapable.

Case managers were soon viewed by many as providing a means for reconnecting homeless mentally ill persons to mental health and other services. "Outreach" became a central concern of case managers, who sought to encourage homeless persons to move into shelters, make contact with service agencies, and turn away from the insecurity of life on the streets. The pendulum was again swinging toward "indoor relief," and the role of case managers was changing accordingly. To this day, the perceived need for case managers continues to grow.

---

she "needs," is a vital part of assessment and is done most effectively in the client's natural environment, whether this is the shelter or a street corner (Rapp, 1987).

### Assessing Clients

The process of learning about clients can best be understood as one of naturalistic inquiry. This process requires the same skills used in effective listen-

*Panel 3–4*

## "Peddling" Psychiatric Services

My model is an itinerant peddler who announces his availability by a sonorous cry, "Fresh vegetables—okra, tomatoes, cabbages," and movement along a well-populated street. Hawking mental health services to a very suspicious, very despondent shelter population requires a similar ostentatious cry in a crowded locale. . . . An ideal place . . . is in the crowded dining hall or up and down the cafeteria line. The message can be something like this: "I'm from the Saint Elizabeth's Hospital Mental Health Team. We're here to make sure no one gets too depressed. A lot of people here look very discouraged and frustrated."

That introduction is likely to bring some nervous jokes: "Yeah. There are some really crazy ones around here. Hey, Joe, they come to carry you off to St. E's!" The clinician-hawker of mental health services responds, "No we are not thinking of carrying anyone anywhere. We know that being without a home and stuck in this shelter has got to be rough and discouraging, and we're here to see if we can help lessen the discouragement just a little. You were teasing Joe, but my hunch is that you worry about what happens to people in this place. You are trying to make light of it, but I bet it is very tough, and I admire your spirit. What keeps your spirit up?"

All this talk should be going on in a public place like a shelter dining room. The clinician should be talking in a loud voice, addressing an entire *ad hoc* group of shelter clients. . . . Moving too soon from a public, informal, *ad hoc* group setting to a more private office setting can be a mistake. The clinician should stay hawking his or her

mental health expertise in that crowded, noisy, hectic shelter dining room or corridor. In hawking your mental health wares, you are powerfully projecting to potential clients a feel for you as a human being, a feel for your attitude toward homeless people, and a feel for your theory of the causes and remedies for mental distress.

This population of homeless people can be expected to be particularly distrustful and wary—harboring memories of many bitter experiences with so-called helpers, who have been disappointments or downright hurtful. So it is unreasonable to expect such distrustful people to come into a private office to see us when we are unknown to them. Quickly and briefly, with gusto and flare and yet with professional dignity we need to display ourselves.

For example, a clinician might say to a group of homeless persons, "I admire you for keeping going in this situation of having no home. I bet you wonder when it is going to be your turn to get some ease in life. Even as a kid you may have been the one to have to worry and take care of your parents and the other brothers and sisters. Maybe it feels like nobody ever takes care of you. So I admire you for keeping going." This speech should be delivered loudly and with the clinician's eye sweeping over a whole group of listeners. Remember that you are wanting, at this first stage, to display yourself and your treatment philosophy in terms meaningful and relevant to homeless people. This is a crucial first stage before you focus on the specific situation of a particular client. If the cafeteria line is long, you should rove along the line

*Panel 3–4*   (Continued)

making this speech several times and then retrace your steps. In my experience, if you have hawked well, on the retracing-your-steps stage, three or four people will grab you and ask to talk to you. In shelters which serve children as well as adults, frequently children have grabbed the clinician and requested help for their parent. At times the child has literally dragged me to the overwhelmed parent.

. . . Telling homeless people that you, the clinician, admire them may seem stupidly Pollyannish and therapeutically counterindicated. . . . Yet, in my experience, such affirmation of the strengths of homeless people by me has enabled homeless clients rather quickly to acknowledge personal problems. For example, a clinician might say, "I admire you for keeping going without a home and living in this shelter." And the homeless person responds, "You admire me? Well, yes it takes a lot to keep going here and avoid getting further messed up. People here meddle and carry tales to the staff and agitate, and it would be easy to lay somebody out. And there is plenty of dope around that it would be easy to get onto. That *was* my problem; now at least I can let the dope alone, but I'm onto booze, and that's why I'm here. You want to hear about it?"

This may be the point for the clinician to ask if the client wants more privacy. He or she may say, "No." Many clients prefer talking about their problems in a relatively public setting; they are not ready to declare themselves patients, which might be the implication of their moving into a private space with the clinician.

As Kathleen Owens continues to discuss drinking problems with the alcoholic guest, she convinces him that she does not blame him for his situation and can understand how he may have come to be a drinker. He begins to fill in some of his personal history, expresses interest in regaining more control over his behavior, and continues to talk.

Something about two ladies from St. E's strutting up and down the cafeteria line of the Anacostia Men's Shelter hawking our mental health wares intrigued this [46-year-old man, a thin, sagging, disheveled, bleary-eyed alcoholic], and captured his attention. He listened a bit more intently. . . . He asked to talk to me and spilled out a uniquely personal account that fit the pattern of the worried child who was trying to take care of a very burdened parent that I had voiced as a "hunch." His early family situation had seen an alcoholic father who abandoned the family, an overwhelmed mother, and the five offspring traumatically being picked up and placed in a receiving home for neglected children.

After talking of all this, this shelter client agreed to go in that very night for detoxification. . . . He is now 5 months alcohol free, has been for 2 months in a foreman's job with a major construction firm, and has graduated from a 30-day intensive alcoholic treatment program and then a 60-day halfway house program. He now has his own apartment and has resumed active parenting of his 5-year-old daughter.

Panel text prepared by Kathleen L. Owens, MSW.

ing, observing, and questioning in any social situation, but with a more systematic method, more comprehensive coverage, and greater diligence in taking notes than is customary in other social situations. Long and Jacobs (1986) classified assessment skills as listening, asking, observing, and recording and provided numerous tips. The following recommendations are adapted in part from Long and Jacobs (1986:2–11–2–19, 4–45, 4–46)

| What to Do | Why |
| --- | --- |
| Observe the shelter as a whole, how guests react to it and interact with each other. | Behavior and attitudes can be understood only in the physical and social contexts that shape them. |
| Observe details, such as how people react to the food, how staff introduce themselves to guests, and how eagerly guests seek to eat or sleep. | Homeless persons can be accustomed to oversimplifying their feelings in response to questions by individuals who do not seem to care. Observing behavior carefully can help to clarify true feelings and concerns. |
| Be flexible in response to what you observe. Change plans or seek out additional assistance when your observations generate new insights. | Assessment is an ongoing process that can lead gradually to improving the delivery of services needed by clients. |
| Listen carefully to the client's statements and repeat them to the client in your own words. | You can only begin to be confident about what the client means if you allow him or her to correct your own descriptions of what was said. |
| Try to imagine the client's feelings; it helps to observe his or her body movements, facial expressions, and tone of voice. | Empathy is a prerequisite to establishing a long-term relationship of trust. Avoid viewing the client as just another needy person. |
| Be aware of your own feelings, particularly how you feel about the client and his or her needs. Be prepared to acknowledge your feelings to the client or to talk about them with a supervisor. | Feelings are a two-way street. The client will be observing you as you are observing him or her. Sometimes it will help to acknowledge your feelings to the client; sometimes it may be better to talk them out with a supervisor or co-worker. |
| Question clients slowly, asking one question at a time, interjecting your own comments and pausing occasionally. | Many clients will not want to tell their whole story immediately, and some of those who do will not be able to tell it all coherently. Relax and use the questioning period as a means for trust-building. |

Follow up initial questions with probes for more detail and explanations of some of your interests concerning the client.

This will show the client that you are listening and will communicate your interest in his or her welfare. The client's initial responses to questions often will lack sufficient detail.

Record information accurately and completely, using a format that is consistent and easy to comprehend.

Case and service records let you reflect on your own actions, prepare for challenges to your service decisions, and assist those workers who may replace you at some point.

### What Not to Do

### Why

Do not criticize or make personal judgments about the client or express your own values about desirable and undesirable behavior.

Unconditional positive regard is the foundation for a relationship of trust. If clients feel that you are judging them on the basis of what they reveal about their behavior, they will not share their experiences with you nor discuss honestly with you how they might change.

Do not express skepticism about a respondent's statements, at least when you are first getting to know them.

Clients will trust you only if you trust them.

Do not include negative personal comments in your notes.

Another service worker may be able to find some positive features in a situation that you reacted to negatively. If so, that service worker may be able to move ahead with the client more constructively.

Observing, listening, and questioning, are some of the multiple methods of assessment which along with written reflections on the results can provide the in-depth information that will improve decision-making about clients. Yet many shelters require a systematic summary of client characteristics and needs that can best be obtained with a more structured assessment method.

Structured client assessments are most likely to occur as part of a shelter intake interview. However, some shelters collect only brief contact information from new shelter users and follow-up with a more detailed assessment when clients request help from service personnel. Information from client assessments is used to develop service plans, to maintain continuity in service delivery as service personnel may change, and, in some shelters, to develop statistical profiles of shelter users.

The Appendix includes a copy of the Long Island Shelter Intake Form, which is a comprehensive case management assessment form that was developed in cooperation with Boston's Long Island Shelter. The form collects background and contact information on shelter guests as well as information about guests' service experiences, needs, and interests in eight key problem areas: residential status, social support, employment, benefits, physical health, mental health, substance abuse, and legal problems. The interview can be completed with most guests in 20 to 30 minutes.

## How to Maintain Rapport with Clients

Successful case managers build an open relationship with their clients and develop a keen sense of their clients' needs. Several principles capture the insights of these case managers and can serve as guides for others (adapted from Rapp, 1992).

| What to Do | Why |
|---|---|
| Do not pressure a client. Build the relationship gradually and let the client determine the pace. | The client should be seen as a partner in developing service and personal goals. Although the pace may seem too gradual to you, the client's personal experiences may lead him or her to see the world very differently. |
| Focus on the client's individual strengths and goals rather than pathology and deficits. | There simply is no other way to build a supportive relationship in which change and progress can occur. Think of the ability to survive homelessness itself as a strength, and use this strength as a starting point. |
| First address the issues raised by the client; you may then be able to get to the issues you believe are important for the client. | For whatever reasons, what the client sees as important issues indicates the current priorities. If these are not respected, efforts to raise other issues will be fruitless. |
| See the community as a resource, emphasizing natural helpers. | Sooner or later, the client will have to manage on his or her own. Drawing as much as possible on natural helpers will help to create the necessary support structure. |
| Retain faith in the capacity of all persons for long-term growth and change. | Dependency in times of stress can be viewed as normal and healthy. Assume that your client would be able to manage better if the extreme stress of homelessness could be reduced. |

| What Not to Do | Why |
|---|---|
| Do not limit your relationship with the client to simply brokering services. | Clients' service needs do not exist in a discrete part of the client. The whole person will determine the success or failure of service provision, so it is with the whole person that you must build a relationship—personal and caring, while still professional. |
| Do not encourage clients initially to focus their energies on achieving unreasonably ambitious goals—finishing college, buying a home, starting a family. | Specifying goals in small parts will lead to more immediate experiences of success. The fear of failure must be overcome step-by-step. But respect clients' own goals and encourage their independent determination of their needs. |
| Do not expect to deliver other services to a client who is drinking uncontrollably. | Drinking must stop before counseling can be effective. Abuse of alcohol or other drugs is far too distracting, not to mention dangerous, to expect the client to be able to focus on other goals (Blumberg et al., 1973). |
| Do not reject clients who are abusing substances; try to get them into a detoxification program. | The client who is abusing substances today may be more ready for progress tomorrow. Always try to maintain a relationship so that future progress can be encouraged. But try to help the client to stop abusing alcohol or other drugs. |

Supportive and mutually agreeable relationships can be sustained with a client if support is provided when it is requested, if the client is treated as an equal in the relationship, if interaction is open and honest, and if some form of regular interaction is sustained. In general, the case manager should not only build with the client a relationship of friendship and trust but also one that is oriented to improving the client's current circumstances and ending their homelessness.

## How to Refer Clients

The case management role is highly dependent on other agencies and on the functioning of the entire local service system for successful performance. The goal for the service system should be to provide a "continuum of care."

A continuum of care exists when clients receive the services they need from multiple agencies without encountering either barriers in moving between agencies

*Panel 3–5*

## Never Too Late for Literacy

One almost illiterate man in his early forties, with a tested IQ of 65, had been a dishwasher for 15 years. His eyesight was poor, but he had no eyeglasses. He was a very suspicious man. With great difficulty, he expressed his dream of wanting to read, get a better job, and learn to have fun with other people. But after receiving from his caseworker a few simple suggestions, he panicked and shipped out of a Skid Row employment agency to another live-in dishwasher job. Several months later he returned with a laminated disk condition, which required immediate surgery. It took much time and assurance to convince him to go to the hospital. The caseworker made repeated visits to the hospital to build a relationship and to discuss simple postdischarge plans, since the man would not be able to work for some time. When the client was abruptly discharged soon after surgery, with no back brace, money, Public Assistance, or a place to live, the caseworker took him for the weekend. A program secretary volunteered to tutor him in reading and arithmetic during her lunchtime, after he had been persuaded that he was not "too dumb to learn." Since his greatest motivation to read was job-oriented, his tutor brought him help-wanted ads and concentrated on the words he could not read. He studied several hours every night; after several months, the caseworker persuaded him to enroll in an Operation Alphabet adult literacy program. His experience in four schools as a child had been so traumatic that he could not sleep the whole night before enrollment in the adult program; so the caseworker arranged to pick him up at his rooming house, take him to school, and introduce him to the teacher. (He said that all that night he had imagined a huge woman with a ruler waiting for him in the hallway of the school.) Fortunately, this was a good school experience; he studied hard and learned how to use the public library. He went on for several months to a work adjustment program, which included remedial arithmetic, and was placed in a small factory as a shipping and receiving clerk. He has been there over three years, has learned every operation in the factory, and has received periodic raises in pay. This whole process leading up to his current job took one and a half years. Meanwhile, he has continued to receive support as a participant in most of the group recreational-cultural activities of the program. (Blumberg et al., 1973:192–193)

Many of the rapport-building principles listed above are reflected in the case of the illiterate guest: (1) The case manager focused on the guest's desire to read and to work, rather than on his fears and inadequacies. (2) The case manager's hospital visits helped to build a strong, personal relationship. (3) The case manager responded to the client's expressed needs and fears and helped build literacy in small steps, beginning with reading want ads prior to a formal literacy program. (4) Client contact occurred in the client's natural environment, even in the hospital. (5) A program secretary and a regular adult literacy program were used as resources for the client, although he appeared to lack local family ties. (6) The client's fears and need for personal support did not shake the case manager's faith in the client's capacity for long-term growth and change. (7) In this case, the drinking problem was under control when the case manager's efforts began.

or discontinuities over time in receiving services. This goal requires that the service network provide services that are comprehensive and easily accessible. Furthermore, persons seeking these services should be able to rely on relationships with individuals, such as case managers, who help to maintain continuity in service delivery and promote communication with service providers. In order to ensure that the services received are actually needed and desired, service requests should be planned with the client and delivered in a flexible manner. Finally, the service responsibilities of each agency should be clear (Bachrach, 1984b; Mechanic and Aiken, 1987).

Of course, no service system actually provides an ideal continuum of care. But case managers should be sensitive to the desirable characteristics of a service system and plan their own work accordingly. Through their own work, case managers can help shape the network's ability to provide a continuum of care.

Effective referral of clients begins to make a continuum of care a reality. Several techniques that follow will help to increase referral effectiveness and are adapted in part from Long and Jacobs (1986:4-32–4-33):

| What to Do | Why |
| --- | --- |
| Know details of each agency's operation and rules. | Bureaucratic organizations expect knowledge of "the rules." Much time can be saved on the phone, and many fruitless client visits avoided, if the case manager knows how the agency operates. |
| Develop personal contacts in all agencies. | Knowledge of the rules only provides half of the knowledge required to interact successfully with service agencies. A personal contact can fill you in on the rest and enable you to proceed in the most efficient manner. |
| Know your client's needs and select referral agencies accordingly. | Both clients and agencies will be more helpful with case managers who can "mix it up" successfully. |
| Prepare clients for referrals and have them bring necessary names and/or documents. | The documentation demanded by agencies often is daunting even to those who can turn to files at home. Inability to document identity and status is a major stumbling block for homeless persons; the single most important step the referral worker can take is to help resolve this problem. |

| What Not to Do | Why |
|---|---|
| Do not treat staff at other agencies as obstacles to be overcome. | You need to be assertive about your client's needs, but do not forget that service agency personnel are likely to be overburdened with many very needy clients. Respect their situation and they are more likely to respect yours. |

There are many obstacles to the success of referral efforts, and these techniques cannot overcome all of them. Fragmentation of agency responsibilities, limited resources, and pressure from more powerful constituents (and their advocates) often diminish the responsiveness of service agencies. Yet individual agency personnel, interacting with individual shelter case managers, can make a difference.

## HOW TO RESPOND TO INTERPERSONAL CONFLICTS

The experience of shelter life will itself shape relations between shelter staff and their guests. Maintaining a pleasant and caring environment is a prerequisite for developing supportive relations with shelter guests. Unfortunately, this may not be an easy task, for conflict is common in large shelters.

---

*Panel 3–6*

### Conflictual Moments in a Large Shelter

9:15: Warning given to Tony B.—damaging furniture, threw chair down stairs.

10:15: George V. and Jim F. were involved in a fight on the first floor. A police car was called to remove George from the island. Both are barred for 60 days. Jim F. is spending the night and should leave in the a.m.

Friday, 8:00 P.M.: A fight broke out at the clothing room between W.E.P. [live-in staff], Randy (who was on duty in the laundry room), and Fred G. It seems that Mr. G. was upset that the laundry room was not open yet. He gave Randy a lot of verbal abuse and an argument broke out between them. Vi stopped the argument. Mr. G. continued to swear and curse. He then pushed and grabbed Randy by the shirt. A struggle followed in which punches were thrown by both men. The fight was broken up by Al who brought Mr. G. to the office. Mr. G. then gave both myself and the detail officer an extremely hard time, swearing and cursing. A police car was called to remove Mr. G.

*Source*: The Long Island Shelter logbook.

---

## Sources of Conflict between Shelter Guests

Why do conflicts occur in shelters? First and foremost, for the same reasons that interpersonal conflicts occur elsewhere, particularly in settings where large numbers of unrelated people are thrust together in close proximity for extended periods. But the many daily frustrations experienced by homeless persons exacerbate the potential for conflicts, leading some to vent their anger on peers, even while others become withdrawn.

One of the major frustrations experienced by homeless persons is their lack of resources. The cost of necessary medicine or transportation may be prohibitive; keeping an appointment may be made difficult by the shelter's own schedule; taking medicine on a regular basis may be impossible on account of storage problems. Some guests may attempt to deal with these frustrations by claiming a particular physical space within the shelter as their own and aggressively protecting that space.

Both untreated mental illness and active substance abuse can lead to unpredictable, conflictual behavior by shelter guests. Although schizophrenics tend to be socially withdrawn, paranoid delusions and occasional aggressive outbursts can occur. Less acute personality disorders often are associated with antisocial behavior. Guests who are intoxicated or high on drugs may become abusive with others, or may be taken advantage of by other guests.

## Managing Conflict between Guests

Whatever its cause, conflict between shelter guests can frighten other guests, even endanger them. Conflict prevents guests from feeling secure in the shelter—the first step in establishing supportive relations with them. Reducing conflict in the shelter, trying to eliminate it, must be given the highest priority.

The best way to deal with the potential for conflict in shelters is to reduce the factors that cause it and thus lessen the likelihood that conflict will occur. But when conflict does arise between guests, effective conflict management can prevent incidents from escalating and reduce the likelihood of recurrent episodes. Long and Jacobs (1986:5-11–5-13) have identified the most relevant conflict management skills for shelter staff.

| What to Do | Why |
| --- | --- |
| Try to defuse conflicts by watching for warning signs, like clenched fists or raised voices. When you notice these signs, try to engage the individuals involved and remove them from the precipitating situation. | The only good conflict in a shelter is a conflict that never happens. It is much easier for individuals to disengage from a troublesome situation before their behavior escalates to the stage of mutual provocation. |
| Assess the situation and the participants: Do you know either participant? Is anyone high on drugs or alcohol or mentally disturbed? Is either person acting as part of, or in reference to, a larger group? | The same behavior can require different responses depending on your relation to the actor, the actor's state of mind, and the actor's relation to others. |

If you know one of the participants or they see you as an authority figure, step toward them to draw their attention (but not too close). Have a backup person go for additional help.

Interjecting a different familiar face into the conflict may be enough to stop some conflicts from escalating. The success of such actions is not assured, however, so be sure that more help is on the way (do not hesitate to contact the police).

Try to create some space between and around the persons in conflict. Ask bystanders to leave the area.

An audience can stimulate conflict directly, through taking sides, or indirectly, by feeding the ego of one or both persons in conflict. If the aggressor focuses his attention on you, you may be able to help him to begin to calm down. And interpersonal space can help to dampen rising emotional tension.

| What Not to Do | Why |
| --- | --- |
| Do not touch the person or come too close to the persons engaged in conflict. Try either speaking quietly, or, if it seems possible and appropriate, much more loudly and authoritatively than the persons in conflict. | In order to avoid aggravating the situation further, respect the personal space of the aggressor. But then try to focus the person's attention on you, and deflect his attention from the other party to the conflict. |

## Sources of Conflict between Guests and Staff

There are additional sources of conflict between guests and staff. Seemingly minor actions can trigger feelings of rejection or hostility. Staff who are perceived as exercising power for its own sake, who demand that "You do this or else," will often elicit hostile responses from guests. Inconsistent responses by different staff to a guest's requests may also trigger hostility. On the other hand, staff may be offended, even angered, when guests speak to them in an abusive way, not recognizing the personal problems or mental illness that may cause this behavior.

## Managing Guest–Staff Conflict

Staff at Boston's Long Island Shelter suggest that adherence to a few basic principles can reduce the frequency of conflict between shelter guests and staff and thus pave the way toward more effective helping relationships.

| What to Do | Why |
| --- | --- |
| Accept guests' opinions, even when they do not take your advice. | It is their life, although it may be hard to see the world as the guest does. Every guest's opinions must be respected, so that trust can be established. |
| Admit to yourself the negative feelings you invariably will have toward some guests on some occasions and find someone else on the staff to share them with. | Repressed feelings can distort your judgment and ability to make decisions fairly. Letting yourself talk about negative feelings and getting some feedback can help considerably. |
| Find out how other staff have responded to a guest's behavior and respect their decisions. | The shelter's specific rules and general principles will become meaningless unless they are applied consistently. Other staff can be the source of new insights or innovative approaches. |
| Record problems in the shelter's logbook. | A written record is the only method to maintain consistent decision-making when guests and staff come and go at different times. |

| What Not to Do | Why |
| --- | --- |
| Do not take personally verbal abuse directed at you. | You will serve as a convenient focus for the general anger and frustrations felt by some guests. |
| Do not whistle to get guests' attention or otherwise appear to be insistent or patronizing. | Respect is a two-way street. When guests believe that staff treat them in a juvenile or uncaring manner, they are likely to reciprocate. And an insistent manner can make persons feel uncomfortable, particularly those who are emotionally troubled. |
| Do not break the rules that guests must follow. | Playing loud music, watching TV after hours, eating in private spaces may be prohibited for guests. If staff do not respect the same rules, it will encourage others to treat these rules as meaningless or simply punitive. |

Do not assume that you always are right.

We all make mistakes, and it is easy to evaluate improperly persons experiencing extreme stress. Be ready to change your opinions and to admit that you may be wrong.

## Summary

When shelter staff respond effectively to interpersonal conflicts, they lay the foundation for cooperative and caring relations between shelter guests and with staff. Handling interpersonal conflict in a manner that is respectful of all the shelter's guests establishes a climate in which individuals are treated with dignity and in which services are delivered responsibly.

## HOW TO COPE WITH STRESS AND BURNOUT

The severity and number of needs that staff confront can result in high levels of stress, disorganization, and ineffective work. A real sense of depression and just plain exhaustion may develop. Some guests may remind staff of the problems they or others close to them have had. Dealing with people who have very limited social skills is draining in itself. In addition, staff may at times feel that they receive little recognition for their work from guests, other staff, or administrators.

Expectations of quick change may be disappointed when working with mentally ill persons and with alcoholics. Many of the problems confronted are chronic; those who have suffered from these problems for years may have lost interest in the most basic actions for preserving personal integrity. You may have to persuade a guest to eat, change into new clothes, take a bath, and the like. Disappointment over an apparent lack of progress can in turn lead to cynicism or withdrawal.

Many other aspects of working with homeless persons may diminish service effectiveness and create frustration among staff:

- Some clients resist help.
- Some clients may leave unexpectedly on trips, and return just as unexpectedly.
- Some clients are very dependent and demanding.
- Some service agencies are reluctant to help homeless persons.
- Some communities may be hostile to homeless persons, the shelters that house them, and the staff that serve them.
- Some family and friends may not be supportive.
- The pay is likely to be too low and the hours too long.
- High initial expectations may be disappointed.
- Means for demonstrating accomplishment may be lacking.
- Funds often are insufficient for service needs (adapted in part from Long and Jacobs, 1986:5-29–5-30).

More basic aspects of one's personality and social relations also cause stress: feeling cynical makes it difficult to make the effort; feeling omnipotent makes it difficult to treat clients on an equal basis; overidentifying with clients makes it difficult to provide help. Commitment to helping homeless persons is sometimes so high among shelter staff that one's own family is neglected and personal health problems are ignored. In the long run, these practices lead to burnout, illness, and interpersonal conflicts that prevent effective service delivery.

In the process of mediating relations between clients and service agencies, some case managers will tend to overidentify with clients, making demands on service agencies that they know are unrealistic. Some case managers will overidentify with service agencies, always acceding to the institutional needs expressed through agency staff and never challenging them to become more responsive to homeless persons. Other case managers may overidentify with the shelter itself, developing an "organizational mentality" and simply trying not to rock their employer's boat.

Many of the personal difficulties in shelter work are unavoidable, but their personal consequences are not. Staff at Boston's Long Island Shelter suggest a few guidelines:

| What to Do | Why |
| --- | --- |
| Do not expect success with all the guests. Recognize the limitations of your resources and value even limited progress by guests. | Some, because of the inner stresses they feel, may return your efforts to help with abuse. Others may simply not cooperate. |
| Prioritize guests' problems and work on the most critical problems first. | You may at times wonder whether your efforts make any difference, but consistency in care and the provision of basic necessities, even just saying "hello" and expressing concern, are important first steps. |
| Discuss guests' demands with other staff and do not be afraid to say no to demands that are unreasonable or that would require you to violate shelter rules. | Some guests may talk day after day about the same issues with the same staff. Guests may try to manipulate staff by making the same demand to multiple staff until they receive a positive response. |

| What Not to Do | Why |
| --- | --- |
| Do not ignore guests' problems, but do avoid being dominated totally by them. Consciously prepare plans | Ignoring problems will lead to becoming insensitive and dictatorial, but a balance between compassion for |

and exercises to maintain some distance from the job.

Do not expect quick achievements. Develop instead realistic expectations for clients by taking satisfaction in small accomplishments and focusing on the work process more than its results. Meet with others to discuss your work and do not blame yourself for failures. Prioritize guests' problems and work on the problems that are most critical first, or, when that is not possible, work on the problems that guests are most comfortable addressing with you.

guests and protective preservation of self is needed. You can sacrifice often and in significant ways, but always take care of yourself!

The problems that homeless persons face are overwhelming; so too, therefore, are the problems faced by shelter staff. "Solving" the problem of homelessness is an unreasonable goal for service workers, but providing tangible assistance to persons who lack so much is fulfilling in its own right. A shelter presents opportunities daily for making a difference in people's lives; plan your work so as to reap the rewards of providing such help.

## CONCLUSIONS

Shelter policies have an important role to play in improving the perceived quality of work. When their caseload is higher, staff will have less time for clients and they will be forced to react to the most critical needs instead of implementing long-range plans and conducting comprehensive assessments; crisis intervention will become the norm. In this type of environment, it is difficult to establish ongoing, supportive relations, and paperwork tends to consume a higher proportion of staff time.

However, even low caseloads and shelter sensitivity to service needs cannot eliminate the potential for staff stress and programmatic problems in shelters. The number and diversity of shelter guests are too great, and the available resources are always too small, to expect continual success. What staff can do is develop an understanding of effective interpersonal styles and seek experience in helping shelter guests resolve a range of problems. Understanding and experience will increase significantly the ratio of successes to failures and will steadily upgrade the functioning of the entire service system.

# Mental Illness among the Homeless

STEPHEN M. GOLDFINGER, ELISE KLINE,
RUSSELL K. SCHUTT, AND EZRA SUSSER

## INTRODUCTION

"She won't give us a date of birth, her Social Security number, or any other information; we just can't get a history." The nurse and the mental health outreach worker were frustrated but concerned. In the shelter, from a distance, "Scarlet" looked almost scholarly: her glasses were balanced precariously on her nose, her greying hair was pulled back severely in a bun, a tailored suit covered her thin frame. She always carried a large stack of books.

Upon closer inspection, it was clear that Scarlet was not studying for an exam. She reeked of urine, she shunned other people, she bound her shoes with duct tape. Outside the shelter, Scarlet would walk down the middle of a busy street without regard for her safety. In the shelter, she stared out the window, tormented by the belief that red cars were following her, beckoning her to prostitution. Throughout the night, she sat on her cot and stared.

Mental illness has many forms, from the delusions of schizophrenia to the paralysis of depression and the dramatic behaviors of some personality disorders. Although Scarlet's schizophrenic symptoms pose particularly difficult problems for care providers, many forms of mental illness complicate the process of regaining residential stability and multiply service delivery problems. And although mental illness may at times lead to noticeably bizarre behavior, more often the pain of mental illness is experienced only on a very personal level. In any case, the response is too often rejection or neglect, frequently followed by further deterioration.

This chapter defines the concept of mental illness, describes the prevalence of mental illness among homeless persons and the causes of variation in prevalence rates, identifies some of the consequences of mental illness, reviews basic diagnostic information necessary for shelter providers, and provides guidelines for responding to mental illness.

## WHAT IS "MENTAL ILLNESS"?

Serious mental illness is most often defined as mental illness that leads to severe and persistent disabilities. Serious mental illnesses can involve disorders of thinking—hearing or seeing things that other people are not aware of, and disorders of feeling—feeling very depressed, very agitated, or both. Disordered thinking and/or feeling can in turn make it difficult to function as other people expect; in severe cases, seriously mentally ill people even have difficulty taking care of themselves.

Identifying serious mental illness and, in fact, defining mental illness are not easy matters. The particular disorders and associated disabilities that are involved in mental illness may not, in themselves, indicate what a clinician would diagnose as mental illness. Paranoid thoughts may reflect real persecution, and depressed feelings may be a temporary reaction to severe loss or stress. Rather, it is the combination of symptoms and their persistence over time in the absence of direct environmental or physical causes that leads a clinician to suspect mental illness.

The American Psychiatric Association (1987) classifies psychiatric disorders in its *Diagnostic and Statistical Manual of Mental Disorders*. The DSM-III-R classifies serious mental illnesses, such as schizophrenia, organic brain syndromes, substance use disorders, mood disorders, and anxiety disorders as "Axis I" disorders. Personality disorders, or long-term behavioral disturbances that impair self-concept and relations with others, are classified as "Axis II" disorders.

However, what might otherwise indicate a basic, chronic personal illness may for some be a response to the severe stress of homelessness itself. Homeless persons experience loneliness, unhappiness, fear, and low self-esteem (Sebastian, 1985). The vast majority of homeless respondents in a Los Angeles study were currently experiencing symptoms of depression indicative of psychological distress and demoralization, yet almost one third of these individuals had no current diagnosis of a major mental illness (Farr et al., 1986).

Many homeless women are fearful, suspicious, and hostile (Surber et al., 1988), partly as a consequence of their vulnerability to, and experience of, physical assault, rape, and theft. Among homeless women, with few personal belongings, social supports, or health care resources, the experience of these crimes can be even more devastating psychologically and physically than is the case with domiciled populations.

It is important to be able to recognize mental illness so that appropriate care and referrals can be provided. However, it is too easy to label troublesome behaviors or aberrant thoughts as "proof" of mental illness. The highly unusual experiences and extraordinarily stressful circumstances associated with being homeless can themselves exacerbate preexisting mental illness and generate symptoms of mental illness. These experiences and circumstances must themselves be seen as part of the problem.

## HOMELESSNESS AND MENTAL ILLNESS

The adverse effects of mental illness on individual choices and behaviors increase the likelihood of becoming and remaining homeless. Persons who are seriously mentally ill suffer from a variety of impairments that decrease normal coping abilities. Primary impairments are the symptoms of the illness itself; they include lethargy, bizarre behavior, avoidance, and withdrawal. Secondary impairments stem from the experience of illness, that is, from the individual's idiosyncratic responses to his or her illness. Such impairments include demoralization, unawareness of handicaps, disturbed social relationships, and unrealistic goals. Tertiary handicaps are a consequence of the negative reactions of other persons to those who are mentally ill, possibly including diminished social networks, unemployment, stigma, and poverty (Bachrach, 1986).

These primary, secondary, and tertiary handicaps dramatically increase the likelihood of homelessness among persons who are mentally ill. Primary deficits may lead to minimal occupational skills or the inability to manage funds; impaired judgment and impulsivity may result in diminished ability to relate to landlords, families, or board and care home operators. The pain and demoralization they feel may result in a wish to escape through the use of drink or street drugs.

The mental health system, often poorly designed and frequently underfunded, may not have the capacity to meet the multiple medical, psychological, and social needs of the mentally ill. Often, psychoactive medications are used as a substitute for ongoing clinical caretaking and case management. Without other supports, mentally ill persons often stop taking their prescribed medication. This may lead to decompensation or increased avoidance, withdrawal, and wariness. Often, the continuity of Social Security or other benefits may be interrupted as the individual fails to show up for appointments. Disorganized behavior tends then to increase further, and a return to stability becomes less likely (Lamb and Talbott, 1986).

Social supports are often affected adversely by mental illness and are likely to be particularly deficient among homeless mentally ill persons. Almost 90 percent of guests in one Boston shelter who had been hospitalized for psychiatric reasons said they had neither family relationships nor friends; almost three quarters of all shelter users reported either no family relationships or no friends (Bassuk, 1984).

These problems appear to be particularly severe among the so-called young adult chronic patients—seriously mentally ill persons, often white and single, between the ages of 18 and 35. Many persons in this age range have never been institutionalized for an extended period, but they find momentary refuge in frequent periods of hospitalization, and then avoid aftercare services. Highly mobile, with over half moving one or more times within the year, these young adults can be volatile, impulsive, demanding, and highly deficient in social skills (Appleby et al., 1982; Kellermann et al., 1985; Schwartz and Goldfinger, 1981).

When serious mental illness occurs in tandem with extreme poverty, adverse consequences are multiplied. Difficulty with the tasks of daily living, recurrent problems in meeting basic survival needs, vulnerability to stress, and lack of motivation put every seriously mentally ill person lacking financial resources at risk of homelessness (Levine, 1984). Even for those who have family or friends who can provide lodging, tensions are likely to mount as the household budget is strained by providing for an unproductive and even possibly episodically violent member; the ill member may also feel a need to escape (Hatfield, Farrell, and Starr, 1984). In the absence of alternative care facilities, long-term or intermittent homelessness is too often the outcome.

Once homelessness occurs, further deterioration in mental health is almost sure to follow. A key goal for shelter staff, difficult though it is to achieve, is to arrest, or at least to slow, this deterioration.

## HOW COMMON IS MENTAL ILLNESS AMONG THE HOMELESS?

Most research on homeless persons has attempted to identify rates of "chronic" or "severe and persistent" mental illness. Numerous studies document high levels of serious mental illness among homeless single adults (Arce and Vergare, 1984). In Boston (Bassuk, Rubin, and Lauriat, 1984) and Philadelphia (Arce et al., 1983), studies identified schizophrenia or major affective disorders (clinical depression and manic depression) among 40 percent of shelter users. About one third of homeless persons in studies that were made from Ohio to Los Angeles evidenced serious psychiatric symptoms (Farr et al., 1986; Roth and Bean, 1986).*

A Los Angeles study focused on life-time prevalence rates. Between 14 percent and 20 percent of the homeless respondents had ever had schizophrenic disorders, 11 percent had suffered from bipolar disorder, 21 percent had had a diagnosis of antisocial personality, and 69 percent had had a substance use disorder. These rates are all substantially higher than in the domiciled population (Farr et al., 1986).

A substantial fraction of the homeless population have been in mental hospitals, although some persons with psychiatric problems avoid hospitalization because of restrictive admission policies by the hospitals and their own conscious dislike of institutions. About 27 percent of the homeless in Los Angeles had been hospitalized at some point in their lives for mental health problems, although only 4 percent of the entire sample had been hospitalized during the previous year. Thirty percent had been treated on an outpatient basis for a mental health-related

---

*Twenty-eight percent of the homeless persons who were surveyed in Los Angeles were diagnosed as having severe and chronic mental illness, but some persons with apparently schizophrenic symptoms did not provide mental health information. When other indicators of severe mental illness were taken into account, the percentage rose to 33 (Farr et al., 1986).

problem at some time in their lives, but just 8 percent had received such treatment within the last 6 months (Farr et al., 1986).

The results of several studies indicate that one third of Boston's homeless have been hospitalized for psychiatric problems, but as many as one third of these persons had not been hospitalized for at least 5 years (Schutt, 1989). Twenty-three percent of Chicago's homeless had been in a mental hospital (Rossi et al., 1986), as had 30 percent of Ohio's homeless (Roth and Bean, 1986).

The rate of mental illness varies across subgroups within the homeless population. Among New York City shelter users, mental disorders were reported by women (37 percent) more often than by men (22 percent) (Crystal, Ladner, and Towbee, 1986). Similar gender differences appeared in Chicago (Rossi et al., 1986) and Boston (Schutt and Garrett, 1986b).

Few studies have attempted to identify the prevalence of psychiatric disorders

---

### Panel 4–1

### Has Mental Illness Become More Prevalent?

Early studies of homelessness on skid row produced a range of estimates of mental illness—probably reflecting inadequate measurement procedures more than actual variation—but overall they suggest that mental illness was less prevalent among the homeless than was true in the 1980s. In his 1963 report, Bogue estimated that 1 in 11 Chicago skid row men had experienced "mental or nervous trouble," that a like proportion were mentally ill, that 9 percent suffered from "chronic mental illness," that 16 percent were neurotic and 4 percent psychotic, that 36 percent had "aberrant" behavior, and that "emotional instability" was a factor in the homelessness of 20 percent. Blumberg et al. (1973) identified 4 percent of Philadelphia's homeless as psychotic, 7 percent as psychoneurotic, and 14 percent as having a personality disorder. Bahr and Caplow (1968:294) neither measured mental illness nor mentioned it as a difference between poor men on skid row and elsewhere; they did find that skid row men had lower levels of self-esteem but that they did not differ in terms of self-estrangement, faith in people, or anomie.*

Bahr and Garrett's (1976) interviewers considered 6 percent of New York City's female shelter users to be "somewhat delusional" and another 31 percent to have "a few bizarre ideas."

Mental illness among homeless persons seems to have become more common in the 1980s. Different studies report that between 20 percent and 50 percent of single homeless adults suffered from serious and chronic mental illness and from 25 percent to 40 percent had ever been hospitalized for psychiatric problems (Arce et al., 1983; Bassuk, 1984; Farr et al., 1986; Lamb, 1984; Levine, 1984; Schutt, 1988; Tessler and Dennis, 1989). Almost two thirds of a Birmingham sample were clinically depressed (LaGory et al., 1990). About half of mentally ill homeless persons also abused substances (Farr et al., 1986; Schutt and Garrett, 1988; Tessler and Dennis, 1989).

*Bahr and Caplow (1968) estimated "sociopathy" with a collection of deviant behaviors and poverty indicators, none of which provides a reasonable direct indicator of mental illness.

among homeless mothers who are living with their children. Bassuk's study of homeless families in shelters in Massachusetts indicated a much lower prevalence of serious mental illness than found among single homeless adults—about 13 percent. This same study, however, found that many mothers suffered from personality disorders (Bassuk, Rubin, and Lauriat, 1988).

## TYPES OF MENTAL ILLNESS

Both the stress associated with homelessness and other threatening circumstances can lead to behavior and thoughts that may appear unusual. What distinguishes mental illness from stress reactions is a combination of relatively intense and persistent symptoms. It is important for care providers to be able to make this distinction between illness and stress reactions so that appropriate assistance can be rendered. Those persons suffering from serious mental illness should be referred to a trained mental health worker, and often can be helped with medication, but the psychiatric symptoms of those persons responding only to current stressful experiences are likely to improve significantly when the source of stress is removed.

A useful distinction can be made between feelings, symptoms, and disorders. Troublesome feelings, such as nervousness, sadness, or even transient depression, are very common, even universal experiences. Such feelings can be termed symptoms when they are very intense, or if they interfere with functioning. If the intense feelings persist and are disabling, and occur in particular combinations, they may reflect psychiatric disorder: *mental illness*.

Psychoses are particularly severe mental illnesses that often involve a confusion between what are personal feelings and beliefs and external reality. Psychotic persons cling to their feelings or beliefs even in the face of objective evidence to the contrary, and may view the world as a terrifying and confusing place. The most common illnesses causing psychosis are schizophrenia, some episodes of manic-depressive illness and major depression, and some organic brain syndromes (including some syndromes associated with severe substance abuse).

### Schizophrenia

Schizophrenia has a particularly deleterious effect on coping skills. Actually a group of related disorders with apparently diverse causes, schizophrenia is characterized by distorted reality testing at some stage and a chronic, often deteriorating course. Symptoms can include delusions and hallucinations that make it difficult to distinguish inner from external reality, and affective flattening, apathy, and poverty of speech—feelings and behaviors that lessen the likelihood of supportive interaction with others.

A thorough psychiatric evaluation by a trained mental health worker is required to diagnose schizophrenia. However, careful observation and listening, and gentle questioning, can help other service staff to determine whether a guest should be referred for such an evaluation.

*Panel 4–2*

## Schizophrenic Delusions

George is 42 years old and from another state. His mother and sister have been dead for several years, yet he believes that the FBI or the CIA has been hiding them somewhere. He has lived sporadically in several states. He always seems to accumulate "evidence" that someone is out to get him. In the South, he claims to have been arrested and jailed for a motor vehicle accident. He denies ever having driven there. He says that someone who looks like him was driving. The lawyer he hired has mysteriously disappeared. He believes there is something "funny" going on. Each day he leaves the shelter in a new "disguise" and will wear layers of clothes until the undermost layer rots next to his skin. He left the shelter after threatening a case manager. He believed the case manager headed an elaborate network of spies with hidden underground systems connected under Boston Harbor to the Massachusetts Institute of Technology and Harvard.

Byron, another schizophrenic guest, is a black man in his thirties who is also a polysubstance abuser (especially alcohol). Emotional reactivity to any kind of interaction is absent. His facial expressions are "flat." Sometimes, when he drinks, he is angry and argumentative. But most of the time he is quiet and withdrawn. Byron will tell an interested listener that he once was a dancer for a famous dance troupe. He will talk about feeling different from other people and how others have picked on him for those differences. Occasionally, he follows other guests, silently copying their motions and gestures. He is unable to answer questions about this behavior, turning away and closing his eyes when asked. He is so quiet that he is almost like a phantom when he follows people. This action has a bizarre quality to it which unnerves people.

Victoria, a 50-year-old white woman, proudly informs other guests that she has been homeless for 8 years. She is homeless "because of Johnny"—Johnny Weismuller, the film star who portrayed Tarzan in the early movies. She is Johnny's woman, and as a result has been persecuted by high-ranking government officials. One night a clandestine group entered her apartment looking for her; in terror, she hid in her closet for days. Somehow, God made a miracle happen. It was as light as daylight in the closet, and she was comforted. Immediately afterward, she left the closet and all her belongings and took to the streets. She has been avoiding her persecutors ever since.

## Major Affective Disorders

The major affective disorders include manic depression (bipolar affective disorder) and major depression. Depression, which is a common occurrence, becomes "major" depression when it involves not only feeling blue but also difficulties with sleeping, eating, physical acts, and concentrating. Bipolar disorder involves both major depressive and manic episodes.

Usually guests having a manic episode come to the attention of the shelter staff because they are up all night, full of energy; they may try to fight with guests or with staff. Their speech may be rapid, with abrupt changes from topic to topic.

---

*Panel 4–3*

**The Mental Status Examination**

Shelter providers can use several questions and procedures to make a preliminary decision about a guest's likely need for a professional evaluation. Rapport must first be established with a client. Then observations and questions from the Mental Status Examination can be used. Observations should include the following: (1) Is the person disorganized, poorly groomed, dressing bizarrely? Are inappropriate behaviors displayed? (2) Does the person manifest false beliefs (delusions), have incoherent thoughts, or believe others can hear his thoughts or read his mind? (3) Do thoughts progress logically, or in no apparent order and in rapid sequence? (4) Are perceptions of the environment distorted by hallucinations of any of the senses? (5) Are observable feelings blunted, flat, or inappropriate? Is the person's mood elevated or depressed? (6).Are insight and judgment impaired?

Some direct questions to the guest can also help in decisions: (1) Are your thoughts going so fast that you can't keep up with them? (2) Have you ever felt as if people were after you or out to get you? (3) Have you ever heard or seen anything that you think might not be there or that others don't see or hear?

---

Grandiose gestures—giving money and belongings to other guests—and flamboyant clothing—colorful, odd garments or excessive make-up—also suggest bipolar disorder. At other times, those persons with bipolar disorders become extremely depressed; on those occasions, they may look exactly like someone with a major depressive disorder. Different individuals may swing between these "poles" only a few times a year, or, rarely, as often as several times a week. Manic depression often can be treated effectively with regular doses of lithium or other medications, but between one quarter and one third of manic depressives have a progressive form of the illness that does not respond to lithium and tends to have a poor outcome.

An individual experiencing a major depressive episode becomes very withdrawn, frequently is tearful, loses weight (or, less commonly, gains weight), and has trouble sleeping. Psychomotor functioning may be retarded, with slowed or monotonous speech and little activity. Sometimes, depressed people become agitated, unable to sit still, pull at their clothes and hair, wring their hands, or pace the floor. Most individuals in this state experience a marked sense of worthlessness and guilt over current or past failures, sometimes of delusional proportions, and may actively think about suicide and death. Some individuals attempt to "drown" their depression with street drugs or cover it up with amphetamines or cocaine.

The possibility of underlying mental illness should always be considered when attempting to lessen drug dependency. Individuals who experience more intense depression or other psychiatric problems when their drug dependence is reduced are likely to return to drug abuse. Providers should be ready to get their

## Panel 4–4

### Bipolar Affective Disorder

George, who is in his late thirties, has been a guest of the shelter for several months. He is extremely critical of the other guests, stating repeatedly that he doesn't belong there and that "it's all a mistake." He tells anyone who will listen that he is an architect, in fact "America's best architect" and has a plan to provide housing for all homeless people.

George did, in fact, study architecture in college. However, in the years since then, he developed increasing difficulty in maintaining any jobs, having last worked 6 years ago. At that time, while working for a real estate firm, he became convinced that he could make himself and the firm the most successful in the field and began to offer clever but unrealistic "deals" to a number of clients. When this behavior was discovered, he was fired. He lived for a time on unemployment benefits, but became severely depressed and suicidal and was hospitalized. Over the last several years, he has categorically refused to take the medications prescribed for him, complaining that they "make his life dull and uninteresting" and that they "impede his gifts." During one incident of depression, he remained at his boarding house, unable and unwilling to show up for his SSI renewal and subsequently lost his disability payments. Shortly thereafter he was evicted and came to the shelter.

## Panel 4–5

### Depression and Drugs

Ireland is a black man in his early thirties who attributes most of his life's failures to cocaine addiction. He is an ex-detective on the police force and did not begin to use drugs until 2 years ago. He has been married several times and blames himself for the failures. When he starts to think about his problems, his depression becomes so profound that he withdraws for days. He self-medicates with cocaine. In other words, when he becomes so down and racked with guilt about his life, he will go out and buy cocaine to either "snort" or smoke. Then, he says, he has enough energy to go on living. At one time, he tried to kill himself by putting his service revolver in his mouth. The only thing that stopped him from pulling the trigger was his little boy walking into the room.

clients some help with depression and other psychiatric problems before this occurs.

Depression can lead to suicide attempts; in fact, the likelihood of suicide attempts appears to be markedly higher among homeless persons than among the general population (Burt and Cohen, 1989). A history of suicide attempts, drug abuse, and social isolation are also associated with a higher risk of dying from suicide. Suicidal thoughts or behaviors should be taken very seriously, and evaluation by a mental health or psychiatric practitioner is essential.

## Personality Disorders

Personality disorders are inflexible and maladaptive personality traits reflecting long-term patterns of looking at, relating to, and thinking about one's world and oneself. These disorders have not often been studied among the homeless, and estimates of their prevalence vary widely, probably due in part to different shelter populations in different cities (cf. Arce et al., 1983; Bassuk et al., 1984).

The personality disorders found most commonly in shelters are the borderline personality and the antisocial personality.

Substance abuse, an unstable life-style, violence, lying, use of aliases, running from the law, defaulting on family or financial obligations, unemployment, and stealing are elements common to life in the shelter world. These may be facets of the antisocial personality.

Another severe form of personality disorder is the schizotypical personality.

---

*Panel 4–6*

### Identifying Major Depressive Illness

The American Psychiatric Association's *Diagnostic and Statistical Manual of Mental Disorders* provides clear guidelines for identifying major depressive illness (American Psychiatric Association, 1987:222–224).

Suspect a major depressive illness if the person: manifests a lowered mood characterized by the following: feeling blue, irritable, hopeless, or sad; and at least four of the following symptoms present almost continuously for at least two weeks:

- sleep disturbance
- eating disorder with significant weight loss or gain
- agitation or motor retardation
- loss of pleasure or interest in usual activities
- fatigue and loss of energy
- feeling worthless and guilty
- difficulty concentrating or paying attention
- preoccupation with thoughts of death or suicidal feelings

The above symptoms cannot be due to schizophrenia or an organic problem.

---

*Panel 4–7*

## Borderline Personality

Marlene has been homeless for the last 6 months and manifests a borderline personality. She has an episodic history of intravenous cocaine abuse. When she is short of money, she will work as an exotic dancer in the most dangerous and rundown part of town. She has short, intense relationships with men and women, although she says she prefers men. These relationships have always ended with her feeling dissatisfied and abandoned. There were several times when her relationships ended and she attempted to reunite with her partner or to punish him by cutting her wrists or putting her fists through windows. She was hospitalized briefly, once or twice, for her suicide attempts. Marlene became homeless when her landlord evicted her following a violent altercation with a boyfriend.

---

This disorder is also a long-term and enduring pattern of responding which is frequently seen in shelters. These guests often are seen as eccentric loners. They do not appear to be involved with any "groups" at the shelter. They may speak in a vague, tangential way, often not getting back to the main point of the conversation. They may also describe some "odd" beliefs. Their eccentricities become more pronounced among larger groups of people and as social anxiety heightens.

Within the shelter setting, the people with borderline and antisocial personalities require the greatest amount of energy in terms of enforcing the shelter rules. Limits and boundaries afforded by the rules always seem to be tested, and guests may go from one staff member to another until they get what they want; consistency and communication among staff becomes imperative.

---

*Panel 4–8*

## An Antisocial Personality

Sam is a 34-year-old intravenous cocaine user who claims that he has AIDS. He is an outrageous liar at the shelter and can be provoked to violence easily. He once went to jail for throwing a prostitute for whom he pimped out of a second-floor plate glass window.

Sam knows how to use the "system" to get what he needs. Once he discovered that he had been accruing Social Security Insurance and hired lawyers until he was made his own payee for several thousands of dollars. He disappeared from the shelter for several weeks and then reappeared, broke and sick. He claims to have spent all his money on drugs and sex. Sam does not appear to worry at all that he may be spreading a deadly virus.

---

*Panel 4–9*

## A Schizotypical Personality

Pat is a "thirtyish" looking young woman. She refused to give her actual age or to tell the interviewer where she has come from (other than saying "the Midwest"). She unties the scarf binding her long, dirty hair, shakes her hair out, and redoes the scarf in a new manner many times during the interview. Pat's answers to questions are vague, and the interviewer keeps wondering what she is leading up to, or trying to say. Pat claims to be involved with, and running away from, a coven of witches on the West Coast. She says that she can still sense their presence. She denied having any hallucinations but later admitted that she was in a psychiatric hospital just once, for a few days.

Transient psychotic episodes complicate the delivery of health services to some persons who are suffering from severe personality disorders. Staff may observe a guest becoming increasingly bizarre, agitated, violent, or suicidal. They may send the guest into a hospital for evaluation only to have the psychiatrist on call either send the guest back that night or call the shelter saying, "What's the matter with you? Sending out this person, who appears fine and is in no distress!"

Such discrepant judgments may occur because the stress of living at the shelter becomes too much for the guest and they decompensate. Then, during the ambulance ride, things quiet down and the drivers tend to be supportive of the guest. With fewer stimuli, the guest may become less psychotic and stressed. The psychiatrist on call sees the guest after a medical clearance (which gives the guest even more time to pull together) and interviews a person who has become perfectly lucid.

### Adjustment Reactions and Stress Disorders

An adjustment disorder is a reaction to a real and identifiable stressor (like eviction, being raped, or losing an important relationship). By definition, this reaction must occur within 3 months of the onset of the stress. Subtypes are distinguished by their predominant symptoms (depressed mood, disturbed conduct, anxious mood, withdrawal) which must be experienced as maladaptive and to have persisted for less than 6 months.

Loss of one's home or lack of a fixed residence in and of itself is a major stressor. A common rule of thumb among shelter workers is that the first 6 months on the street are traumatic; after that, a person begins to adapt to street life. Adaptation to street life often means learning negative ways of coping. Drug use is common as a means of coping with stress. Another means of adapting is by selling sexual favors in order to survive. Invariably, these modes of "adaptation" increase the risk of robbery, rape, infection, and even greater trauma.

Street life is especially dangerous for young women, many of whom already have suffered rape or childhood abuse and may reexperience these traumatic events as recurrent or intrusive memories or dreams. There also may be intense psychological distress if the person is exposed to situations or events which resemble or symbolize that original circumstance. Symptoms may develop after a few months or years and may result in self-destructive behavior, such as substance use disorders.

Panic disorders and phobias are severe types of anxiety disorders that appear occasionally among homeless persons. Panic disorders occur unpredictably and often without a clear stimulus and can last anywhere from minutes to hours. Phobias involve an irrational fear of a particular object, activity, or situation that leads to attempts to avoid the feared stimulus and to anxiety attacks upon encountering that stimulus.

## RESPONDING TO MENTAL ILLNESS

Many features of shelter living contribute to poor mental health and impair health improvements. But the system of mental health services outside of the shelter often provides little assistance; in fact, some features of that service system increase the prevalence of homelessness among seriously mentally ill persons. In order to help those guests who suffer the torments of mental illness, shelter staff must themselves be ready to lend a hand.

Improving mental health service delivery in shelters requires an understanding of how shelters and the surrounding service system may impede service delivery and how these impediments can be overcome. It also requires a sensitivity to the homeless mentally ill person's reactions to their illnesses and to their experiences, and a willingness to find strengths in these persons that can be used to cope with the mental illness.

---

*Panel 4–10*

### Adjustment Disorders

Martini is 19 years old. She has lived on the street for several years, since her mother's boyfriend raped her and her mother threw her out. She has recurrent nightmares of these events and sometimes in settings similar to the rape she gets flashbacks. She says her younger brother describes feeling the same way about things and also has intrusive thoughts popping into his head. She thinks he was raped, too, but he denies this.

Martini has a boyfriend but finds that she needs to get high before she can loosen up enough to have sex with him. He is an active drinker and often uses cocaine. He has been encouraging her to use coke since she gets depressed and it gives her a boost of well-being.

---

---

*Panel 4–11*

## Guidelines for Identifying Anxiety Disorders

1. Suspect an anxiety state if the person manifests the emotional and physical symptoms of anxiety: feelings of severe apprehension or terror, fear of going crazy or losing control, and fear of dying.
2. Confirm by observing, listening, and collecting additional information.
3. Based on your findings, identify the problem:
   a. Anxiety caused by stress
   b. Panic disorder
   c. Phobic states
4. If the anxiety is accompanied by the following, it is probably not a primary anxiety state:
   a. A thought disorder or impaired reality testing—probably psychosis
   b. Fluctuating consciousness, disorientation or memory impairment—probably organic brain syndrome
   c. Persistently lowered mood and physical, behavioral, and cognitive symptoms of depression—depression (anxious or agitated)
   d. Physical symptoms—possibly a physical disorder

*Source*: Bassuk, Carmen, and Weinreb, 1990:150.

---

## Problems in Mental Health Services

Although many homeless persons have had contact with psychiatric hospitals or outpatient services, these contacts tend to be less than adequate to meet their needs. Barriers to mental health care for homeless mentally ill persons include preclusive admission policies, inadequate services, geographically determined responsibility, inappropriate expectations, and the social distance between providers and the homeless (Bachrach, 1984b).

Because of the policy of deinstitutionalization and the legal definition of patients' rights, psychiatric hospitals have encouraged brief periods of stay and relatively strict admission criteria. And because they arrive under less favorable circumstances—brought by the police, lacking the support of a family member, dependent on a public facility—the homeless are less likely to be accepted (Appleby and Desai, 1985).

When they are discharged from psychiatric hospitals, often after just a few weeks, the homeless again fare poorly. Nearly 80 percent of the initial number of undomiciled admissions at a large Chicago hospital (not all the same individuals) were discharged as undomiciled (Appleby and Desai, 1985); only 30 percent of the formerly institutionalized homeless interviewed by Rossi et al. (1986) reported discharge planning prior to release, and two in every five went immediately to a shelter or to the streets. Nearly two thirds (62 percent) made no contact with a Community Mental Health Center after their discharge (Rossi et al., 1986).

---

*Panel 4–12*

### Sporadic Hospital Use

He [a 19-year-old male] had been kicked out of his own house; they had gotten a restraining order to keep him away. He had been a [psychiatric] inpatient and outpatient. . . . [He] said he was hyperactive and had mood swings—"ups and downs"—and got going real fast when he was working. . . . He had been on medication, but had not taken it in a year.

*Source*: Terry, 1986:18–19.

---

Homelessness may be precipitated by hospitalization for a first psychotic episode. Some patients refuse to participate in discharge planning, are unable to maintain a stable lifestyle, and then begin a cycle of progressive deterioration and episodes of homelessness in synchrony with rehospitalization, discontinuation of medication, and further rehospitalization (Levy and Henley, 1985).

Adequate community-based care is often lacking. Many homeless mentally ill persons lack case managers or family members to provide them with assistance in the community; they miss appointments, go into crisis once again, and then must return to a hospital for treatment. The need for mental health services often is not seen as a high priority while these persons are in the community. Even when clearly indicated, many referrals are not completed because of inadequate facilities, exclusionary admitting criteria, and time-consuming processes (Barrow and Lovell, 1982, 1983).

Conflict over service responsibilities can further complicate the provision of mental health services, particularly to homeless persons (and others) who suffer from substance abuse or other medical problems in addition to mental illness. A substance abuser who is mentally ill may be rejected by a psychiatric facility on account of the substance abuse and be refused admittance to a detoxification facility because of the mental illness. Mental retardation or organic brain disorders in combination with mental illness and substance abuse can lead to the same result. Each agency has a "valid" reason for rejecting the potential client, leaving him or her to return to the streets or a shelter (Goldfinger and Chafetz, 1984).

In addition to these structural barriers, the homeless persons' attitudes can prevent effective engagement in psychiatric care. Some homeless persons dislike intake interviews and other proactive treatment efforts (Arce and Vergare, 1984); some deny mental illness as part of a coping strategy (Drake and Adler, 1984). The younger, psychiatrically impaired homeless who have never been institutionalized are often angry and particularly prone to denying their mental illness (Segal and Baumohl, 1985). Even when low-income housing and social services are available, patients often migrate toward "the crevices of the city," avoiding mental health care (Appleby et al., 1982; Drake and Adler, 1984).

*Panel 4–13*

**Employment**

Regular employment is not a reasonable alternative for many mentally ill homeless persons. Among New York City shelter users with psychiatric problems, 62 percent confronted at least two barriers to employment, such as being over 65, abusing alcohol, having physical impairments, lacking employment experience or a grade school education, or having a jail record. Only 26 percent of those without psychiatric problems confronted two or more of these employment barriers.

*Source*: Crystal et al., 1986.

In the absence of adequate mental health services, jails may be used to control the mentally ill. One study of county jail inmates referred for psychiatric evaluation found that 39 percent had been living on the streets or in missions or SROs. The misdemeanors with which they are charged may be a reflection of their illness, rather than of criminality *per se* (Lamb and Talbott, 1986; see also Solarz, 1985).

To varying degrees within shelters and on the streets, homeless persons experience chaos and unhealthy living circumstances, lack regular friends and personal privacy, are physically assaulted, and are socially stigmatized. Within shelters, the usual consequences are high levels of social tension and personal

*Panel 4–14*

**Safety and Psychosis**

Safety becomes an issue when guests become so psychotic that they do not take care of themselves. Some guests become infested with lice, crabs, or maggots. Some stop eating and suffer from rapid weight loss or eat out of trash bins and run the risk of food poisoning or rat bites. Some guests are so driven by their fearful delusions and hallucinations that they may hurt themselves or others. One guest was frightened that the television in the lounge was televising his thoughts and that the other guests were going to hurt him. He became so agitated that he threw an ashtray at the TV; it missed, bounced off a wall, and hit another guest in the head. Nursing staff attempted to have the guest hospitalized in a psychiatric facility. The psychiatrist on call felt that the person had calmed down and was no longer a threat to himself or others. He was released to the streets in a few hours and was back at the shelter trying to gain entry again.

depression. For those who already suffer from serious mental illness, these problems are multiplied.

The rapid spread of AIDS now contributes significantly both to the generation of homelessness and to the hazards of shelter living, particularly for those who are mentally ill.

## Improving Service Delivery to Mentally Ill Persons

Much good can be done for homeless persons who are suffering from serious mental illness while they are still in shelters. By focusing on individual guests' needs, the particular shelter's social milieu, and a variety of means for eliciting help from the service system, shelter staff can begin to make a difference.

### Guidelines for Work in the Shelter

Mental illnesses appear in many forms and often without clear distinguishing characteristics. Most illnesses affect the personality and cognitions of people in a way that results in wide individual variation. And with the exception of some well-established drug therapies, the appropriate response to most mental illnesses often is in dispute, and, in any case, varies from individual to individual.

The guidelines for responding to physical health problems can be both specific to particular problems and detailed in their instructions (see Chapter 7). This degree of specificity and detail is neither possible nor desirable in the case of mental illness. Instead, response guidelines are phrased in general terms, so as to emphasize the common features of mental illness and the typical needs of persons who are mentally ill.

---

*Panel 4–15*

### Mental Illness and HIV Infection

Some guests pose safety and ethical problems for shelter staff. One guest, a young woman, was dually diagnosed as a chronic schizophrenic and a polysubstance abuser (alcohol and intravenous cocaine were her drugs of choice). She was sexually active and provocative. She was also HIV positive.

At the shelter, she was so disorganized that she got down on all fours and said that she was a dog. She exposed herself to guests and staff and invited them to have intercourse with her. Staff became increasingly concerned about her behavior—that she would infect others and that her continued substance abuse would escalate the development of her AIDS-related illnesses. Each time the professional staff sent her to a psychiatric hospital for assessment, however, she was back at the shelter within a few days.

---

| **What to Do** | **Why** |
|---|---|
| 1. Learn about social relations and prevailing attitudes in the shelter before starting direct service work. Examine staff and guest feelings about mental health care and the service system staffs' orientations to homeless clients. | Mental illness may be stigmatized by both groups, making a direct approach to discussing mental illness inappropriate. Mental health programs may be seen as a means to improve treatment or to lengthen stays in the shelter. Staff may seek to use mental health workers to help remove troublesome clients from the shelter. Understanding these fears and perspectives is the first step to working around them and beginning to change them. |
| 2. Provide direct assistance when guests experience personal crises, even while making arrangements for professional care. | Whether a guest is escaping an abusive interpersonal relationship, attempting to end drug or alcohol dependence, or contemplating suicide, a sympathetic and supportive staff member who takes the time to care about the guests's problems can lay the foundation for a long-term, beneficial relationship. |

---

*Panel 4–16*

## A Gradual Approach

The subculture in a transitional hotel for homeless women made it clear that conventional approaches to initiating contact with mentally ill women were likely to meet with little success. Mental illness was highly stigmatized, and psychiatrists were seen as both intrusive and threatening. Therefore, when a psychiatrist was added to the hotel's mental health team, he initiated contact with the community by running the weekly bingo game. The game created a friendly, nonthreatening atmosphere that drew more residents than any other activity. It also allowed the psychiatrist himself to become a guest of the hotel and to be treated with hospitality rather than feared. After the bingo-playing psychiatrist became a familiar and accepted figure in the hotel, women who had avoided him at first began to seek treatment, and staff could assume that referrals would not cause shame (Susser, Goldfinger, and White, 1990).

3. Reach out to "hard to reach" patients who refuse to be treated elsewhere. Use a gradual approach to build rapport; if necessary, postpone treatment of flagrant symptoms and, instead, simply provide a place to sit quietly, or to talk and be heard out respectfully, or to socialize with others.

An overly aggressive attempt to discuss psychopathology may recall earlier negative treatment experiences. Trust-building takes time, often in direct proportion to the severity of the mental illness.

4. Mental health workers in shelters need to view the process of assessing and recruiting clients for treatment as part of an ongoing process of negotiation that is of value in itself. Be willing to chat with clients about issues important to the client, without focusing, at least initially, on treatment issues. Proceed to more comprehensive treatment in a gradual way.

When clients are respected as active participants in defining the nature and level of intervention needed, they will be more likely to take an active role in facilitating whatever treatment they accept.

---

*Panel 4–17*

## The Utility of a Label

One psychiatrist used a letter to the SSI office as the basis for discussing mental illness with a patient who was willing to take medications but not to accept that she had a psychiatric problem. She insisted that she received SSI because of a knee injury, and wanted an increase in payments as she could hardly survive on the meager amount. Together with the psychiatrist, she composed a letter to the SSI requesting an increase. In the process, she acknowledged that the letter would have to state that she had a mental disability, whether or not this was true, and composed her own description of her disability. This proved to be the opening for a frank discussion of mental illness, and the nature of schizophrenia, after which the psychiatrist and the patient "agreed to disagree" as to whether the patient had schizophrenia. After that point, treatment proceeded with more explicit goals, such as improved hygiene, but still without insisting that the patient accept that she had a psychiatric diagnosis (Susser et al., 1990).

5. Assess resistant clients by gathering information gradually. In
emergency shelters, short conversations may provide a means for
such information collection,
whereas in shelters with day programs or other treatment-oriented
activities, task-oriented group interactions may provide the best
setting for gradual assessment.
Outreach workers may find that
the most reliable assessment can
occur at settings outside of the
shelter. Use this information to
develop a portrait of guests' problems and strengths.

6. If involuntary hospitalization is
required, try to accompany the
patient through the admission
process, visit the patient frequently, and bring gifts that the
patient will appreciate. Help the
patient maintain social ties in the
mental health community or elsewhere in the community.

The shelter or outreach worker has the
opportunity to observe guest behavior
as it occurs, rather than through re-
constructions after-the-fact. Episodes
of drunkenness, indications of drug
abuse, lethargic or otherwise depressed behavior can indicate fundamental problems more reliably than
direct questions. The resulting mental
health portrait can help staff make appropriate referrals for additional services and provide service agencies
with information necessary to establish eligibility and determine service
needs.

Involuntary hospitalization can be a
traumatic experience; its negative impact can be lessened by providing social support. Many guests are so
discouraged by life circumstances that
they have a tough time believing they
can be helped. During and after an
episode of hospitalization, they may
need help in order to keep appointments and take their medications.

---

*Panel 4–18*

### Arranging for Hospitalization

Shelter staff may have to hospitalize guests when they become so disordered that they represent a threat to others, are suicidal, or are clearly unable to take care of them- selves. If staff are worried about the behav- ior of a guest, calling the emergency unit of a psychiatric or medical hospital is appro- priate. The staff should speak to a psychi- atric nurse or psychiatrist on call for more information about sending the guest in. It is always a good idea to send a referral note along with the accompanying police or ambulance attendants. The note should list all the reasons for referring this guest, such as the behaviors the staff have observed, as well as the identification of the guest. Indi- cate whom the emergency room staff should call if they want further information.

7. Be willing to adopt unusual treatment strategies when working with the most difficult clients, such as those dually diagnosed with substance abuse and mental health problems.

8. Maintain an atmosphere of caring and mutual respect in the shelter; intervene directly to set appropriate limits to violent or disruptive behaviors. When guests are escalating toward violent behavior, separate and move them toward a quiet area. If necessary, ask police to intervene and place a violent guest in protective custody. A verbally abusive guest may need to be removed from the shelter.

If they are to succeed, treatment plans must be of interest to the patient. Years of rejection, even abuse by service agencies, can result in resistance to traditional, direct treatment strategies.

Safety is one of the most fundamental human needs, and one that is most often violated by life on the streets. A shelter that cannot protect its guests from violence is not really a "shelter" at all. Promoting safety may at times require punitive action to a few guests, but the good of the large number of peaceful guests must be the paramount concern.

---

*Panel 4–19*

### Through the Back Door

A 56-year-old woman in a hotel for formerly homeless women had a combination of chronic alcoholism, severe liver damage, atypical psychosis, posttraumatic stress disorder, and diabetes. Her only intimate relationship was with a pimp who sold and injected drugs; but efforts to educate her about the risk of AIDS and to treat her for her illnesses had failed, partly because she did not keep appointments or follow medical advice. The treatment team then decided to pursue the one area in which she expressed genuine interest—resolving feelings about her family of origin, especially the grandmother who had raised her. She was deeply touched by these efforts, and later was willing to confront her drinking and her sexual behavior.

Another example concerns a homeless young man in a large municipal shelter. He was episodically violent, used drugs, had an uncontrolled seizure disorder, and was at very high risk for HIV infection. Much of his childhood, and almost all of his adult life, had been spent in institutions, mainly jails, hospitals, and shelters. In spite of some appealing qualities to counterbalance these factors, it seemed highly unlikely that, in the near future, any supportive residence would accommodate him. Even in the shelter, he was unwelcome and was periodically evicted. Therefore, contrary to the program philosophy of serving as a bridge to housing rather than an agent of "social control" in the shelter, an approach was developed to foster his long-term social adjustment in the shelter.

---

*Panel 4–20*

**When Barring Becomes Necessary**

Elmer was an impulsive man who often stayed at the shelter after going on a "crack run"—smoking crack for days or weeks at a time. When he was high, he had a very short fuse: he might blow up and start screaming at other guests. Some of the other guests were equally impulsive and violent. One evening in an argument over beds, Elmer attempted to assault another guest. Staff separated Elmer and the other person. They then called for the policeman on duty. The officer escorted Elmer from the shelter and he was not allowed back in for 2 months.

---

9. Maintain a regular daily routine in the shelter: such basics as meals and showers should be provided at predictable times.

A daily routine can be reassuring, even therapeutic, by providing stability and predictability for people whose lives are characterized by uncertainty and, at times, chaos. This can be one of the chief mechanisms whereby shelters provide emotional support.

10. Enforce shelter rules. Occasional exceptions may be necessary, but all staff and guests should know what the rules are and that they will be applied fairly and consistently. Prohibitions against weapons, alcohol, and drugs are particularly important. Sexual activity in the shelter also is a commonly prohibited activity, as it tends to upset both guests and staff.

Structure and adherence to shelter policy promotes a certain degree of safety for shelter guests. When staff do not follow through in enforcing rules it is not uncommon to have guests complain about how lax things are getting in the shelter. It is not uncommon to hear guests and staff reminiscing about the "good old days" when so-and-so worked at the shelter: "Why, then you'd never see such-and-such kind of behavior." Structure and consistency are twice as important when a person's general lifestyle is marked by transience and chaos.

11. Maintain appropriate interpersonal boundaries with shelter guests. Shelter staff should discuss and even write out a behavior code for themselves.

Many homeless persons, particularly women, have a long history of victimization. Some women may have found that, in the past, flirting was necessary for survival on the streets or even in their families and may still behave in a seductive manner. Some women may try to use such techniques to get attention or favors from shelter staff.

| What Not to Do | Why |
|---|---|
| 1. Do not play favorites. Maintain a consistent, caring approach to all shelter guests. Although feelings about different guests inevitably will differ, do not let these feelings interfere with providing the most appropriate care to all. Above all, do not be tempted to exploit guests socially or sexually. Seek help if this seems to be happening with yourself or with other staff. | Staff have a number of sources of power over guests: they may control entry, they assign beds, they distribute clothes, they set limits on guests' behavior. Abusing this power means destroying the possibility of maintaining fair and supportive relations with all the guests. Guests should know that even if they behave seductively or provocatively, staff are not going to respond in a way that subverts the "helper" role. |
| 2. Do not try to avoid hospitalizing seriously ill patients at all costs, even if they resist the idea. | Some seriously ill psychiatric patients require "asylum": a safe refuge in which they are free from the immediate threat of psychiatric and physical harm. When the community cannot provide such refuge, an institution may be the answer (Bachrach, 1984a; Goldfinger, 1990). |
| 3. Do not overemphasize the importance of physical security and discourage other staff from adopting a "police" approach to their jobs. When a guest's aggressive actions are under control, try to learn about his or her concerns and needs. | Security is a paramount concern in a shelter, but an overemphasis on security can lead too quickly to neglecting the needs of guests for emotional support and understanding. Violent acts require immediate preventative action; the potential for violence requires a longer term prevention strategy. |
| 4. Do not tuck a guest into bed who is talking about suicide and then turn out the light. Do not assume that "it's just the alcohol talking." | Talk by a guest about suicide should always be taken seriously. Contact a mental health professional immediately and keep in touch with the guest. |
| 5. Do not jump to conclusions about guests' psychological problems or needs. | Even mental health professionals can have difficulty diagnosing persons who are traumatized by street living or suffering from substance abuse. Labeling a guest as mentally ill may be regarded as a withdrawal of support and preclude additional efforts to help. |

## Guidelines for Work Outside the Shelter

Shelters simply cannot provide a suitable environment for the long-term treatment of mental illness. The primary goal of staff should be to minimize the length of time that their guests spend homeless by helping them to move into more permanent housing and to develop supportive connections to the regular service system. Although this is not an easy task, several strategies can help.

1. *Advocacy.* Advocacy is a standard component of general case management services. When advocating for homeless clients, staff must be prepared to target agencies that provide clothing, housing, and physical health care as well as mental health services. Advocating first for basic needs may make it easier later for guests to trust you and allow you to help them make connections with mental health service agencies.

2. *Demystify the illness and the system.* Educate the resident about his or her illness and about the service system, so that he or she can approach service agencies with as much knowledge, expertise, and "clout" as possible. First, help clients to describe what others think is wrong with them in words that are most effective in securing entitlement, program, or other desired services. Reading the DSM-III-R together can be helpful. Second, discuss how service agencies are structured and the barriers to receiving services from them. Discussing previous experiences and reading agency regulations may help.

3. *Use sociopathy constructively.* Clients often must be taught ways to "outwit" the system in order to overcome arbitrary and discriminatory actions that lessen their ability to secure needed services. Seriously mentally ill individuals may need to be able to creatively answer job interview questions covering the time periods when they were hospitalized. A jacket and tie or a dress may have to be added to the client's wardrobe.

---

*Panel 4–21*

### Advocating for "Veterans"

Many clients in a 200-bed Manhattan women's shelter have enrolled in a mental health care program, ostensibly in order to get a more regular supply of soap, toilet paper, and other necessities. After they began to attend the program, some clients asked for help in other areas, such as obtaining welfare or negotiating with the shelter bureaucracy. When the program had gained credibility as an advocate in these areas, the team offered to help clients to extract needed services from more threatening systems, such as hospitals and clinics. Treatment for mental illness was then presented as another entitlement, countering the prevailing view among the women that it was a form of punishment. In fact, posters in the shelter advertised the mental health program as an entitlement analogous to veteran's benefits, available only to "veterans" of the mental health system.

---

*Panel 4–22*

## Taking On the System

One homeless man had been consistently denied Social Security Disability payments despite clear clinical evidence that he did, in fact, suffer from a major mental illness of sufficient duration and disability to qualify for the aid. By discussing his previous application attempts, he and his clinician were able to clarify the ways that he had participated in providing the system with grounds for rejecting his application.

Together, they rehearsed how he would approach his next application process and how he would answer various questions that might occur: "I am schizophrenic and have been diagnosed as such three different times at three hospitals; I have not been able to work since my diagnosis, and I have only $1,100 in total savings. I believe that I qualify for SSI benefits."

---

4. *Develop peer support*. Develop peer groups that can provide ongoing support as case managers and treatment sites change. Such groups can help clients to navigate welfare and other agencies, engage in outreach to recruit new members, and may even develop unique treatment approaches based on their members' needs.

5. *Expand services*. The effort to serve the homeless mentally ill cannot be limited to shelters, nor can it rely solely on traditional mental health providers. Community care programs for the homeless mentally ill should include street outreach, on-site rehabilitation, and psychosocial clubs (Kellermann et al., 1985). Those individuals who seek to deliver mental health services to homeless persons can help others to understand the need for these services.

A good starting point for additional community-based services is a drop-in center that allows clients to begin to relate to staff and others as friends, without pressure, while receiving basic survival services (receipt of mail, public aid

---

*Panel 4–23*

## Transferring Street Skills

A group in a women's shelter categorized the skills needed to be a good panhandler. These included understanding the neighborhood, "sizing up" potential givers, and having a convincing story. Clients then applied these skills in negotiating for carfare in the shelter, learning the criteria for getting carfare, sizing up the worker, and showing the worker the necessary appointment slips. (Screaming had previously been the preferred technique.) Later, the same skills were used in applying for welfare.

---

**Panel 4–24**

**A Support Group**

A formerly homeless woman in New York originated groups in hotels and shelters where women with drinking or drug problems could discuss their experience of homelessness as well as their addictions (White, 1988). With the exception of the leader, group members were not abstinent. These groups became a "pretreatment" option for those who were not yet ready for treatment. Over time, many women who attended the groups developed the motivation needed to give up alcohol and/or drugs.

---

advocacy, money management, mental health referrals, paralegal services, and casual labor service) (Segal and Baumohl, 1985).

## CONCLUSIONS

Many staff members in shelters agonize over the appropriate approach to take to psychiatric problems among their guests, because this decision forces them to confront a basic service dilemma: Should shelters make the greatest possible effort to help guests directly, ministering to their mental health and other needs or should they seek only to reconnect guests with extant service systems, no matter how difficult that may be?

It is a cruel dilemma. Successful efforts to deliver services in shelters inevitably tend to "institutionalize" the shelter function, or the "shelter industry" as it is often called. When guests become used to the security of shelters, aided by the comprehensive array of services, staff members then see their functions as comparable to service jobs in permanent service agencies, and other service agencies feel less responsibility for the shelter users. The result is less pressure to end the state of homelessness itself.

On the other hand, shelter users who suffer from serious mental illness face an array of problems that compound the already devastating effects of homelessness itself. Shelters are often their last resort, but the troubled behavior of some guests may make it difficult to continue to welcome them within the shelter, whereas the passive withdrawal of other guests can lead to increasing isolation from everyday life. Even those guests who are willing to seek services from the regular service system are likely to encounter expectations that they cannot live up to and rejection of their claims. Shelter staff have little choice but to reach out to these guests and try to establish supportive connections. The avoidance behavior among some of the seriously mentally ill homeless simply makes such outreach all the more necessary.

# Homeless People with Alcohol Problems

"Have you ever had problems due to drinking?" "Do you have any history of a drinking problem?" "Have you ever been admitted to a detox or treatment program because of your drinking?" Jimmy has heard these questions in one form or another a hundred times or more for the past 5 years, and he has come to regard these, as well as his answers, as part of a ritual for admission to a shelter for the homeless.

Jimmy, who has been homeless over 5 years, accepts drinking and drunkenness as a fact of his life. "The doctors told me 9 years ago that booze would send me to an early grave unless I laid down the bottle," he tells the caseworker during intake at a New York shelter for homeless men. "I've been on the wagon; I've been in detox; I've been in programs and hospitals; I've been in jail—I've done it all," he confesses. Now, at age 51, he has been separated from his wife and two children for over 12 years, and his case records show that he has been hospitalized at least five times over the past 24 months for liver disease and alcohol-related accidents. His caseworker says that, "In a way, Jimmy has given up. We see people like Jimmy every day at this shelter."

Although Jimmy may not typify all homeless alcoholics in cities in the United States, his case serves to illustrate how drinking and alcohol abuse play major roles in the personal problems of the homeless. In fact, research studies over the past 50 years estimate the prevalence of alcoholism as somewhere from 20 percent to as high as 50 percent. For example, recent studies conducted in Boston (Garrett and Schutt, 1989), Denver (Atencio, 1982), New York (Barrow and Lovell, 1982), and Oregon (Multnomah County Social Services Division, 1984) estimate that from 30 percent to 50 percent of the homeless have a problem with alcohol abuse or alcoholism. Figures based on similar studies in Ohio (Roth and Bean, 1986), Baltimore (Fischer and Breakey, 1987), Milwaukee (Rosnow, Shaw, Concord, Tucker and Palmer, 1985), Phoenix (Brown, MacFarlane, Paredes, and Stark, 1982), and Los Angeles (Ropers and Robertson, 1984) estimate the prevalence somewhat lower at 20 percent to 30 percent.

Regardless of the variation in prevalence, the fact is that a significant proportion of the homeless is afflicted with alcoholism and related problems. These problems complicate efforts at intervention, as well as compound the health risks already faced by the homeless. Thus, it is important that those who work with the homeless understand the nature of alcohol abuse and alcoholism, how these problems are manifested among the homeless, and the types of services available to them.

This chapter addresses five topic areas: (1) alcohol and the homeless; (2) alcoholism and alcohol-related diseases—what they are and how to respond to them; (3) screening clients for alcohol problems; (4) detoxification; and (5) recovery and rehabilitation services. Each sections combines generic information with research and program literature on the homeless.


## INTRODUCTION

The stereotypical image of the homeless alcoholic is probably the skid row derelict drunk in an alley or doorway of an abandoned building. Although there remains some truth to this stereotype, homeless people show a diversity, including those with alcohol problems, that was not seen in earlier decades. In the 1940s through the 1960s, profiles of homeless alcoholics characterized them as predominantly older, white males, who were divorced or separated, were high school dropouts, and had high rates of physical disabilities and, above all, lengthy histories of alcohol abuse (Bahr, 1965; Bogue, 1963; Straus, 1946). Today, the composite profile looks very different (Fischer, 1989; Garrett, 1989; Koegel and Burnham, 1987; Ropers and Robertson, 1984):

- The vast majority are males in their thirties to early forties.
- Racial composition varies by city, but in most more than one half are nonwhite or of Hispanic origin.
- Half or more have a high school education.
- Approximately one out of every two has never been married.
- From 30 percent to 60 percent have impaired health, mostly related to alcohol abuse.

In addition to changes in social composition, it is also clear that the problems of homeless alcoholics are more complex than ever. For example, current studies indicate that from one quarter to one third of those with alcohol problems also suffer from psychiatric impairment (Fischer, 1989; Fischer and Breakey, 1987), and that as many as one in every four has a history of drug abuse (Fischer and Breakey, 1987). Other studies help to refine this profile. Thus, a Los Angeles study of the homeless (Koegel and Burnham, 1987) reported that psychiatrically impaired alcoholics show a different social and health profile than those who are "pure alcoholics," and a Philadelphia report (Shipley, Moor, and Shandler, 1987) indicated substantial background differences among alcohol/drug abusers versus those with only an alcoholic disorder. In sum, homeless alcoholics are not so easily stereo-typed as they were in the past. Responding to the needs of this diverse population is now a major challenge to the helping professions.

## The Skid Row Subculture

Alcoholism and alcohol abuse among the homeless is best understood not as an isolated personal pathology, but as part of a larger subculture that is both permissive and tolerant of heavy drinking practices. Although skid row (or skid road in the west) is shrinking in many cities owing to urban renewal, elements of its drinking subculture remain intact. For many alcoholics, drinking is an impor-tant context for social interaction with others, which makes the alcoholic less isolated than other types of skid row inhabitants (Garrett and Bahr, 1973, 1976).

Classic skid row studies (Bahr, 1965; Bogue, 1963; Peterson, 1955; Rubington, 1958, 1968; Wiseman, 1970) provide a detailed picture of drinking patterns and social interaction. For both alcoholic and nonalcoholic drinkers, drinking is a primary context for social interaction. Early studies (Peterson, 1955; Rooney, 1961; Rubington, 1958, 1968; Wiseman, 1970) indicate that much of the drinking on skid row takes place in structured group situations, such as in "bottle gangs" or in skid row bars. For skid row women, however, group drinking is less common (Garrett, 1970).

Contrary to popular belief, only about one in four alcoholics on skid row drinks primarily wine (Bogue, 1963), preferring instead beer or whiskey. Neverthe-less, virtually all skid row alcoholics admit to buying fortified wines (so-called because they have had extra alcohol added) for reasons of economy. A veteran alcoholic on Chicago's West Madison Street skid row explains why: "Your cheap wines—we call 'em rot gut down here—gives ya' a good drunk for your money!" (Garrett, 1965:5). Wine drinkers, however, often have curious beliefs about the effects of fortified wine, such as "It thickens the blood," "brings out the devil in people," or "gives you diarrhea" (Garrett, 1971:112). Yet, because fortified wines have popular appeal to alcoholic derelicts, some cities, such as Portland, Oregon, and more recently Seattle, have sought to restrict their sale on skid row.

On skid row or off, not all homeless people are drinkers. In fact, available research indicates that about 15 percent are teetotalers, and nearly one third are light or controlled drinkers (Bahr, 1965; Bogue, 1963). Among heavier drinkers, however, consumption far exceeds conventional drinking practices. A Chicago skid row study, for example, reports that nearly 6 of every 10 alcoholics indicated an average weekly consumption of not less than seven pints of whiskey or the equivalent, and more than half of these estimated consumption at 10 or more pints. In fact, nearly 4 of every 10 heavy but nonalcoholic drinkers estimated consump-tion in excess of seven pints weekly.

## Alcohol as a Factor in Causing Homelessness

Although the term *skid row* implies a marked downward mobility, evidence from research indicates that the vast majority of the homeless have followed a horizontal rather than a vertical pathway to homelessness. Thus, most of the

---

*Panel 5–1*

**The Homeless Veteran Alcoholic**

By his own admission, Ken is an alcoholic. "I'm at rock bottom now," he says, "and I know I need help bad—what am I gonna do?"

But life was not always this low for Ken. Raised in a working-class community near Boston, he says there is nothing unusual about his early life; that is, until his father was killed in an automobile accident. "My dad, he was a heavy boozer sometimes. Maybe you'd call him an alcoholic, too. But we had good times and all the things that kids want." In high school, Ken had a lot of friends and played baseball on the school team in his sophomore year. But he also had his fling with drugs and drinking: "A lotta kids did dope and booze. We'd do grass a lot. Coke wasn't a big thing then. Grass and wine, maybe some beer, if I could get it—that's all." But, these did cause some problems for Ken. "I had a few scrapes," he admits. "We got pulled over by a cop. We'd been doin' grass and drinkin' and he saw a bottle." Another time, the police arrested Ken and others at a beach after a fight broke out. Both incidents led to juvenile probation for Ken.

After graduating from high school, Ken took a job as a carpenter's apprentice through connections with a family friend. "I was good with my hands, I think, and I was hopin' to get into construction work—good money in that, you know." But Ken also had some problems when his boss suspected he was high on marijuana on the job. Later, Ken was fired when he failed to show up for work. "I guess I was drinking the whole weekend and felt like hell on Monday." One week later, he received his draft notice to report for military duty.

Ken says he did not mind basic training. "It helped me straighten out my life and I got along with everybody okay." After 9 months of duty at a base in New Jersey, Ken was sent to Vietnam. He had troubles almost from the day he arrived: "It was pure hell, like nothing you ever seen, man. It got so I'd do anything I could get my hands on. You don't know what I seen. It messed me up. Druggin' and drinkin', I wasn't the only one. It's hard to talk about it." Ken confesses that he had run-ins with the military police in Vietnam, but he was returned stateside and later given an honorable discharge, but not before being hospitalized "for being messed up and all strung out."

Since discharge from the Army, Ken

---

homeless come from working-class or impoverished backgrounds, rather than from high social class status (Bahr, 1970; Bogue, 1963; Garrett, 1987). On the other hand, research on the life histories of homeless men and women shows that they have experienced a marked pattern of disaffiliation in the years preceding their homelessness. This disaffiliation process involves a "disengagement" from the groups, such as family, friends, church, co-worker, and voluntary associations, that function to link people into normal, mainstream society at any level of social class. For alcoholics, this disaffiliation pattern is especially pronounced (Bahr, 1965; Bahr and Caplow, 1968; Bahr and Garrett, 1971, 1976; Garrett, 1970).

What role does drinking play in the "skid careers" of the homeless alcoholics? Does heavy drinking or alcoholism precede homelessness or does alcoholism have

---

*Panel 5–1*   (Continued)

has had trouble in adjusting to life on his own. He forgets how many jobs he has held—working as a dishwasher, at a laundry, in a warehouse facility, and others. "I either up and quit or I'd get drunk and just not go back." He also took college classes using veteran's benefits, but dropped out within 2 months. Now 38 years old, Ken says drinking is his main problem, and that he cannot get it under control. Twice he has been hospitalized because of accidents that happened when he was drinking, and he has been at detox more than a dozen times in the past few years. Although he has never been married, Ken makes it clear that "I ain't gay or anything like that. I just can't get my life together, man, that's all."

Ken has been homeless for about 3 years. Although he receives benefits from entitlements, he makes his way on the streets and at Boston-area shelters, preferring to spend his money on alcohol and personal things. There are risks in his lifestyle: "It's dangerous on the streets," he warns. "I got rolled more than once when I was drinking. You don't know who to trust." Neither does he trust many of the agencies where he can get help for his drinking and personal problems; and even

though he acknowledges he needs treatment, he never accepts their advice or referrals. "I got fed up with the VA. Red tape. They don't understand—I don't need their help." Now that he has lost touch with his sister, he is alone. "I got no one to help me out."

When Ken is drinking, every day is like the one before. "I sleep out—the Common, the South End, it depends. Maybe I hit the Night Center or maybe Pine Street. Just depends on how I feel." Drinking is the first order of the day, and it begins with a stop at a package store for some wine. "I get a bottle and maybe hang out at the Common. I meet up with some of the guys. We have a few hits. We just hang out." If he can keep food down, he visits a downtown fast-food chain for something to eat and coffee. "Sometimes you get bounced if you stay too long, so then I walk around, check things out, maybe meet up with someone. That's all." By nightfall, Ken is always drunk. "Last night," he explains, "I guess I was down in the street. There was rain and somebody took me to that Center. I need help bad, I think." But Ken refused to be taken to the hospital, and today he is sitting in the Public Garden with his bottle.

---

its onset as a consequence of homelessness? Available evidence suggests that for the majority of homeless alcoholics, the onset of heavy drinking precedes homelessness itself. Early studies reported that for about two thirds of the homeless men (Bahr, 1965; Straus, 1946) and women (Garrett, 1971) alcoholics on skid row, a heavy drinking pathology preceded homelessness. Evidence from a more recent Los Angeles study of inner-city homeless alcoholics, however, suggested that as many as 80 percent show symptoms of alcoholism before they become homeless (Koegel and Burnham, 1987). Thus, although the skid row and homeless subculture is permissive toward heavy drinking, most alcoholics who become homeless have already experienced the onset of a drinking pathology.

## A PRIMER ON ALCOHOL ABUSE AND ALCOHOLISM

The homeless are not alone in their problems with alcohol. Yet, although they constitute only about 5 percent to 7 percent of the estimated 18 million Americans who suffer from a drinking problem, their risk is disproportionately high—at least four times greater, on the average, than in the general population. Moreover, even though all alcoholics run high risks of developing alcohol-related diseases, a recent Los Angeles study (Koegel and Burnham, 1987) found that homeless alcoholics also have higher morbidity rates than other types of alcoholics. Thus, a fundamental understanding of alcoholism and of the health consequences of chronic drinking patterns is an essential part of the knowledge required for responding to the needs of the homeless.

### Alcohol and Alcoholism

Ethanol, which is contained in beverage alcohol, is one of several alcohols produced through a process of fermentation of fruit or cereal substances. Although ethanol is an intoxicant, it is less toxic than other alcohols, such as methyl alcohol ("wood alcohol"), since the body converts it into harmless substances, carbon dioxide and water. Of course ethanol is not consumed in its pure state, but instead is ingested through intake of beverage alcohol, such as beer (3 percent to 6 percent ethanol), wine (12 percent to 14 percent) or distilled spirits (40 percent to 50 percent). Regardless of beverage, however, ethanol is a highly addictive substance which can create a chemical dependency and changes in the body if it is consumed in excess over an extended period of time. This characteristic of ethanol has led some professionals to label alcohol a *drug*, in the same sense that cocaine or heroin are called drugs. In any case, physical dependency on alcohol is the hallmark of what we term *alcoholism* or *alcohol addiction*.

Alcoholism is also more than an addiction to alcohol, since it always causes problems in the personal and social functioning of the alcoholic. Thus, defining alcoholism is not easy, since it involves many dimensions, and professionals often disagree among themselves as to its definition. So, too, are there differences in viewpoints about the causes of alcoholism.

The medical model interprets alcoholism as a progressive disease having physiological determinants. Some of those who support the medical model believe that it is an innate body chemistry or genetic disposition that makes some people vulnerable to the effects of alcohol. Others believe that long periods of heavy drinking trigger the disease process by stimulating biochemical changes. In either case, alcoholism constitutes an addiction requiring medical treatment, especially during the withdrawal period. Continued sobriety requires total abstinence.

Another conception of alcoholism is the psychological model. Once again, although psychologists differ on which psychological factors are causally important, they tend to agree that alcoholism is a consequence of an underlying personality disorder. Given effective therapy, the psychological factors compelling the alcoholic to drink can be modified such that the patient can sustain sobriety.

Behavioral psychology, however, takes a different viewpoint. In fact, the behavioral therapist is even reluctant to use the word *alcoholism*, or to imply that it is a disease *per se*. In its place, they see "problem drinking" as caused by environmental factors that bring rewards for heavy drinking. Although there are different types of behavioral therapy, they all converge on the premise that behavior is controlled by its consequences. Thus, if the rewards for heavy drinking are manipulated so that they are no longer pleasing, the drinking pattern can be modified. This approach has been controversial, since it implies that alcoholics (or problem drinkers) can return to sociable drinking patterns.

Sociologists, on the other hand, approach alcoholism from a very different perspective. They are almost never interested in individual behavior, focusing instead on factors rooted in culture and society, such as drinking customs or social attitudes toward alcohol use, that promote and sustain heavy drinking practices. One common sociological perspective sees heavy drinking and alcoholism as a consequence of strains built into society that place social stress on some groups more than others. Those who are more vulnerable to this stress, for example, people in high-stress occupations, the economically disadvantaged, or groups who have become disenfranchised from mainstream society, run substantially higher risks of becoming alcoholics. In a sense, then, alcohol serves as an escape from tensions or personal failure.

A second set of sociological theories, however, sees alcoholism as a consequence of social groups, such as family, friends, co-workers, and even the community at large, who label drinkers who exceed customary drinking practices as *deviant*. This label of disapproval sets in motion social and psychological processes that sustain abusive patterns of drinking. Neither of these two viewpoints, however, is linked directly to treatment of alcoholics. Instead, sociologists dwell on manipulating social factors that can reduce stress, promote less risky drinking practices, or that modify social attitudes toward drinking and alcoholism.

Finally, the most eclectic viewpoint by far is one advocated by Alcoholics Anonymous (AA), which acknowledges the possibility of medical and genetic vulnerability, as well as the influence of psychological and sociological factors. Alcoholism is also viewed as a spiritual failure, in which the drinker loses touch with the moral, or even religious fabric of life. Although the AA model holds that alcoholism is a progressive disease that is based on uncontrollable drinking, it also sees alcohol itself as the root of the problem. Put simply, there is no alcoholism without alcohol! For this reason, AA advocates complete abstinence as the cornerstone of recovery. Therapy entails an intensive peer-group relationship, in which AA members help one another to stay sober. Today there are over 50,000 AA groups with an estimated membership of more than one million, making it the most popular treatment approach (Maxwell, 1984:2–3).

Although staff, case managers, and administrators of shelter programs, even counselors in detox centers, need not become experts in theories or causes of alcoholism, it is important to appreciate that there is no single answer or approach to the alcoholism problem. This holds true for alcoholism among the homeless, as well as for other populations. Instead, there are different levels for understanding these causes, and thus different approaches to treatment. In fact, it is also clear that alcoholism is not a single disease.

*Panel 5–2*

## AA and the Homeless Alcoholic

Unquestionably the most widely advocated treatment for alcoholics is Alcoholics Anonymous or AA. Founded in 1938 by two alcoholics who felt they needed each other's support for continued sobriety, AA's approach involves self-help through peer-group association and spiritualism. The AA preamble to its *Twelve Steps and Twelve Traditions* (1991:i) provides the best description of how the organization works.

> Alcoholics Anonymous is a fellowship of men and women who share their experience, strength and hope with each other that they may solve their common problem and help others to recover from alcoholism. The only requirement for membership is a desire to stop drinking. There are no dues or fees for AA membership; we are self-supporting through our own contributions. AA is not allied with any sect, denomination, politics, organization or institution; does not wish to engage in any controversy; neither endorses nor opposes any causes. Our primary purpose is to stay sober and help other alcoholics to achieve sobriety.

The fundamental credo of AA lies in its Twelve Steps, which lead members from a self-acknowledgment that they are "powerless over alcohol" and that their "lives had become unmanageable," to a final step of spiritual awakening and a dedication to carry the AA message to other alcoholics. Today, almost every modern treatment approach includes an AA component, and it is universal among programs serving homeless alcoholics. AA meetings are held, oftentimes nightly, at detox centers, shelters, hospital and community-based programs, and even at county and city jails. One alcoholic informant explains how AA touches the lives of the homeless on San Francisco's skid row: "AA is a part of life down here. If a guy is a drunk and living on the streets, you know all about it. Almost every drunk on Mission Street has probably been to meetings at one time or another. A lot of places, they make you go to AA if you want to stay there."

In their national survey for the National Institute of Alcohol Abuse and Alcoholism, Wittman and Madden (1988) pointed out that AA is a cornerstone of recovery programs for the homeless with alcohol problems. Especially in residential settings, AA augments individual and group counseling approaches, and depending on institutional emphasis, even spiritual recovery. "Even if they return to drinking—and most do," explains a case manager at Boston's Long Island Shelter, "our guests get acquainted with AA. It opens up a service to them when they leave us. . . . It can make a difference in their lives—someday."

Alcoholics on skid row, however, do not always seek out AA to help support their periods of sobriety (Bahr, 1965; Bogue, 1963; Henshaw, 1968; Wiseman, 1970). Comments from a veteran alcoholic on skid row in Los Angeles offer some clues as to why: "Man, it makes no sense to me, you know? You trade stories on how low you sunk. I mean, everybody is in the same place down here. . . . And, you get guys in AA who sit through a meeting, then head out for a bottle."

Yet, for alcoholics who are in transition from a recovery program to an independent living situation, AA represents an important bridge to a new life. "I got a break when I left the program—I got a job in the shelter," a recovering alcoholic in Boston explains. "And AA helps keep me improving myself. I go three times a week—it's my whole social life, you might say. When the time is right, AA is always there!"

## Types of Alcoholism

Most people today are accustomed to hearing alcoholism referred to as a disease. Nevertheless, it is only in the past three decades that the disease concept of alcoholism has taken hold. Although massive public education programs by government agencies and private organizations, such as AA or the National Council on Alcoholism, have furthered this cause, it is E. M. Jellinek and his now classic work, *The Disease Concept of Alcoholism* (Jellinek, 1960), that laid the groundwork for this formulation. Jellinek noted, however, that there are different types of alcoholism syndromes. He used Greek letters to delineate his typology.

The *Alpha* type is a purely psychological dependence, in which alcohol is used to "deal with life" and to remove inhibitions or to escape from stress. Thus, alcohol helps to remove the drinker from psychic pain. Presumably, once the stress is removed, the dependence on alcohol weakens or disappears.

In the second type, *Beta*, alcohol is used to lessen physical not psychological stress. Among people who live in subcultures, such as skid row, the military, or other occupational lifestyles where drinking customs are permissive, even prized, heavy drinking can lead to chronic physical problems, such as gastritis or liver disease. Thus, continued drinking helps relieve physical stress.

The *Gamma* type is most commonly seen in North America. This syndrome manifests a configuration of social, psychological, and medical symptoms that become progressively worse as heavy drinking continues. It involves a physical dependence that is characterized by a "loss of control" or uncontrollable drinking. The disease concept is most closely associated with the Gamma type of alcoholism.

In contrast, the *Delta* type reflects not a "loss of control" over alcohol, but instead an "inability to abstain." Thus, this type of alcoholic has become physically dependent on alcohol, mostly because drinking customs promote regular and sometimes heavy alcohol consumption. More commonly seen in such countries as France or Chile, this type of alcoholic can experience severe alcohol-related diseases, as well as major withdrawal symptoms if they are forced to abstain. This, too, fits Jellinek's notion of the disease concept of alcoholism.

Finally, what Jellinek called the *Epsilon* type is characterized by episodic or spree drinking. In this type of alcoholism, there may be periods of abstention or moderate drinking, yet these are punctuated by prolonged drinking bouts or "benders" that usually result in physical and emotional exhaustion. During these benders, there is often acute health risk because of heavy consumption over a short period of time. Although drinking patterns are irregular, overall consumption of alcohol among spree drinkers may exceed that of the conventional chronic alcoholic. Some studies of skid row (Bahr, 1965; Bahr and Caplow, 1968; Blumberg et al., 1973) report that this type of alcoholism is evident in nearly one out of every three homeless alcoholics.

## Progressive Symptoms of Alcoholism

One of Jellinek's (1946) first studies, based on some 2,000 alcoholics in AA, charted the progressive signs and symptoms of alcoholism found in the Gamma type. Although there were observed variations in the appearance and patterning of symptoms, there were also remarkable similarities.

The road to alcoholism seems to begin with a prealcoholic phase where the drinker gradually shifts from social or convivial drinking to one where alcohol offers relief from normal stresses that virtually all people encounter. As the pattern of relief drinking continues, an increase in tolerance for alcohol develops. This process can last from several months to as long as 2 years or more, yet directly observable signs of alcoholism are absent.

In the early stage of alcoholism, which Jellinek calls the *prodromal phase*, warning signs begin to appear. The most important of these is the onset of alcoholic *palimpsests* or *blackouts*, which involve temporary periods of memory loss. The person may appear to be normal in behavior, yet later cannot recall events that have occurred during the blackout period. Other warning signs also appear: occasional feelings of guilt about drinking behavior, gulping the first few drinks, sneaking drinks so that others at social gatherings do not notice, and an increasing preoccupation with alcohol. Increased blackouts foreshadow the onset of true addiction. This phase, Jellinek noted, can last anywhere from several months to 4 or 5 years, depending on the physical, psychological, and social circumstances of the drinker.

The middle or crucial phase of alcoholism is marked by a loss of control over drinking. Thus, once consumption begins, there is a persistent physical demand for more alcohol. It continues until the drinker is too sick or too intoxicated to ingest more alcohol. This physical craving can be triggered even by taking a single social drink. Other symptoms signal complications in both personal psychology and the social life of the drinker: steady increase in consumption; pronounced excuse-making for drinking; job loss or instability; changes in family habits and personal relations; persistent remorse and self-pity; feeble attempts to change drinking habits, including periods of abstinence ("going on the wagon"); geographic escape; and onset of regular morning drinking.

Heaving drinking continues to undermine the alcoholic's health. Neglect of proper nutrition brings the onset of alcohol-related disorders, and hospitalization for an alcoholic complaint is likely. The disease process, thus, is in full motion.

In the late or chronic phase, physical and psychological debilitation escalates. Prolonged benders, together with disregard for personal health, lead to impairment of thinking and an inability to accomplish even simple mechanical acts without alcohol. An estimated 1 in 10 alcoholics will develop alcoholic psychoses, and most alcoholics experience attacks of tremors, anxiety, or indefinable fears, which can usually be reduced by drinking. These are signals of a loss of tolerance for alcohol. As drinking takes on a compulsive character, alcohol-related diseases become a major hazard to the alcoholic's health.

Finally, it should be noted that Vaillant (1983) offered convincing scientific evidence that Jellinek's conception of alcoholism as a progressive disease is indeed the case. Although Vaillant reported that the patterning of symptoms does not show the orderliness described by Jellinek, his results indicated essentially two outcomes of alcoholism: recovery through abstinence or death.

## Alcohol-Related Diseases

During the early phases of alcoholism, symptoms of the disease are primarily behavioral or nonphysical. However, if alcoholism remains untreated, the effects of long-term heavy drinking on the body's organ systems eventually create medical complications that dramatically change the character of the disease. Although the onset of these secondary diseases depends on a number of factors—extent of drinking, nutritional habits, even genetic disposition—it is usually these alcohol-related disorders that ultimately bring the alcoholic to a premature death. Among the homeless, health risks to the alcoholic are especially acute. Compared to the non-abuser, alcoholics have four to seven times higher rates of liver disease; twice the rate of trauma; two to three times the rate of seizure disorders and other neurological impairments; twice the rate of nutritional deficiencies; and at least one and one-half times the rate of hypertension, chronic pulmonary disease, gastro-intestinal disorders, and arterial disease (Fischer and Breakey, 1987; Ropers and Boyer, 1987a; Schutt and Garrett, 1986b).

## Pancreatitis

Chronic heavy drinking can cause an acute inflammation of the pancreas, a gland that makes digestive juices which are needed to break down starches, fats, and proteins. Inflammation of the pancreas can disrupt normal digestive processes. Symptoms of acute pancreatitis are nausea, periods of severe vomiting and diarrhea, and almost always intense upper abdominal pain that extends through to the back. The skin becomes cold and clammy, and in severe cases the drinker may go into shock.

Acute pancreatitis requires treatment and abstinence from alcohol. If alcohol abuse continues, it almost always leads to a chronic form of pancreatitis. Although pain may not be so severe, symptoms similar to the acute form will recur. Diabetes can develop as a consequence of the impaired capacity of the pancreas to produce and release insulin.

## Liver Disease

Alcoholic liver disease is one of the most serious medical consequences of chronic heavy drinking. In fact, cirrhosis, the most serious form of liver disease, ranks as the fourth leading cause of death after age 45. It is uncommon after age 65, since relatively few people with cirrhosis survive to that age. Three types of liver disease are associated with alcohol consumption.

*Acute Fatty Liver.* This condition is often the first step in the development of a more serious stage of liver disease. Because of the disrupting effects of alcohol on the digestive system, acute fatty liver occurs as deposits of fat accumulate in healthy liver cells. Onset of this disorder develops when approximately one third to one half of the total caloric intake is in the form of alcohol. In fact, this condition can occur in any drinker who has consumed large amounts of alcohol over a short period. Acute fatty liver is reversible if alcohol consumption is stopped.

*Alcoholic Hepatitis.* Far more serious is alcoholic hepatitis, which often has its onset following a prolonged drinking bout. Although hepatitis is not unique to alcoholics, it has a very high incidence among alcoholics.

In alcoholic hepatitis, there is an acute inflammation of the liver and cell damage. Jaundice, that is, a yellow-look to the skin and to the whites of the eyes, is the most observable sign of hepatitis. This yellowing comes from bile, manufactured by the liver, which is circulating in the bloodstream in excessive amounts. Other symptoms include: loss of appetite, periods of nausea and vomiting, fatigue and weakness, mild fever, and some weight loss. Although hepatitis is reversible in some alcoholics following abstinence, it can become fatal for others. It carries a mortality rate ranging from 10 percent to as high as 30 percent.

*Cirrhosis of the Liver.*   By far the most serious form of liver disease is alcoholic cirrhosis, which involves a permanent, irreversible damage or scarring of liver tissue. Oftentimes, alcoholic hepatitis is a forerunner of cirrhosis. Thus, during screening or intake of homeless clients, those who report having suffered hepatitis should also be suspect for cirrhosis. More than 50 percent of patients who continue to drink after being diagnosed with cirrhosis will be dead within 5 years. Until the 1970s, liver damage common to alcoholics was not seen as a consequence of alcohol *per se*, but rather was due to long-term nutritional deficiencies. Evidence since then indicates that alcohol itself plays the major role.

Cirrhosis afflicts the drinker with a number of medical complications. Put simply, the liver is impaired to a degree that it cannot perform normal functions. Toxic substances that are removed in a healthy liver now circulate in the bloodstream. This can cause complications elsewhere in the body, including the brain and intestinal system.

Early symptoms of cirrhosis can go unnoticed: gradual loss of appetite, occasional nausea, and abdominal pain. As the disease progresses, however, more pronounced symptoms appear, such as jaundice and accumulations of fluid in the abdomen, which can cause a protruding of the stomach. Other complications can also develop, such as bleeding from varicose veins in the throat or from similar dilated veins in the stomach.

### Cardiovascular Disorders

Chronic heavy drinking is now believed to be the direct cause of a condition known as *alcoholic heart muscle disease* (AHMD). The onset of AHMD is most commonly seen in men who have had at least 10 or more years of excessive drinking. In its severe condition, this disorder entails abnormal functioning and enlargement of the heart muscle, so that even mild exertion can cause extreme shortness of breath.

Alcoholic deterioration of the heart can also create irregularities in rhythm, which, in some cases, can even lead to sudden death. Less severe cases involve palpitations of the heart (sometimes referred to as *holiday heart*), which are not uncommon after prolonged drinking bouts. Although this symptom may not indicate a fatal condition, clients should receive appropriate medical follow-up.

Since alcohol elevates certain fat levels that are linked to hardening of the arteries (or arteriosclerosis), chronic excessive drinking can increase substantially the risk of heart attack. In addition, heavy alcohol consumption is also linked to hypertension or high blood pressure.

## Anemia

By far the most common blood disorder among chronic alcoholics is anemia. Although there are different types of anemia associated with alcoholism (e.g., iron-deficiency anemia, spur cell anemia, etc.) these represent a combination of medical complications brought on by prolonged heavy drinking and by poor nutritional habits that are especially characteristic of middle- and late-phase alcoholics. For this reason, alcoholics undergoing treatment, especially during the detoxification process, are often given therapeutic doses of vitamins. One form of anemia, spur cell (so named because under the microscope the red blood cells appear spur-shaped), is associated with the final stage of alcoholic liver disease.

Thus, anemia's relationship to alcoholism is part of an overall debilitation of the body. Chronic fatigue, lack of appetite, and pallor of the skin are generalized symptoms. This run-down condition also leaves the alcoholic open to common diseases and infections, in part owing to a depressant effect of alcohol on the immune system. Common ailments, such as colds or flu, take longer to clear up for chronic alcoholics, and thus they run a higher risk of developing pneumonia. Since heavy cigarette smoking often is associated with chronic problem drinking, there is also an elevated risk of chronic obstructive lung disease and head and neck cancer.

## Disorders of the Nervous System

Contrary to the popular conception, alcohol has a depressant effect on the central nervous system, and, except in small doses, does not act as a stimulant. In fact, acute alcoholic intoxication brings about mild delirium; thinking is blurred and both recent memory and higher mental functioning are altered.

Alcoholism involves the gradual development of a physical dependence on alcohol. This dependence or addiction signals a loss of tolerance for alcohol. In simple terms, chronic drinking patterns bring about a change in the way in which the body metabolizes alcohol, as well as altering its effects on the nervous system. As tolerance increases, it takes more alcohol to achieve the same intoxicating effect that lesser dosages had earlier in the drinking career. After years of heavy drinking and the onset of alcohol-related diseases (liver disease, in particular), alcoholics experience a reverse tolerance for alcohol in which only a few drinks will bring about intoxication.

*Withdrawal Syndromes.* Physical dependence can carry acute health risks when drinking is stopped. Early withdrawal symptoms can be expected within 8 to 9 hours or less. Symptoms during this early withdrawal include tremulousness, anxiety and edginess, rapid heartbeat, irritability, and loss of appetite. Nausea and vomiting, insomnia, and a generalized weakness are also common symptoms. Withdrawal following a prolonged drinking bout is also likely to carry a giant hangover headache, which has in earlier times been cured by the morning drink (referred to by some alcoholics as the "hair of the dog that bit you"). Many alcoholics are compelled to take a morning drink so as to avoid these early symptoms of withdrawal.

If abstention continues beyond a 48- to 96-hour period, these symptoms begin to escalate. Flushing of the face, sweating (especially at night), increased body temperature, and elevated blood pressure occur. These symptoms may subside over the course of a few days, but sleeplessness, irritability, and edginess can persist for a few weeks or longer. Although early withdrawal symptoms may not necessitate immediate medical attention, the alcoholic requires close observation during this period. This is especially true of late-phase alcoholics, since they may have a higher risk of developing complications during withdrawal. If acute symptoms persist or worsen after a 3- to 4-day period, it may indicate the onset of delirium tremens, more commonly called the *DTs*.

*Acute Alcoholic Hallucinosis.*    About one of every four alcoholics suffering withdrawal syndrome will experience alcoholic hallucinosis. Because homeless alcoholics in general tend to be more debilitated and to have more extensive histories of alcohol abuse than those from other contexts, this percentage may be higher. Among those experiencing this syndrome, symptoms usually appear within the early phases (24 to 48 hours) of withdrawal. The symptoms, which are easily mistaken as a primary psychiatric disorder, include hallucinations, both visual and auditory. The patients will see and especially hear things that do not exist in reality, and also they are very likely to suffer terrifying nightmares. Although hallucinations represent misperceptions, they seem real to the alcoholic and they are likely to act upon this distorted reality. Because hallucinations usually have a paranoid theme, that is, a perception that someone or something is threatening them, the client needs to be watched carefully, since this can lead the alcoholic to do harm to their person or to others. However, alcoholic hallucinosis does not necessarily require immediate medical treatment, providing the alcoholic is in a safe environment and that symptoms do not persist for an extended period. In a majority of cases, acute hallucinosis will subside within the first week of withdrawal.

*Alcoholic Seizures.*    Convulsive seizures, often called "rum fits" by alcoholics, are not uncommon during the first 12 to 48 hours of withdrawal, and if abstention continues should disappear within a week. Typically, these seizures, known as "grand mal," involve violent muscle contractions, rhythmic movement of the limbs and body, eyes rolled back into the head, and unconsciousness. Seizures, which can be terrifying to witness, usually last a few minutes, and when consciousness is regained, the victim is disoriented and stuporous for an extended period. Although not common, some alcoholics can experience successive seizures with almost no intervening period of quiet.

  Even though seizures are not in and of themselves immediately life-threatening (indeed, they are common among alcoholics experiencing withdrawal), it is important that other causes for the seizures be eliminated and it should be noted that about one of every three alcoholics who suffer seizures will eventually progress into DTs. For this reason, medical referral of the alcoholic following the seizure should be made.

*Delirium Tremens.*    By far, the most dangerous consequence of withdrawal is the onset of delirium tremens (DTs), which in the past has carried a mortality rate as high as 20 percent. Although DTs still pose an extreme risk to life, this mortality rate is not as high today.

DTs have two major types of symptoms. On the one hand, delirium involves hallucinations, disorientation to reality, and confusion. On the other, the alcoholic experiences uncontrollable nervousness and agitation, marked shaking or tremulousness, and the vital signs show elevated blood pressure, rapid pulse, and fever with profuse sweating. These symptoms are similar, at first, to early withdrawal signs, but in DTs these become considerably more pronounced. To the alcoholic, full-blown DTs are a fate almost worse than death, where they may see snakes crawling on their bed, creatures on the floor, and hear terrifying voices or sounds. Although the duration of acute attacks vary by individual factors, symptoms subside within 3 days in the majority of cases (and in mild cases, within a day).

Although there is no specific cure for DTs, close observation of the alcoholic and medical care are necessary. The monitoring of vital signs is important, together with supportive care to reduce anxiety and prevent exhaustion. Most medical authorities recommend medication to control blood pressure and pulse.

### Summary of Withdrawal Symptoms

Sooner or later all shelter workers will encounter a guest who is experiencing withdrawal symptoms from alcohol dependency. The severity of these symptoms will vary with the individual and health-related factors of the drinker. Withdrawal can range from the classic hangover to a full-blown case of delirium tremens. If the alcoholic or alcohol abuser is in the early stages of the disease process, withdrawal may consist of only minor symptoms which subside without treatment. As the illness progresses, however, there is a greater likelihood that withdrawal symptoms will be more severe.

*Minor Withdrawal Symptoms.* Fine tremors, mild sweating, some disorientation, and possible convulsions (seizures) are seen. This period can last from shortly after the last drink to between 24 to 48 hours after the last drink.

*Major Withdrawal Symptoms.* Major symptoms (such as delirium tremens) can begin from 24 to 48 hours after the last drink.

*Marked Tremors.* In the early stages, tremors can be observed in the upper body extremities, but can gradually involve the entire body, including voice projection.

*Elevated Vital Signs.* The temperature will increase to 99–100 degrees or slightly higher. The pulse will increase to 110 or greater. The blood pressure also rises and can go to 150/90 or greater. It is the assessment of vital signs that offers the most accurate predictor of mental and physical agitation.

*Hallucinations.* Both auditory (voices or sounds) and visual hallucinations are possible. These are extremely frightening, often consisting of threatening voices

---

### Panel 5–3

### A Case of the DTs

Any alcoholic who has been drinking heavily for 10 years or more will tell you that the DTs is serious business. "The first time I seen it happen to a guy I thought he was gonna die on the spot," said a 42-year-old homeless man in Seattle, who has himself experienced early withdrawal symptoms. "He was like seein' things comin' at em and he grabbed this board and started jabbin' it all around and screamin' like crazy. He was scared as hell and so was I. That look on his face was unreal. . . . We all knew what it was—he had a case of the DTs."

But, if DTs are frightening to watch, they are even more horrifying to those who experience them firsthand. "It was worse than death," according to a 52-year-old alcoholic woman in New York, who indicated that she nearly died during withdrawal. "I felt things crawling on me—spiders, bugs, I don't know what it was—and I felt helpless. I was shaking, I heard things and my skin was like it was on fire. I can't remember all of it, but I remember that feeling: pure hell!"

Although there is no accurate way of telling who will eventually go into DTs, the following characteristics seem to increase this risk (Kinney and Leaton, 1987:147):

1. Daily drinking with heavy consumption (two quarts of wine or a fifth of whiskey, e.g.) during a bender of a week or more prior to abstinence.
2. A history of chronic drinking for at least 10 years.
3. An experience with convulsive seizures and/or DTs during a previous period of complete abstinence.
4. Early withdrawal symptoms, including the onset of seizures, that do not improve over time.
5. Recent abuse of other drugs, sedatives in particular, which can complicate the withdrawal syndrome.

Because one or more of these factors seem to increase the risk of DTs, clients who indicate that they have been drinking heavily before admission to a shelter should be screened for these factors. This is especially true of first-time guests who are unknown to shelter staff. Once identified, these clients should be monitored closely. If a client with these risk factors is already exhibiting early withdrawal symptoms at intake, arrangements should be made for transfer to a detox or medical setting.

---

and terrible sights, such as rats and spiders crawling up one's legs. The person can alternate rapidly from hallucinations to reality.

*Profuse Sweating.*   As the mental and physical agitation increases, so does the sweating (diaphoresis). Extreme sweating as well as inability to keep food and fluids down during this period often leads to dehydration and complications resulting from dehydration.

*Sleeplessness.*   The person is consumed by restlessness and agitation. Since this can last for up to 4 to 5 days, it can be exhausting. This period is usually followed by a deep sleep from which the person wakes clear-headed, but without much memory of what went on over the past few days.

*Seizures.*   If not brought under control, seizures at this time can be life-threatening. (See emergency care for seizures in Chapter 7, pp. 172–173.)

## Emergency Response Procedures

Unfortunately, alcohol abuse often comes to the attention of shelter staff not after a careful assessment but in response to a medical emergency. It is how the shelter responds to these potentially life-threatening emergencies that determines whether supportive relations with alcoholic guests can be established and treatment programs begun.

| What to Do | Why |
|---|---|
| Withdrawal (minor). Suggest detox or recovery program. | The person may be open to this suggestion at this time. |
| Be supportive but not enabling. | Being nonjudgmental and supportive can help the person "hear" your suggestion for treatment. |
| If there is no nausea, offer a hot meal and a bed. | Many alcoholics do not eat when they are drinking and are thus malnourished. A hot meal, but not a large one, will be of benefit. |

| What Not to Do | Why |
|---|---|
| Do not be judgmental or "preachy." | Alcoholism is an illness, not a character flaw. There is no such thing as "pulling yourself up by the bootstraps" here. All that is accomplished is to create guilt and fear, neither of which will be helpful or successful in getting the alcoholic into treatment. |
| Do not offer a large amount of coffee. | Coffee is a stimulant. It will not help to sober a person up. Coffee will only succeed in keeping the person awake at a time when he or she would probably be asleep as a natural result of the anesthetic effect of alcohol. |

| | |
|---|---|
| Do not tuck the person into bed and forget about him or her. | It is entirely possible that the person will progress to a more serious form of withdrawal. As the anesthetic component of the alcohol works its way through the system, the person may experience such events as vomiting and aspirating during sleep. In extreme cases, such as overdose, the person may stop breathing. |

| **What to Do (Major DTs)** | **Why** |
|---|---|
| Transport the person via ambulance to the nearest hospital as quickly as possible. | Delirium tremens is an emergency! If it is not treated, the person is at risk of death from cardiac arrest (heart stops), respiratory arrest (breathing stops), hyperthermia (very high body temperature), and uncontrolled seizures. |
| Keep the environment as calm as possible. | This protects the person from additional stimulation that would increase an already agitated state. |
| Keep the area well-lighted. | This helps to reduce visual hallucinations. |
| Stay with the person and monitor behavior. | To protect the person from agitated behavior. |
| Speak in a low voice and be reassuring. | To help reduce anxiety and fear and to offer support. |

| **What Not to Do** | **Why** |
|---|---|
| Do not move the person to the hospital without qualified help. | The person is in very serious danger at this time. Transportation needs to be done by trained people who can anticipate and respond to possible reactions to movement. |
| Do not attempt to take a temperature by mouth or rectally. | In case of severe tremors, the thermometer is at risk of breaking and causing harm. |
| Do not offer liquids or food. | Food or fluids will increase nausea and the possibility of vomiting. |

## ALCOHOLISM SCREENING

There is seldom a difficulty in identifying stereotypical skid row alcoholics during intake at shelters or social service centers. Their appearance alone is a dead giveaway. Some of the "stigmata of chronic alcoholism" include: bloated appearance with a protruded abdomen; an overall debilitated look; reddening of the skin in the face and neck; acnelike lesions; and possibly even an enlarged or bulbous nose. The problem with relying on physical recognition, however, is that most homeless clients with alcohol problems are not stereotypical skid row alcoholics.

Identification of clients who have drinking and other drug problems helps to single out those who may require treatment. This process is called *screening*. In shelter settings, screening at intake is important so that clients with substance abuse disorders can be identified and referred to appropriate agencies where they will undergo evaluation by qualified professionals.

Numerous screening instruments have been devised that effectively identify alcohol and other drug abusers (see Lettieri, Nelson, & Sayers, 1985). Some are relatively complex batteries of items, such as the Addiction Severity Index or ASI (McLellan, Luborsky, Woody, & O'Brien, 1980) that must be administered by trained interviewers (McCarty, Argeriou, Krakow, & Mulvey, 1990). Still others, such as the Quantity-Frequency-Variability Index (Cahalan, Cisin, & Crossley, 1970) or the Alcohol Dependence Scale (Horn, Skinner, Wanberg, & Foster, 1984) are principally research tools used in surveys. However it is accomplished, shelters and other agencies serving large numbers of homeless clients should adopt a screening method to identify those with alcohol and other drug problems.

### Michigan Alcohol Screening Test

One of the most widely used screening instruments is the Michigan Alcohol Screening Test (MAST). First introduced by Selzer (1971) and associates, it includes 25 questions, answerable with a yes or no, that can be used in a structured interview or that can be completed by the respondent. The items touch upon self-perceptions of drinking behavior, alcohol-related misbehaviors, and medical and psychological problems resulting from alcohol use. Examples of MAST items are: Do you feel you are a normal drinker? Have you ever awakened the morning after some drinking the night before and found that you could not remember part of the evening before? Have you ever gotten into trouble at work because of drinking? Have you ever been told you have liver trouble? Cirrhosis?

Past experience with MAST has shown it to be a valid and reliable instrument on a number of populations. Two variations of MAST have also been introduced. The *Brief MAST* uses 10 of the original items and the *Short MAST* (SMAST) contains 13 items that have been found to be as effective as the longer version. In their major study of Baltimore's homeless, Fischer and Breakey (1987) used the SMAST to single out alcoholics from nonalcoholics.

## CAGE

One of the most efficient alcoholism screening devices is a 4-item test known as *CAGE*.

1. Have you ever felt you should cut down on your drinking?
2. Have people annoyed you by criticizing your drinking?
3. Have you ever felt bad or guilty about your drinking?
4. Have you ever had a drink first thing in the morning to steady the nerves or get rid of a hangover (an eye-opener)?

CAGE is easy to administer, is less intimidating than lengthy questionnaires or inventories, and has been shown to be highly reliable in identifying alcoholics. Two or three affirmative responses indicate a high index of suspicion; four affirmative responses indicate alcoholism.

## "Do It Yourself" Index

An alternative to standardized screening tests, and probably the most widely used by shelters and social service centers, is to develop a few questions that provide self-report information about the client's drinking. This approach also seems more sensible for processing clients in an alcohol treatment setting, such as detox centers, since there is already strong evidence that drinking has been a problem. Moreover, this "homemade" index enables agencies to tailor items that remain sensitive to factors peculiar to a specific setting or type of client. Regardless of context, however, it should be understood that an answer to a single item is less important than the overall configuration of responses.

A number of items can be used. For example, a self-classification item gives an approximate idea of the client's drinking:

> Thinking back over the past 3 months, how would you describe your drinking? Quite a lot, moderate, light, or do you drink at all?

Although this direct approach may raise doubts as to "truthfulness" and accuracy, some studies reported that these types of items may be just as valid as more complex measures that try to quantify drinking behavior. Moreover, virtually all varieties of information about drinking given by clients are self-reports, which also carry a risk of distortion (Garrett and Bahr, 1974).

Similar items take a "problem" approach:

> Do you feel you have any problem with drinking? Yes, no, or not sure? Follow-up item: What kind of problem has this been? Job, family, health, legal, or something else? Have you ever been treated for a drinking problem? Yes, no? Follow-up item: Where were you treated? Alcohol treatment program, AA, outpatient clinic, VA, detox?

Items that collect specific information about drinking patterns are also widely used, such as:

> Thinking back over the past (3 months), about how often did you usually drink? Daily, few times a week, about once a week, less often, or do you drink at all?

When did you have your last drink? How much did you drink then? What beverage(s) did you drink?

An example of how this approach can help in screening homeless clients for alcohol problem is seen in the Intake Form used by Boston's Long Island Shelter for the Homeless (see the Appendix). As developed by the authors, this battery of seven items singles out clients who should be referred for clinical assessment. In addition, this instrument constitutes a beginning point for collecting additional information about the client's drinking that will be useful to case managers and treatment professionals. For agencies who compile aggregate data about the clients they serve, these items can be designed so that they are usable in a data base.

## DETOXIFICATION: A FIRST STEP TOWARD RECOVERY

In years past, the homeless alcoholic lived a life that was like a broken phonograph record; the same events were repeated over and over, almost without interruption. The repetitive cycle of drinking, drunkenness, and sobriety, albeit temporary, was typically punctuated with stints in the jail or the "drunk tank," stops at a skid row mission for a meal and religion, visits to a municipal shelter for a rare bath, handout clothing, and an overnight stay, and sometimes even a period in the dreaded "alcoholic ward" at the city hospital, if life took a turn for the worst.

Early research literature is rich with insights into the lives of chronic homeless alcoholics and the institutions they visited on their drunkenness-sobriety circuit. None are more illuminating than Wiseman's (1970) study of how the homeless derelicts circulate on a skid row "loop" in a western city or Rubington's (1973) classic analyses of the drinking culture, the life and times of the chronic alcoholic and the steps of an alcoholic relapse. Elsewhere, both Peterson's (1955) study of the skid row wino and later Spradly's (1970) offered descriptions of the wino subculture and the humiliation of sobering up in a Spokane "drunk tank." Pittman and Gordon (1958) documented the revolving-door phenomenon of the chronic police case inebriate in a midwestern city, where chronic alcoholics clogged up the court system at enormous public cost. Similar reports (Chicago Committee on Alcoholism, 1955; Garrett, 1965) cited case studies or statistics that show a single alcoholic could account for as many as 15 or more arrests in a year's time. In the 1960s, a National Task Force found that over half of all police arrests were for public drunkenness, most were on skid row (President's Commission, 1967). At times, processing public inebriates has been so routine that one study reported that magistrates in a Canadian court spent, on the average, less than 60 seconds per defendant (Giffen, 1963).

Although homeless alcoholics still face a perilous existence today, there have been dramatic changes in both the number and the quality of "stops" on the drunkenness-sobriety circuit. Moreover, enlightened public attitudes toward alcoholism, the emergence of aggressive outreach efforts and intervention strategies, new treatment alternatives, and, no less important, legal reforms offer possibilities of returning homeless alcoholics to stable, alcohol-free lives that were virtually

*Panel 5–4*

## Can You Trust the Homeless Alcoholic?

In the 1960s, Howard Bahr and associates conducted a major study of the homeless on New York's famed Bowery. At the time, the Bowery was home to more than 10,000 homeless people, an estimated one third of whom were alcoholic derelicts. As part of this study, the investigators undertook a special analysis of the data to see if homeless respondents gave accurate answers to questions included on the study's interview schedule. Using information culled from respondents' case folders, they were able to compare answers given in the interview to corresponding information collected by case workers during client visits to a men's shelter. They also compared this analysis to data collected from a group of working class men who had similar social characteristics but were not homeless.

The investigators' findings were revealing; first, because they showed that about one in every three homeless men did not give accurate answers, that is, their responses in the interview did not agree with the information contained in their case folders. But, even though the comparison groups fared somewhat better, their agreement rate was not significantly higher. The authors concluded that, although the information provided by some homeless clients did sometimes show inconsistencies, the respondents themselves are no more likely to provide "mis-information" than comparable clients.

But what about information on drinking problems and alcohol consumption? Answers to questions about life history facts—education, jobs, marital status, and so forth—are one thing, but items on a client's drinking and alcohol problems are quite another. In fact, survey researchers and clinicians alike have always treated such questions with special sensitivity, since these involve intimate, personal disclosure. Moreover, alcoholics and problem drinkers, in particular, have a denial system in place that can distort self-disclosure statements.

A second study on New York's Bowery, this time conducted by Garrett and Bahr (1974) during the 1970s, focused specifically on the quality of information about drinking practices supplied by shelter clients. The study differed from the first because both men and women were included, and because it compared self-classifications of drinking (e.g., heavy, moderate, or light) with objective information about alcohol consumption supplied by the client elsewhere in a lengthy, 2-hour interview. Presumably, if a respondent indicates a self-classification of, say, "light drinker," he or she will also report objective information about the amount consumed over a time period (e.g., three or four glasses of wine per week) that matches this self rating. Although the methodology was complex, the study's conclusions are very relevant to those who gather information about drinking problems from homeless clients.

1. Homeless women almost always reported consistent information about their drinking behavior and problems; that is, their self-appraisals of drinking matched assessments based on objective reports of consumption patterns. This held true of all types of drinking patterns—heavy, moderate, or light.

*Panel 5–4*  (Continued)

2. On the other hand, self-ratings by homeless men were less consistent with objective assessments. But, unlike the pattern seen in the women, these inconsistencies increased with level of drinking. In other words, self-ratings of drinking among heavy drinkers were far more inconsistent with objective information than for moderate or light drinkers, respectively. This same pattern held true for nonhomeless men, even though their consumption was not, on the average, as high as among the homeless.

3. Among those of either sex where disagreements were noted (about one third of the men and about 20 percent of the women), a pattern also emerged. Women were just as likely to overestimate their drinking problem as they were to underestimate it. But, for the men, virtually all disagreements were in the direction of underestimating the full extent of their drinking. This pattern was most pronounced among heavy drinkers. The authors concluded that among the homeless, women's responses to questions about their drinking, including self-perceptions (which are typically accepted at face validity), are less likely to be distorted than among their male counterparts.

Both studies drew attention to the importance of careful information-gathering from clients about their drinking during intake or counseling interviews.

1. Basing opinions or decisions about the client's drinking problem should never be done on an answer to a single question, that is, short of the client disclosing a history of alcohol abuse. Instead, this assessment should be done on the basis of clusters of items about drinking practices, effects on health, or personal problems. As a rule, questions should be asked that make clients think about their drinking. Thus, instead of asking, "Do you have a drinking problem?" consider a more open-ended approach, such as, "How about your drinking? What's it been like in the past?"

2. The homeless with alcohol problems are sometimes debilitated owing to the effects of chronic drinking. This debilitation can take its toll on memory recall and accuracy, particularly among older chronic alcoholics. During withdrawal symptoms disorientation and confusion often make the alcoholic an unreliable respondent.

3. About one in every four shelter clients manifests a dual diagnosis of both alcohol abuse and psychiatric disturbance. These cases require special skill and patience. Establishing a strong rapport with the client can be unusually important in these interviews.

4. Many chronic alcoholics are heavy users of social service agencies, and thus they are accustomed to dealing with case managers and counselors. In fact, many are remarkably fluent in the professional terminology for alcohol-related disorders. This can give a false impression that they have insights into their drinking problem. Experience in working with alcoholics also suggests that these insights are oftentimes shallow. As one chronic alcoholic explained, "Talk is cheap when I deal with my social worker!"

nonexistent years ago. It is instructive to review in detail the first step in the recovery process: *detoxification*.

## Detoxification Centers

The initial phase of the recovery process begins with detoxification, which historically has been the local jail or "drunk tank" for most homeless alcoholics. With the passage of the Uniform Alcoholism and Intoxication Treatment Act (the Hughes Act) in 1971, however, an impetus to decriminalize public intoxication statutes and to develop alternatives to incarceration for public inebriates helped to establish detoxification (or detox) centers. These facilities, staffed by qualified medical personnel and sometimes well-trained paraprofessionals, were designed to handle police case inebriates that might otherwise be processed through the criminal justice system. Although the detox center approach is now well-established throughout the United States and Canada, some have observed that these centers constitute nothing more than a new station on the loop for homeless alcoholics (Fagan and Mauss, 1978). A Minnesota study (Neuner and Schultz, 1986), for example, found that virtually every homeless alcoholic in a sample of 43 had multiple admissions to detox centers in a single year, including one man who had accumulated 147 admissions. Data reported in the nationwide Health Care for

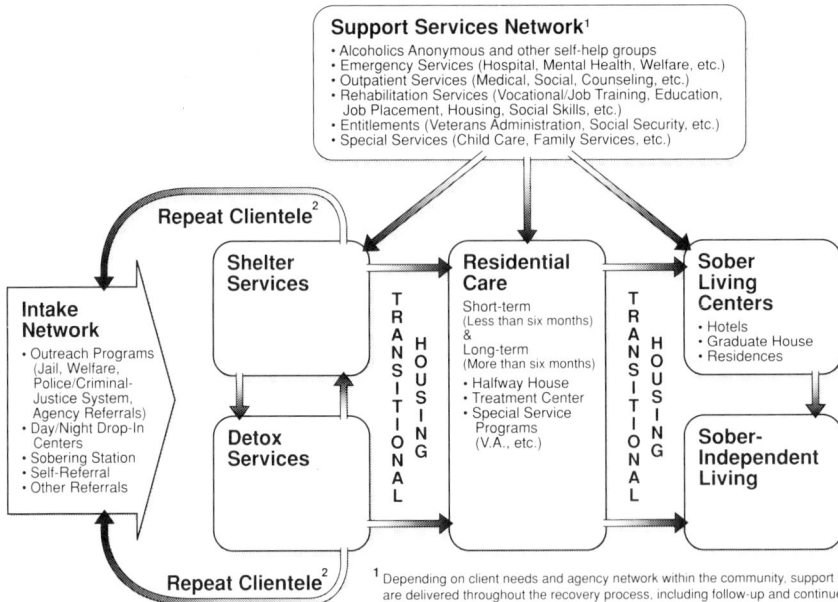

**Figure 1.** Recovery Process for the Homeless with Alcohol and Other Drug Problems

the Homeless project (Wright and Weber, 1987), as well as in other studies (Fagan and Mauss, 1978), confirm that detox now plays a central role in the alcoholism cycle of the homeless derelict. In fact, one project report (Wright, Weber-Burden, & Lam, 1987:3) drew upon a case study of a 39-year-old informant to illustrate a prototypical street alcoholic, in which the subject reported as many as 480 admissions to detox over a 9-year period, exclusive of the visits when he was turned away!

---

*Panel 5–5*

### Networking the Homeless Alcoholic

For many homeless alcoholics, networking public and private agencies can become a way of life. Although shelters, detoxification centers, hospitals, and rehabilitation agencies provide for the alcoholics' basic needs and oftentimes delay their demise because of alcohol-related diseases, they also play a role in sustaining the drinking cycle of the alcoholic.

Just how much time do homeless alcoholics spend in public and private agencies? One study conducted at a social service center on New York's Bowery in the 1970s found that about half of a sample of 57 alcoholic women spent more than 275 days each year in shelters, hospitals, and residential care facilities. "It's what keeps me alive," said one respondent. "The shelter is my home," remarked one 63-year-old alcoholic, "and it is the only way I can have my cake and bottle, too!" (Garrett, 1973).

Neuner and Schultz (1986) reported data on networking of private and public agencies by chronic alcoholics and the estimated cost of providing services. The case of "Nick" illustrates a common pathway for many alcoholics.

| | |
|---|---|
| Hennepin County Detox | 115 days |
| Ramsey County Detox | 69 days |
| Outstate Detoxes | 10 days minimum |
| Court Appearances | 5 days |
| Bell Hill | 13 days |
| Adult Correctional Facility | 49 days |
| Hennepin County Medical Center | 24 days |
| Salvation Army | 1 day |
| Adult Detention Center | 3 days |
| Shelters and/or Drop-ins | 20 days |
| Total | 317 days |

How much did all of these services cost? Of the 43 chronic recidivist alcoholics studied, the estimated total annual cost to the public system exceeded $22,800 per client. The authors concluded that, "based on an estimated population size of four hundred twenty-five active chronic clients, the total expenditure based on these figures is $9,707,829 per annum" (Neuner and Schultz, 1986:22).

*Source:* Adapted from Garrett and Schutt, 1987c.

Despite high recidivism, detox centers preserve a human dignity in the recovery process, however temporary, that is not possible through the jail system. In place of the stigma of criminal confinement, detox facilities offer instead safe places to sober up for those experiencing withdrawal. Even for those who return to their drunkenness cycle (which in some programs is 9 out of every 10 clients), medical services during detox help to delay the onset or progress of alcohol-related diseases.

In addition to detoxification services, these centers also create opportunities for intervention that can lead the alcoholic into long-term recovery. Most detox centers maintain counseling or case management personnel who refer patients to appropriate agencies for long-term recovery. Bill, a 47-year-old recovering alcoholic who was homeless in Boston for 8 years, explains how his tenth detox admission put him on the right track:

> I was on this five-day bender when the police, they brought me to detox. I had a rough time with the withdrawal—bad case of the shakes and everything, couldn't keep food down for two days. By the third day, the counselor, he met with me again and said I could get help if I wanted. I said "maybe," but right then all's I wanted was to get back on my feet again. . . . Well, that night they got me to go to the AA meeting. I was thinkin' donuts and coffee, but not AA. The next day, the counselor and me met again, and said he would really like to see me straighten out my life. I heard that story before and never wanted to deal with it. But now the time was right, I guess. Sometimes it's that way. . . . I stayed in this dormitory a few days—transition lodging, they called it—and a few days later, I got into a program. It ran almost a month, and when I finished it I felt better than I had for 15 years. . . . Anyways, the program hooked me up with a [recovery] house on the South Shore, I got a job, been working steady, been dry for almost three years, and now I'm trying to get my life back together again.

Although Bill's story illustrates how intervention and referral at the detox level can offer a pathway to long-term recovery, it also signals high recidivism rates and the difficulties in connecting homeless clients to other treatment agencies. One study (Finn, 1985), examining referral patterns of some 20 detox programs serving public inebriates, found that 17 centers indicated that only one in four clients accepted referral for continued treatment. The percentage of clients who accepted referrals, however, seemed to vary widely (see Table 1).

The type of care involved in the detoxification process itself as well as the emphasis placed on referral of the client to a second-level treatment depend on the approach used by the detox center.

Table 1.  Referral Patterns of Detox Programs

| Program | Percentage accepting referrals |
| --- | --- |
| St. Louis Harbor Light | 10 |
| CASPAR (Cambridge/Somerville, MA) | 28 |
| Seattle detox | 30 |
| Manhattan Bowery Detox (New York) | 40 |
| DRC/P Philadelphia Detox | 50 |
| Hooper Detox Center (Portland, OR) | 75 |

Sources: Fagan and Mauss (1978); Shandler and Shipley (1987); Wittman and Madden (1988).

## Medical Detoxification

In this approach, detoxification is administered in a medical facility or hospital under the direct supervision of qualified staff, including a physician and a nurse. Most medical detox facilities operate a 3- to 5-day program, which is sufficient to stabilize blood pressure and pulse for the vast majority of patients. The key to this approach is medical management, which involves monitoring vital signs, careful attention to nutrition, close surveillance of withdrawal symptoms, and emergency medical assistance if required. In the medical approach, it is common to administer drugs, such as tranquilizers (the benzodiazepines). This helps to relieve many of the common symptoms of withdrawal, such as sleeplessness, anxiety, and restlessness, as well as some of the physical problems (Mendelson and Mello, 1985).

One advantage of this model is that physical examination of the patient helps to discover alcohol-related diseases that might otherwise go undetected. A disadvantage of this quick withdrawal regimen is that the patient who leaves detox after 3, 4, or 5 days is likely still to be very shaky, with lots of tranquilizers in his body. When the medication leaves his body, it can be difficult to maintain abstinence. A 7- to 10-day detoxification period is likely to lead to better results.

Although the primary emphasis is medical management, most programs also have counseling and alcohol-education components, as well as convenient access for patients to Alcoholics Anonymous (AA) meetings. Oftentimes, medical detox programs are linked to larger rehabilitation organizations for the homeless through a working agreement to take nonpaying patients or "welfare cases," in which the state or city pays a standard fee, regardless of true costs. The Philadelphia Diagnostic and Rehabilitation Center, for example, has a cooperative agreement with several nearby hospitals willing to take homeless clients, as well as access to a state medical assistance program that covers costs (Shandler and Shipley, 1987:55–56). CASPAR, a comprehensive services program in Cambridge-Somerville, Massachusetts, actually operates its own medical detox program, accepting only hospital referrals and police case inebriates (Wittman and Madden, 1988:10). Regardless of organizational arrangements, medical detox programs are costly to operate. Nevertheless, they continue to be the dominant approach used by treatment programs, constituting about two thirds of the detox centers nationwide (NIAAA, 1983).

## Social or Nonmedical Model

Initially developed in Canada during the 1960s (Sadd and Young, 1987), the social model rejects the use of medicine or drugs. In place of medical supervision, this approach substitutes a supportive social environment to help the client endure withdrawal from alcohol. Social detox centers are typically staffed by counselors (many of whom are recovering alcoholics themselves), Emergency Medical Technicians (EMTs), and a nurse. Clients are monitored closely for signs of complications during withdrawal, and their vital signs are taken at periodic intervals. Emergency medical treatment is usually available through an arrangement with a nearby hospital. However, statistics indicate that only about 1 in 20 clients will develop medical complications (Mendelson and Mello, 1985).

Although these facilities are rarely elaborate, consisting of private or semiprivate rooms for patients, a lounge or recreation area, they provide a clean, comfortable environment for waiting out the detoxification process. Clients capable of keeping food down are offered three solid meals, as well as snacks and a generous selection of liquids. The social detox model, however, places emphasis on getting the clients to accept a referral to another treatment agency for follow-up care appropriate to their needs. Thus, counseling plays a major role in the program, and AA meetings are typically required of patients. Because the social model is far less expensive to operate, and because these facilities are often situated in low-income districts, these detox programs are taking on a major role in serving the homeless.

Which of the two models is best? Answers to this question reflect a heated debate among alcoholism treatment professionals. In defense of the medical model, for example, Mendelson and Mello (1985:327) have this to say: "It is regrettable that for a time, custodial care at bargain rates may again replace effective medical treatment of alcohol withdrawal." Sadd (1985:15), on the other hand, who completed a comparative study of medical and nonmedical detoxification services in New York, concluded that: "for the majority of the public inebriates in our sample, non-medical detoxification is as safe as medical detoxification."

### Sobering-Up Stations

These facilities are a cross between social detox and drop-in centers. Usually situated in or near districts with high concentrations of public inebriates, this outpatient approach provides a safe and supervised place to regain complete or partial sobriety. Usually staffed with an EMT or nurse, and case managers/counselors, these facilities offer minimal services. Beds, showers, and meals are not provided. Coffee and snacks, however, are usually free for the asking. In some sobering-up stations, security rooms or holding cells are available to handle potentially violent or involuntary clients. Virtually all of the clientele are walk-in or police case inebriates, who stay for a few hours to as long as 7 or 8 hours, depending on their mood or level of intoxication.

Although sobering stations might be called "halfway measures," they contribute nonetheless to the support services available to the homeless with alcoholic problems. At the very least, they get derelicts off the streets, free from victimization or exposure to the elements, and they provide still another intercept point where some can be successfully referred for follow-up care. At the same time, they divert the homeless alcoholic from the criminal justice system.

## RECOVERY AND REHABILITATION SERVICES

The delivery of services to the homeless has never been a simple task for a number of reasons. First, almost every client has multiple needs that begin with financial assistance, affordable housing, and food. This picture is even more complicated for the 40 percent who require treatment services for a drinking problem, many of whom also suffer from serious physical and psychiatric disorders. Second, by their very nature, the homeless are mobile and unstable in their residential habits, which makes the planning of treatment and recovery programs a difficult process (Breakey, 1987). Simple medical advice, such as "take two aspirin, go to bed, and get plenty of rest," is more difficult to follow for homeless clients. Third, homeless clients often resist becoming involved in treatment services, partly out of fear of what to expect and partly because they have a mistrust of many service providers (Breakey, 1987). Wiseman's (1970:240–241) study of skid row alcoholics, for example, concluded that most homeless alcoholics want to be "cured of alcoholism" and to seek out needed social and medical services, yet there is often a distrust even a hostility toward their benefactors that prevents them from doing so.

Although these and other factors create obstacles in planning and delivery of services, the vast increase in the numbers of homeless in this decade have also brought about renewed determination and creative solutions to serving the needs of the homeless, and especially those with alcohol problems. The starting point, however, rests with devising strategies that will funnel clients into the service network.

## Outreach Services

The successful delivery of services to the homeless with alcohol problems depends on locating clients in need of those services. Historically, many agencies, however well-intentioned, have taken a relatively passive approach to attracting clientele. Placing service institutions in areas of high concentrations of public inebriates, such as skid row districts, offers visibility and easy access, yet fails to overcome the mistrust of service providers and the inertia for seeking help that are barriers for many homeless alcoholics. One early exception is the Salvation Army, who have since the turn of the century taken aggressive measures to rescue drunkards, such as New York's "Boozer's Day patrol" that combed lower Manhattan on Thanksgiving and other holidays looking for public inebriates (Stoil, 1987).

Today inventive outreach strategies are far more common. In fact, even agencies with a passive approach to outreach have taken on a new look. Drop-in centers, which have always been a part of the service network on skid row, act as a catchment area for referring clients to detox, shelter, and medical services. In Boston, for example, a Night Center was implemented in 1987 near the downtown district close to the habitat of many street alcoholics. Although it functions like most drop-in centers, its operating hours, from 7 P.M. to 7 A.M., are keyed to times when most homeless alcoholics are vulnerable to victimization and, during cold months, hazardous weather. Staffed with a director, counselors and a nurse, the Night Center makes referrals for emergency shelter, detox and medical services in cooperation with local shelters and the Boston City Hospital. Van service provides immediate transport of referrals to their destinations.

Many agencies, however, utilize aggressive outreach programs. In the 1960s, the Manhattan Bowery Project, precursor to the Manhattan Bowery Corporation (MBC), pioneered outreach teams. Today, Mobile Outreach Teams patrol New York's streets in vans contacting homeless people in need of help. Team members

---

*Panel 5–6*

## Police Responses to the Homeless Alcoholic

Although detoxification centers have removed some of the strain public inebriates place on the criminal justice system, police still must deal firsthand with drunks found in doorways, in parks, or on the streets. Moreover, one recent National Institute of Justice study (Finn, 1985) found that restrictive admission policies at many detox or shelter facilities and limited bed space oftentimes make it difficult for police to sustain a cooperative relationship with community agencies that are serving the homeless and/or the alcoholics. In fact, jail lock-up, however inhumane, is sometimes the only place available.

One approach for solving this dilemma has been for police and sheriff departments to form a network or coalition with service agencies so that the two function as a team. Here is how it works:

1. Law enforcement and community agencies, such as detox centers, shelters for the homeless, mental health organizations, City or County Emergency Medical Assistance organizations, initiate meetings so that each agency understands the role of the other agencies in serving target groups (e.g., public inebriate, homeless, or mentally ill). Collectively, these representatives try to develop an integrated or team approach that will enhance services to target groups, and simultaneously solve organizational problems. Thus, for the police, the problem is how to divert public inebriates from the criminal justice system; for the detox center, the issue comes to be how to funnel public inebriates into detoxification services. In Los Angeles, for example, a task force was set up comprising even the District Attorney's Office, the Fire Department, and the Superior Court. The important point is that representatives carry the power to commit their organization to implementation of the resulting agreement (Finn and Sullivan, 1988). Civil statutes can play a major role in both facilitating or hampering the development of these networks. It is important, therefore, that all parties understand what existing laws will permit or require.

2. Written agreements on the roles and responsibilities of each relevant organization are drawn up. This tends to avoid misunderstandings and to assure that the police and community agencies are careful to commit only those services that they are truly prepared to offer. Some organizations even provide written instructions and policies to their staff. Thus, the Washtenaw County (Michigan) Sheriff's Department prepared instructions on how to handle

---

are trained in using skills to establish trust and rapport with the homeless on the street, as well as in needs assessment and case management. Their mission is to bring homeless individuals to essential services, such as detox, emergency shelter, or medical services. The Midtown Outreach Program, which includes psychiatrists, nurses, and social workers, actually brings social and health services to homeless men and women in shelters or where they live on the streets. Services are delivered by two types of teams: street workers and mobile psychiatric outreach teams (U.S. Conference of Mayors, 1987). Evidence of MBC's success is seen in the number of contacts who reject help. Of the 7,700 Bowery men, for example, who

*Panel 5–6* (Continued)

persons requiring psychiatric services (Finn and Sullivan, 1988).

3. Programs for continued evaluation of the network should be worked out to help sustain cooperation, to ascertain problems that were unanticipated in the original agreement, and especially to document the value of the network. Thus, in Montgomery County, Pennsylvania, where a Mental Health Emergency Ambulance was implemented, it was found that the network saved police 218 hours in just 1 month (Finn and Sullivan, 1988).

4. Cross-training approaches help to promote better communication within police-agency networks, as well as improve skills in handling target groups by both police and agency staff.

In Oregon, police academy classes make visits to the Hooper Detox Center in Portland to observe operations (Newton and Duffy, 1987). Social workers train police and police train social workers in handling the homeless and inebriated in Madison, Wisconsin. In San Diego, courses at the regional police academy train cadets on how to use the County's Inebriate Reception Center (Finn and Sullivan, 1988).

Finally, two examples illustrate how network agreements can serve the homeless. San Diego County contracts out the operation of its Inebriate Reception Center, which has a capacity to serve up to 80 clients. San Diego Police are required to transport all public inebriates to the Center. Most of the 25,000 police referrals are homeless. Usually, police spend not more than 7 minutes, on the average, to negotiate the Center, as opposed to approximately 1 hour it would take to book the case for jailing (Finn and Sullivan, 1988). At the same time, this arrangement has enhanced the Center's outreach efforts.

In Boston a similar network has been implemented, involving the city's largest shelter, the Pine Street Inn. Although the shelter is privately operated, police are instructed to bring the homeless and public inebriate to Pine Street at any hour of the night. A precinct captain keeps officers abreast of guests who have been barred by Pine Street because of a past history of violence or psychiatric problems. The Department of Welfare pays for an off-duty police officer to work at Pine Street, which helps keep order in the shelter and prevents inappropriate referrals. As one patrolman explains it, "this has made our life a lot easier. Everybody wins—the police and court system, Pine Street, and most of all, the homeless." A staff member at Pine Street agrees: "We have a good working relationship with the Boston Police, which helps our efforts at outreach."

were contacted during a recent year, only 3,000 refused to accept any help whatsoever (Wittman and Madden, 1988:36).

A somewhat different strategy is used by New York's Women in Need Alcoholism Outpatient Clinic (WIN), which is a comprehensive treatment program that was implemented in 1987. Substantial numbers of disaffiliated or marginally homeless women are known to reside in lower and midtown Manhattan "welfare hotels" (Bahr and Garrett, 1971, 1976), about one-fifth of whom have serious drinking problems (Garrett and Bahr, 1976). Thus, WIN's outreach efforts include repeated visits to hotel lobbies, as well as to other locations (public parks, detox and

*Panel 5–7*

**Case Managers and Counselors Can Make a Difference**

Case managers and counselors experienced in working with alcoholics are usually realistic about how their clients use the social services system. A caseworker serving homeless women in New York City's Department of Social Services says she is always nervous about connecting clients with a referral: "Getting the client, especially the alcoholic, to accept referral services is hard enough. Getting them to go to the services is something else again." A Boston counselor at a detox center agrees, but adds, "the sad part is that when I am successful in getting the patient interested in a referral program, the waiting period is so long that many tire out and return to the streets and, in case you didn't guess, back to drinking." And, in Seattle, a worker in the Department of Social and Health Services complains that "the bureaucracy can be a killer at times. The homeless can get caught up in paperwork, waiting periods, evaluation of eligibility. . . . It makes it hard to work with homeless clients, especially those with a health or drinking problem. Sometimes they just disappear."

These types of client problems are common in the delivery of services to the homeless, and especially those with alcohol problems. Several studies (Garrett and Schutt, 1986; Schutt and Garrett, 1988; Wright et al., 1987) indicated that although

alcoholics rank high on service utilization patterns, such as shelters and detox centers, they are also unreliable when it comes to keeping appointments and following-through on referrals (Schutt and Garrett, 1988). For example, at Cornhusker Place, a comprehensive agency serving predominantly homeless alcoholics in Nebraska, an estimated 40 percent of postdetox patients do not follow-up on referrals (Wittman and Madden, 1988:17).

Although the problem of client attrition can reflect problems in the design of delivery systems in the organization itself, there are details that case managers, counselors, and other staff members can monitor or oversee that will make a difference in successfully linking the alcoholic with needed services. Here are a few points that should be kept in mind:

1. Negotiating a referral with a client requires more than providing the agency's name and address, and then leaving to chance that the client will connect with the agency. Two principal reasons for client attrition or drop-out are: the client's needs and agency services do not match, and the agency and client fail to connect (Mandell and Schram, 1985). Thus, it is important that the worker assess the needs of the client carefully, as well as obtain accurate information about the agency (Garrett and

rehabilitation units) where women can be contacted. Counselor teams speak with women about substance abuse problems and try to link them into WIN's rehabilitation services (Wittman and Madden, 1988:80–85).

Other outreach efforts show similar ingenuity. In Boston, for example, outreach services are comprised of both private and city units. Mobile lunch wagons circulate through districts where the homeless spend daylight hours, serving coffee, soft drinks, and nourishing meals on the streets. Both the city and the Pine Street Inn operate mobile vans that pick up willing clientele for transport to detox,

---

*Panel 5–7*   (Continued)

Schutt, 1987a, b). This also enables the worker to help structure client expectations about the next level of treatment or service, as well as to alleviate underlying anxiety and apprehension.

2. Provide the client with a write-up of the referral, including details, directions, and especially a contact person in the referral agency. Sometimes this personal connection can be made during a session with the client, which helps to cement a bridge between the client and the agency prior to arrival.

3. No less important is to make certain the client leaves with all the required documents necessary for intake at the referral agency. "The bureaucracy can be a killer at times," as one observer comments, and nothing can be more disheartening for the client than to be rejected or delayed at intake because of missing paperwork. In one instance, a New York study (Garrett, 1970) traced a homeless alcoholic woman through a series of referrals over a year-long period. Not once was a successful connection made, that is, except with the police when she was arrested, and with the hospital following a suicide attempt.

4. Transportation arrangements are crucial, especially with an alcoholic client. Experienced personnel in detox centers, for example, know how important trans-

portation service is in moving the client to a program for extended care, since sober alcoholics suffer a "postdetox" syndrome that makes them edgy and nervous. This makes them highly vulnerable for a relapse. Many organizations, however, maintain a van or shuttle service to move clients to other agencies. This also offers a double bonus, because the driver can serve as an advocate in place of the case manager that provides social support to the client at intake.

5. Finally, always make it a point to follow-up with the referral agency after the client intake is completed. This can provide valuable feedback information for future referrals, as well as work out any unanticipated barriers with the present client (Mandell and Schram, 1985).

Recovery programs that offer comprehensive services for the homeless with alcohol problems are much less likely to have difficulties in moving clients to other programmatic services within their own organization. On the other hand, most agencies do not enjoy this luxury and must instead utilize services through networking arrangements. In either event, it is important to remember that case managers or personnel involved in direct services can themselves make a difference in successfully linking clients to a referral.

---

shelter, or medical services. At Bridge Over Troubled Waters, which serves homeless and runaway teenagers (many of whom have substance abuse problems), outreach workers are deployed in a "mobile clinic" to try to link clients into needed services.

In Santa Monica, California, a coalition approach to outreach was developed in 1986, consisting of four teams from different agencies. Teams specialize in a service area: case management and advocacy for the homeless with substance abuse or psychiatric problems; mental health services; and medical care for all homeless individuals. All teams are mobile, visiting appropriate sites, such as jails, hospitals, or other agencies that will provide contact with prospective clientele. Team members work with clients to link them to services, and follow-up case management is made for an extended period (U.S. Conference of Mayors, 1987: 31–34).

This brief survey is only illustrative of the types of outreach services that are possible. In general, however, it should be said that successful outreach efforts depend in part on knowing the target clientele. This includes an understanding at different levels: profiles of their service needs, their habitats, the community institutions they frequent, and even the subculture that influences their lives. The population of homeless alcoholics is a puzzle of many parts. Although they are more diverse than they were in decades past, their lifestyles and drinking patterns, as well as their social relationships, are rooted in a subculture that is to some extent different from that of other homeless clients.

## Comprehensive Services

The multiple needs of almost all homeless clients require a variety of short- and long-term services. Yet, although alcoholic and psychiatric disorders represent critical needs for as many as three out of every four homeless clients seen at shelters (Garrett and Schutt, 1986), the homeless themselves rank other requirements, such as housing, entitlements, jobs, or food well ahead of their perceived need for alcohol or psychiatric services (Ball and Havassy, 1984). Thus, participation in treatment programs is unlikely unless these basic needs are fulfilled (Breakey, 1987).

Comprehensive programs contain multiple components that serve the basic needs of the homeless, including vocational training, education, employment or job placement, and preparation for independent living. At the same time, clients are linked into services for alcohol or psychiatric treatment. There are two principal approaches: full-service and coalition or cooperative agreements.

### Full-Service Agencies

Comprehensive services can be offered within a single or autonomous program or through interrelated components of a larger parent organization. For example, Detroit's Mariner Inn provides virtually all of its services on an in-house basis, including support for basic needs and a 4-step recovery program. Clients are given help in planning for independent living arrangements and are linked into jobs. On the other hand, efficient delivery of services can also be achieved by individual programs in a larger organization (Wittman and Madden, 1988). For example, in Massachusetts, CASPAR contains a medical detox facility, emergency shelter care, outpatient clinical services at Cambridge Hospital, a drop-in center, half-way house facilities that include treatment services for both men and women, and a graduate house offering transitional, independent living for those leaving recovery houses.

Full-service organizations have important advantages. Moving clients through the recovery system is uncomplicated and usually free of bureaucracy. Case management is often made easier, since services remain under the same organizational umbrella. In this type of setting, communication among staff members on clients and services is easily facilitated, which helps to improve overall organizational effectiveness. On the other hand, these agencies are very costly to operate, more complex to staff, and require leadership skilled in human and health services management.

## Coalition Approach

Comprehensive services for the homeless with alcohol problems can also be achieved through coalitions of independent agencies, both public and private. Different arrangements are possible. For example, in Multnomah County, Oregon, the Public Inebriate Service Network integrates state, county, city, and private agency funds to provide programs for inebriates in Portland's downtown area. Services include a detox and sobering-up centers, residential treatment centers, an alcohol-free housing program, and a special program for Native Americans with alcohol problems (Wittman and Madden, 1988). This approach is also unique in that the network plays an advocacy role in lobbying for ordinances and legislation to support its programs. The Task Force on Public Alcoholism, for example, brought about a ban on sales of fortified wine in the downtown Portland area, which had the effect of dispersing public inebriates from this area.

Coalitions or cooperative agreements can also exist on a smaller scale. At Boston's privately operated St. Francis House, where about half of the clientele have alcohol and substance abuse problems, a state-funded team of mental health professionals visits the facility four times weekly to coordinate psychiatric care. At the same time, medical services at St. Francis is operated by a team funded by the Johnson/Pew Health Care for the Homeless Program. Case managers at St. Francis perform a follow-up on their clients who are being served at other agencies.

The principal advantage of the coalition approach are, first, that quality services can be offered system-wide that are rarely possible within a single agency. Teams of physicians, psychiatrists, nurses, and social workers are costly to staff, yet under coalition arrangements offer a breadth of professional services that few single agencies enjoy. Second, coalitions can strengthen the internal effectiveness of other agencies within the network. Again, St. Francis House is a case in point. The addition of medical and mental health teams makes it possible to achieve greater success with alcoholic clients. Moreover, interagency coalitions can help to widen the clientele served by some agencies, which can enhance their evaluation profile and oftentimes improve financial support. A third, though less obvious advantage, is that the coalition approach engages a community of services, not just a single organization. This is best illustrated in the Portland approach. Thus, coalitions can broaden the base of citizen, and especially political and professional, support for alcoholism treatment and prevention services, both for the homeless and the community at large.

The risks, however, are obvious. Coalition agreements must be worked out in detail, and even then failure of a single agency can jeopardize an entire network.

---

*Panel 5–8*

### The Salvation Army Harbor Light:
### A Model Program Serving the Homeless with Alcohol Problems

Many agencies serving homeless clients with alcohol problems have received national recognition for their exceptional comprehensive programs. Among the most known are Philadelphia's Diagnostic and Rehabilitation Center, the Manhattan Bowery Corporation (New York), the Cambridge-Somerville Program for Alcoholism Rehabilitation or CASPAR (metropolitan Boston), and the Public Inebriate Services network (Portland, Oregon). Yet there is probably no organization that can match the long tradition of dedication and service provided by the Salvation Army, which has its origins in the United States in the 1880s. Recognizing that the public inebriation-jail cycle offers no hope of returning alcoholics to permanent sobriety nor does it offer pathways to physical and spiritual recovery, the Salvation Army founded community centers that provide rehabilitation services. Today, it operates more than 150 facilities nationwide (Stoil, 1987).

During the 1940s, the Salvation Army introduced its Harbor Light centers, which are comprehensive rehabilitation programs specifically designed for the needs of homeless alcoholics. This network now includes 31 centers (Stoil, 1987). Recently, a NIAAA-sponsored national survey, directed by Friedner Wittman, singled out the Harbor Light network as among 15 exemplary programs serving the homeless with alcohol problems (Wittman and Madden, 1988). Harbor Light in St. Louis illustrates the comprehensive approach to alcohol/drug-treatment recovery.

Four levels of recovery are provided at the St. Louis Harbor Light. Level I consists of a 30-bed detoxification unit that accepts walk-in and referral patients, including police case inebriates and referrals from two vans that cruise the skid row district of St. Louis. A staff of 11 aides, all recovering alcoholics, is supervised by an RN or a licensed vocational nurse (LVN), and medical backup is provided by a nearby hospital. About one in five detox patients ac-

---

Cutbacks in state or municipal funding in detox facilities, for example, can cripple the flow of clients into other treatment services, or impair the efficiency of the network. In other instances, organizational changes, such as those in leadership or in the institutional mission in one or more agencies in the network, can have a major impact on service delivery.

## Components of the Recovery Process

Recovery programs for the homeless with alcohol problems utilize a variety of service components. Program designs differ, of course, according to a number of circumstances: treatment philosophy and objectives, funding support and assets, staffing situation, variations in target clientele, and other factors unique to the community setting. Nevertheless, it is instructive to review some of the common components in recovery programs.

---

*Panel 5–8*  (Continued)

cepts assistance in Level II or a collateral service.

The second level is a 28-day residential program serving up to 44 men and women and staffed with a clinical director and three counselors. Some 50 hours of programs cycle residents through courses on daily living skills, meetings, and both group and individual counseling sessions. The goal of this program is to remotivate clients to engage in independent living and to acquire sills needed for self-sufficiency. Approximately two of every three clients complete Level II programming.

Level II engages clients in job-seeking and locating safe, alcohol-free housing. Two full-time counselors search for suitable jobs and appropriate housing. The program has required activities, including attendance at AA meetings. Most Level III participants live at the Harbor Light facility (averaging about 30 days), and about three of every four are successful in locating both a job and permanent housing.

The final level, open to those who did not locate either a job or permanent housing, is a residential hotel offering alcohol/drug-free living to 185 men and women (not all of whom have been homeless). Rent varies from $170 to $360 monthly, including meals. Although strictly enforced house policies govern residents, there are no organized programs, except for weekly AA meetings and spiritual classes. Average stay at the hotel is from 4 to 6 months. The residence is operated without any public funding.

St. Louis Harbor Light also offers other programs, such as emergency shelter and drop-in services, a hold-over program for chronic alcoholics (who complete detox, but do not enter Level II), facilities for elderly pensioners, and more. But, like other recovery programs with comprehensive services, Harbor Light's physical plant is hard-pressed to serve clients drawn from St. Louis's estimated 10,000 homeless, about 40 percent of whom are estimated to have drinking problems.

*Source*: Adapted from Wittman and Madden, 1988:57–62.

---

## Residential Care

Although shelters play a crucial role in the service network for the homeless, their primary contribution is temporary housing, emergency services, and screening clients for referrals. Clients who are chronic alcoholics almost always require primary care in residential facilities. In fact, because alcoholics are oftentimes physically and psychologically debilitated, their length of residence in recovery programs is usually longer than with other types of clients, ranging from 3 to 6 months or longer. Although programs differ in their approach to primary care (e.g., group and individual counseling, spiritual recovery, AA, etc.), the recovery process is sometimes tiered into a series of steps or phases. Some examples illustrate how this operates.

At Nebraska's Cornhusker Place, residents in the extended care program go through four phases over approximately a 6-month period. The first phase involves evaluation, developing a treatment plan, counseling, and attendance at AA meet-

*Panel 5–9*

## A Handbook for the Homeless Alcoholic in Treatment

Many organizations serving the homeless develop brochures and flyers that provide general details about their program, which are useful in advertising services to potential clients, referral agencies, and to the general public. But S.T.A.I.R., a comprehensive recovery program in Boston serving primarily homeless alcoholics, has developed a handbook on alcoholism and health specifically for their clientele. Authored by Suzanne Gunston, S.T.A.I.R.'s Nursing Coordinator, and funded locally through the John Hancock Mutual Life Insurance Company, the handbook covers a variety of topics that are especially relevant to the homeless alcoholic: How alcohol affects body organs; alcohol and infection; nutrition; lifestyle problems, such as exposure, lice, scabies, ringworm; detox and withdrawal syndrome; and how to obtain health care if you are homeless.

The section on nutrition and alcoholism is illustrative of the approach taken in the handbook (Gunston, 1988:5):

Malnutrition is one of the most common [among the] several complications of alcoholism. Often when a person is drinking he has loss of appetite, nausea, vomiting, diarrhea or he may simply forget to eat. When a person is homeless, food may not be available to him at a time when he might feel like eating. Poor nutrition contributes to problems with proper functioning of almost all body functions.

It is important for those who drink and for those who are in recovery to understand that improved nutrition is one of the most important parts of recovery. Improved nutrition is within the reach of almost every one who is willing to follow a few simple rules:

1. Try to eat breakfast. Breakfast foods are most often high in thiamine (cereals, breads).
2. Try to eat three meals daily. This will provide a variety of food nutrients. Soup kitchens are available to serve three meals daily to the homeless. (Weekly schedules of soup kitchens in the Boston area [are] appended.)
3. Keep in mind that foods which are high in thiamine are very important. These foods include green leafy vegetables, broccoli, breads and cereals, nuts (including peanut butter) and pork. A diet providing a variety of foods usually will include enough thiamine.
4. Drink an adequate amount of nonalcoholic fluids. This will prevent dehydration.
5. Do not eat food which is old or discarded. This may result in infection or "food poisoning."
6. Although vitamin supplements may be helpful, it is more important to begin improving eating habits.

S.T.A.I.R. reports that clients do in fact read the handbook, and that they often question staff about some its comments. "It provides clients with concrete guidelines about how they can help themselves, both during treatment and once they leave S.T.A.I.R., and it helps to orient the patient to our program," explains the author.

Although the handbook is a small part of the overall details of a recovery program for the homeless alcoholic, it is one that is worth trying. Since production costs are modest, it is sometimes easy to locate funding in the private sector, such as local businesses or community groups. This, too, has a payoff, since it broadens the base of community support for services to the homeless.

ings. A second phase provides for medical and physical examinations, and the final two phases stress independent living skills and preparation for reentry into the community. A similar sequence is used at Detroit's Mariner Inn: (1) basic intake services; (2) medical examination, therapy, and alcohol education; (3) education and work skills; and (4) employment and preparation for alcohol-free, independent living (Wittman and Madden, 1988).

Half-way houses, which are usually situated in neighborhood settings, provide a similar type of program. Although these facilities can take various forms, they involve group living circumstances where house residents continue their commitment to sobriety through AA, group, and individual counseling programs. At the same time, residents are able to restore a sense of independent living and community life through outside activities, such as jobs, volunteer work, recreation, and other activities.

In New York's Women in Need program, an outpatient clinic approach is used to provide treatment services to clients who either live in their own apartments or in housing provided by the program. Different types of housing are available. These include residential houses with accommodations for families, a dormitory-style facility for emergency sheltering, a building with studio units, and transitional apartments for women who are about to move to permanent housing. At the same time, residents become involved in WIN's Alcoholism Outpatient Clinic (Wittman, 1987).

### Alcohol-Free Living Centers

Long-term housing is as crucial to the recovery process as treatment itself. However, most early efforts at rehabilitating homeless alcoholics failed to link clients to long-term housing opportunities. At best, recovering alcoholics could look forward to locating an affordable single-room occupancy (SRO) hotel on or near skid row, which left them vulnerable to relapse and eventually to repeat the alcoholism-homelessness cycle.

Alcohol-free living centers (AFLC) constitute a relatively new approach in the network of recovery services for homeless alcoholics. Although usually operated by larger agencies offering comprehensive services, AFLCs provide low-cost rental units in an alcohol-free environment. Other than AA and house meetings, AFLCs do not usually sponsor in-house programs. Some residents, however, may be involved in outside programs, such as outpatient clinics or support services, depending on their personal needs.

Both the philosophy governing the operations and the living arrangements vary by program. A 1986 NIAAA-sponsored study in California found that facilities range from small, single-family homes in urban and suburban settings to larger hotel operations, such as San Francisco's Arlington Hotel, which offers alcohol-free SROs (see Chapter 8). The number of residents in AFLCs ranged from 6 to as high as 174 (Korenbaum & Burney, 1987). Residency periods vary by house member, some staying less than a year and others up to 3 years or more. Some operations include residency limits; others do not.

Wittman and Madden's (1988) national survey of recovery programs spotlights

---

*Panel 5–10*

## House Rules for Alcohol-Free Living Centers

There are many issues that need resolution during the planning stages of an alcohol-free living center. Who is the target population? How will they be selected? How long can they remain residents? What support service should be offered? How will the housing be financed?

For residents, however, day-to-day living is governed by rules that represent mandates for continued occupancy. Although each house can take on its own "personality" and unique dimension, there are rules that are common in many alcohol-free living centers:

1. Total abstinence from alcohol and drugs is required of residents both on and off the premises. Violation of this rule is grounds for immediate eviction.
2. Guests and visitors of residents are not permitted to bring in or to consume alcohol or drugs on the premises.
3. All residents must participant in household duties and upkeep as determined by the house manager and/or group consensus.
4. Each resident is expected to pay rent promptly. Delinquent rent can be grounds for eviction. However, a resident will not be forced to vacate because of temporary hardship; each such case will be considered separately.
5. Vandalism, destruction of house property, theft, verbal, or physical abuse will not be tolerated; a violation is grounds for eviction.
6. Residents are expected to respect the rights of others and to abide by reasonable standards of conduct that do not unnecessarily disturb others.

*Source*: Adapted in part from Korenbaum and Burney, 1987.

---

some innovative approaches to alcohol-free housing. For example, Oxford House, Inc., organized in 1976 in the District of Columbia, represents a self-help approach to establishing AFLCs (see Chapter 8). The Sullivan Lodging House Realty Trust, a program of Boston's Pine Street Inn, charges rents in its three AFLCs, but funds used to acquire housing are secured from a combination of donations by private individuals, corporations and businesses, and community organizations, as well as public funds. Shelter administrative staff play an active role in managing the AFLCs.

### Support Services

Throughout every phase of the recovery process, support services to the alcoholic can make an important contribution to sustaining sobriety and returning to independent living. This is especially true of the homeless, who often require follow-up medical treatment, vocational and educational programs, and revitalization of social and living skills.

Service agencies for the homeless now give major attention to these needs, either by providing in-house programs or through linkages to public or private agencies. Vocational training and work experience are especially emphasized. For example, the Manhattan Bowery Corporation's Project Renewal begins with an intensive orientation period about work, family, and independent living skills, followed by participation in MBC's work projects. Arrangements can also be made for work in housing rehabilitation projects and in community or neighborhood jobs. Participants benefit from a "paycheck" approach to therapy, and some remain with MBC as members of their organization.

In Maine, the York County Alcoholism Shelter operates a certified bakery and institutional cooking vocational training program, where shelter trainees learn the trade, including handling customers' delivery of products to local businesses. Profits benefit the shelter, which also operates maintenance and building trades vocational programs (Wittman & Madden, 1988).

In the Work Experience Program at Boston's Long Island Shelter, some guests from the shelter enter a vocational rehabilitation program that includes jobs that support the shelter operation. Housing is on a live-in basis, and participants work as counselors and in operational services (food preparation, housekeeping, etc.). Participants also receive support services that help prepare them for independent living, reliable work habits, and sustained sobriety.

At Detroit's Mariner Inn, recovering alcoholics receive both vocational and educational services. Thus, in addition to work experience, some residents are offered high school classes and others are encouraged to pursue college study. The underlying philosophy is that basic skills are essential to solid job performance and advancement, as well as to personal living skills and habits.


## CONCLUSIONS

Research studies and practical experience with service delivery have now built an enormous knowledge base about the homeless with alcohol problems. It is clear that the composition of this population has become more diverse in the past two decades, that their health and personal problems are more complex than ever, and that their numbers continue to increase. At the same time, services for the homeless and attention to those with alcohol problems have also improved over this same period. Detox centers now divert many public inebriates from the criminal justice system; aggressive outreach strategies have improved efforts to bring clients to needed services or to bring services to clients; a broad network of primary recovery programs for the homeless is in operation; and service approaches to rehabilitating the homeless alcoholic now address housing strategies, job training and work experience, and other support services that contribute to sustaining sobriety and reintegrating the alcoholic into a stable lifestyle.

Although this network of services requires expansion to meet the needs of a

*Panel 5–11*

## Where Do I Go From Here?

Everybody who works along Canal Street seems to know Minnie. "She walks up and down the street to the bridge and back at all times of the day and night," said a Chinese businessman who runs a corner convenience store. "She'll stop in a doorway to have a hit of her pint along the way, rest a minute, then she's on her way with her sacks and cart. But, she's harmless—she hurts nobody," explained a bank clerk who occasionally gives Minnie his spare change.

Minnie is one of New York's countless homeless alcoholics, who cycle in and out of emergency shelters when street life takes a turn for the worse. "I get by," she says defiantly. "I go to the shelter only when I have to, for a shower, a night's sleep in a bed, but I don't like being around all those women. And those rules . . . and those social workers. . . ."

Minnie's problems began when her husband, Vern, was killed in the Korean War. "We was never married actually," she admits, "but we was the next closest thing. My Vern never came home to me and I've been lost without him." Her last job, among a dozen she has held in 10 years, was a waitress in an all-night diner in lower Manhattan during the 1960s. She explains her life as a fall from the "good life":

"I've had it all taken from me. Lost it all. We was comfortable, my Vern and me—good job, nice apartment, a good life. But Vern never returned . . . and what was I to do. I never worked before, I had no family here. I got to drinkin' in those days. It helped me feel good, but I never did hold a job for long. The bottle and me, we'd lose the job within a month."

Now 64, Minnie has lived on the streets for nearly 15 years, spending nights in abandoned buildings and warehouses, endless days in the subways, and occasional nights at New York's Port Authority Building. In warm weather, she fashions a shanty from cardboard and produce boxes she collects in Chinatown and retreats to a private spot she knows near the Manhattan Bridge. "I'm real comfortable and I like my privacy. I get me a pint and I sleep like a baby." She admits openly that her life revolves around her drinking. "People are good to me—they give me money, they buy me drinks, and that keeps me going."

But Minnie has also spent much of the last 10 years in hospitals. This year she was hospitalized four times, twice for complications that are due to liver disease and once for injuries she suffered from falling on the street. The fourth is the worst of all. She was hit by a truck as she was crossing Canal Street. Doctors say she may not walk again. And now Minnie asks, "Where do I go from here?"

---

diverse clientele, future efforts must also address solidifying political and economic commitments at the local, state, and federal levels. Housing remains a crucial issue for the recovering alcoholics, as with other types of homeless people, lest they repeat the homelessness-alcoholism cycle. Emphasis on vocational training and job placement is no less important, since continued sobriety and a stable lifestyle depend on the ability of the recovering alcoholic to be self-supporting.

# 6

# Homeless People with Drug Problems

Although alcohol abuse remains as the nation's number one drug problem, public concern over the abuse of other drugs—marijuana, heroin, cocaine, and more recently "crack"—has been far more intense over the past two decades. Media stories that focus on the link between drugs and crime, the gang violence associated with narcotics trafficking, the health risks of drug use, or the epidemic of "crack babies" among others offer convincing evidence that drugs and drug abuse destroy individual lives and families and cost the American economy billions of dollars.

## INTRODUCTION

America's homeless, though often stereotyped as textbook alcoholics, have not been spared as victims of the drug epidemic. Many of the so-called new homeless have cycled through the permissive drug culture intrinsic to street life in inner cities. As a homeless teenager who "belongs among the street people" of Hollywood Boulevard in Los Angeles explains it, "Drugs are what happens to kids when they come here . . . and you just get involved." For others, drug abuse functions as an antecedent of homelessness, contributing to the person's inability to cope with the general environment. "We see homeless men who are classic examples of a 'fall from grace,'" as one Boston detox counselor commented. "Married, good job, and a home—they lost it all to their habit, to drugs."

Since drug abuse also affects substantial numbers of homeless people, this chapter will address (1) the nature and extent of the drug problem among the homeless; (2) provide an overview of basic information about drugs relevant to service providers; and (3) outline health factors that are related to drug use, especially the crisis of AIDS.

## PREVALENCE OF DRUG ABUSE

Evidence on the prevalence of drug abuse among the homeless is not nearly as extensive as findings on alcohol abuse (Milburn, 1990). One reason for this is that many studies combine alcohol and other drugs into the category of "substance abuse." Although substance abuse is a commonly used term for chemical abuse or dependency, lumping both alcohol and drug abusers into a single category precludes making distinctions between these two groups. This is particularly unfortunate, since there are oftentimes social and clinical differences between alcohol and other drug abusers that both researchers as well as service providers need to understand.

Available estimates of the prevalence of drug problems among the homeless vary widely. For example, studying a nationwide sample of homeless subjects in the Health Care for the Homeless program, Wright and Weber (1987) reported that 10 percent—about 1 in 10—reported a history of illicit drug use. Similar results are reported in Los Angeles (Farr et al., 1986) and Oregon (Multnomah County Social Services Division, 1984). Other estimates are well above this figure. For example, Robertson, Koegel, and Ferguson (1989) estimated that one in five homeless teenagers in Hollywood were drug abusers. Even higher estimates are reported in Boston (Mulkern and Spence, 1984b), San Diego (Wynne, 1984), and New York City (Division of Substance Abuse, 1983). All told, summaries of these studies by Fischer (1989) and Milburn (1990) suggest that estimates of drug use among the homeless range from as low as 3 percent to as high as 55 percent, with the largest concentration being from 10 percent to 33 percent.

### Patterns of Drug Use

Gathering information about a client's drug use is more complicated than collecting information about alcohol use. Clients or respondents are oftentimes more reluctant to disclose specifics of their use of illicit drugs precisely because this identifies illicit acts. Moreover, unlike ethanol or beverage alcohol, there is a relatively large menu of substances—narcotics, depressants, stimulants, cannabis, inhalants—available to drug abusers, which further complicates efforts to discern patterns of drug use accurately. For these and other reasons, relatively few studies on drug abuse among homeless people provide an in-depth picture of consumption patterns.

Available reports, however, offer some clues about the "drug of choice." Studies in San Diego (Wynne, 1984), St. Louis (Morse, Shields, Honnecke, Calsyn, Burger, and Nelsen, 1985), and Boston (Robinson, 1984) note that marijuana is the most widely used illicit drug among the homeless in these cities, followed by cocaine and heroin. For example, as many as 46 percent of homeless drug abusing

## Panel 6–1

### Prevalence of Drug Problems among Homeless People

Although shelter workers and other service providers need not become experts on the epidemiology of drug abuse to be effective at their work, it is nevertheless helpful to understand that the prevalence of drug abuse among homeless clients, even at the local level, can vary dramatically. If you are serving a young homeless population, say 18 to 25, you are more likely to encounter drug problems than in older groups, since drug use is more common among youth in general than it is in people 35 years or older. Yet, it is also true that the prevalence of drug abuse varies according to the setting (e.g., shelters, clinics, soup lines, etc.) where information is gathered, as well as by the assessment technique (e.g., self-report, psychiatric examination, standardized scale, etc.) used to identify drug problems.

Pamela Fischer, at The Johns Hopkins University Medical School, offers an especially in-depth look at the variations in prevalence rates of alcohol, drug, and mental health disorders among homeless people. Her work is based upon a review of dozens of research studies conducted at the national, state, and local levels within the past decade. Findings on drug abuse illustrate how the prevalence rates vary among the homeless population (Fischer, 1989:363) (see Table 2).

Although there are numerous factors that can explain these variations, including study methodology, the overall data compiled by Fischer show that prevalence rates tend to be higher in clinical/hospital and shelter settings than in other sites, such as SRO hotels, food/services settings, or in street surveys. Shelter settings tend to col-

lect a wider cross-section of homeless people, whereas the SRO hotel populations are "semihomeless" and often made up of elderly, fixed-income clientele who are less likely to be drug users. In food services, such as soup kitchens, there is likely to be a bias in favor of higher functioning homeless individuals, in contrast to hospital settings that often serve homeless patients precisely because they are drug or alcohol dependent.

Fischer also noted substantial variations in drug abuse prevalence according to technique of assessment (Table 3). In these results, records review and self-reports yield the widest range of prevalence rates. Yet, as Fischer noted, identifying drug abuse (and other disorders) by these assessment methods entails diverse criteria that can lump, for example, one-time users with clinically diagnosed drug addicts. Neither are psychiatric examinations, which yield lower estimates of drug abuse, free from biases, since clinicians often lack specific training for working in settings where homeless clients are typically found. This also may affect clinical judgments.

Overall results from Fischer's literature review are instructive, first, because they demonstrate that some methods of identifying homeless drug abusers yield higher prevalence rates than others; second, some service settings evidently attract higher numbers of drug abusers; and third, they serve as a reminder to service providers that statistics on drug abuse can vary dramatically from one agency setting to another, even within the same community.

*Source*: Adapted from Fischer, 1989.

Table 2.  Estimates of Drug Problems
by Data-Collection Site

| Site (number of studies) | Percentage of prevalence |
|---|---|
| Clinical/hospital (13) | 1.9–70.0 |
| Shelter (51) | 1.0–61.2 |
| SRO hotel (4) | 12.5–31.0 |
| Food and service sites (4) | 3.0–43.0 |
| Service users (2) | 1.7–2.3 |
| Street (7) | 14.0–48.0 |
| Total (60) | 1.0–70.0 |

women in San Diego reported using marijuana; 21 percent specified tranquilizers, and 13 percent indicated cocaine (Wynne, 1984). In contrast, the Boston study revealed more modest figures: 8 percent reported marijuana use, less than 1 percent sedatives, and less than 5 percent cocaine. Polydrug use, that is, the abuse of more than one drug substance, is also reported in some studies (Bassuk et al., 1984; Corrigan and Anderson, 1984). In fact, the concomitant abuse of alcohol with other drug substances, especially cocaine, marijuana, and sedatives, is not uncommon among some homeless people with a history of substance abuse (Fischer, 1989). Dockett (1989), for example, found that 16 percent of Washington's homeless who indicated they had a substance abuse problem had in fact a dual problem with both alcohol and other drug substances.

Still other reports offer information about the regularity of drug use. The study by Stark (1985) of the homeless population in Phoenix revealed that nearly 1 in 5 used drugs 1 to 9 days each month, on the average, and that nearly 1 in 20 reported usage in excess of 20 days per month. Similar results are reported in Oregon (Multnomah County Social Services Division, 1984), where 11 percent of the homeless were identified as daily users. A New York City report (Division of Substance Abuse, 1983) indicated that as many as 32 percent of a New York City sample of homeless respondents could be classified as "serious drug abusers."

In sum, overall findings suggest that the drug problem among the homeless varies by city, region, and site and there is some evidence that drug use is more prevalent among the homeless than nonhomeless groups (Fischer, 1989).

Table 3.  Estimates of Drug Problems by Assessment Method

| Assessment method (number of studies) | Percentage of prevalence |
|---|---|
| Psychiatric examination (6) | 1.0–23.1 |
| Standardized scale (9) | 8.0–48.0 |
| Prior/current treatment (4) | 6.0–14.0 |
| Records review (19) | 1.7–70.0 |
| Self-report (25) | 2.0–61.2 |
| Provider assessment (3) | 2.3–38.0 |
| Total (66) | 1.0–70.0 |

## Characteristics of Drug Abusers

Several studies permit a glimpse of the social characteristics of homeless drug abusers; these findings parallel those reported in studies of drug abuse in the general population. For example, drug abuse is more characteristic of homeless men than women. Ladner, Crystal, Towber, Callender, and Calhoun (1986) reported in their New York study that 28 percent of the men were identified as drug users; this compares to 3 percent for women. Similarly, Rosnow et al. (1985) found that male drug abusers outnumbered women in Milwaukee by two to one. In fact, the extensive literature review of Fischer (1989) showed that most studies report homeless men as more likely than women to be drug users. After examining 67 studies on the homeless population, Fischer (1989:367) found that prevalence rates for drug abuse in men ranged from a low of 3.4 percent to as high as 61.2 percent; for women this range was substantially lower (9 percent to 26 percent).

Age, too, is correlated with drug use, as it is in the general population. Robertson's report on homeless teenagers in Hollywood indicated that as many as two of every five were drug abusers. Ladner et al. (1986) found that a majority of the homeless drug abusers in New York were under 30 years old. Findings from these and similar studies are consistent with the report by Koegel and Burnam (1987) who found that homeless alcoholic males in Los Angeles resemble the traditional stereotypes of older men on skid row, compared to those with alcohol and other drug disorders, who tend to be younger. Observations by a case manager at a Los Angeles treatment facility support this link: "Older men are much more likely to be your straight alcoholics. In younger clients, we see other drug problems, especially cocaine and crack."

Evidence from other studies note a relationship between drug abuser and race/minority status. In a New York study (Ladner et al., 1986), for example, minorities were nearly four times as likely as nonminorities to be identified as a drug abuser. Similarly, Milburn and Booth (1988) found that the use of illicit drugs was higher among black men in Washington's homeless population.

Finally, it is also clear that drug problems are correlated with alcohol and mental health disorders among the homeless. In the national Health Care for the Homeless (HCH) program, Wright and Weber (1987) found that slightly more than 40 percent of the drug abusers who visited HCH sites also gave evidence of mental illness. Moreover, nearly 6 of every 10 of the male and nearly half (46 percent) of the female drug abusers were also identified as alcohol abusers. Similar results are reported in other studies (Arce et al., 1983; Farr et al., 1986).

## A PRIMER ON DRUGS AND DRUG ABUSE

In an era where drug use has become one of the nation's most pressing social problems, everyone should make an effort to become informed about the drug problem. Oftentimes, "tough talk" by politicians and police obscures the fact that drug abuse is also a serious public health issue. Understanding drug abuse as a

*Panel 6–2*

## The Street Homeless of Washington: A Snapshot of Alcohol and Other Drug Abuse

In 1988, Kathleen Dockett, a professor of psychology at the University of the District of Columbia, undertook a study of Washington's street homeless. Because street homeless are more difficult to locate and count than those who are in shelters and other fixed locales, as the U.S. Census Bureau discovered in its 1990 Census, the researcher used meal sites as an occasion to interview some 186 subjects. Informants estimated that as many as 93 percent of Washington's street homeless utilize free meal services.

Although this study was an effort to gather a wide variety of data useful in assessing the service needs of Washing-

ton's homeless, the results on respondent history of alcohol and drug abuse are instructive, since they offer profiles that typify the homeless population in many urban centers (see Table 4).

Although these data show that alcohol problems are more common among Washington's street homeless, as with the homeless in most cities, the most striking difference in the two profiles is the age when a substance abuse problem began. Note, however, that more than one third of those with other drug problems experienced difficulties at age 17 or less—more than twice the percentage in the alcohol group.

*Source*: Adapted from Dockett, 1989.

Table 4.  Abuse Profile of Street Homeless

|  | Percentage | |
|---|---|---|
|  | Alcohol | Other drugs |
| Ever had a problem | 76 | 31 |
| Age when problem began |  |  |
|   17 and under | 15 | 35 |
|   18–25 | 55 | 38 |
|   26–35 | 14 | 26 |
|   36 and older | 16 | 1 |
| Average age of onset | 25 | 21 |
| Number of times hospitalized or in detox |  |  |
|   None | 48 | 67 |
|   Once | 16 | 16 |
|   Twice | 15 | 10 |
|   Three or more times | 21 | 7 |
| Percentage indicating they need help with their problem | 26 | 22 |
| Percentage receiving help in last 6 months | 35 | 24 |

public health problem should be seen as a cornerstone of successful drug education, prevention, and treatment efforts.

Because drug abuse is a reality of working with homeless populations, this
section provides a brief overview of commonly used illicit drugs and their effects
on the body.

## Dependence on Drugs

Popular as well as professional literature on drug problems are filled with
terms like *chemical dependency, substance abuse, addiction, drug dependent, chemical
abuse,* and, of course, just plain *drug abuse.* In lay circles, these terms are often
interchangeable; in self-help groups, they can function like "buzz words" that all
insiders know. In the professional community, too, labels change over time; what
used to be "drug addiction" is now "drug dependency." In fact, sometimes new
labels or buzz words carry a political message, as in the label, "alcohol and other
drugs," which helps to erode commonly held beliefs that alcohol is not connected
with today's drug problems.

Although service providers working in shelters or similar organizations need
not be fluent in medical discourse about drugs, it is helpful for them to understand
the distinctions among various key terms.

Certain drugs can bring about a condition known as *psychological dependence* or
*habituation.* Although professionals themselves have different definitions of this
concept, psychological dependence involves a compulsion or craving for the drug
to achieve a psychological state, to avoid discomfort, or to relieve stress. In this
respect, the drug is reinforcing or rewarding to the user. Cocaine, for example,
carries high potential for developing a psychological dependence; this potential
appears somewhat less for marijuana.

On the other hand, *physical dependence* is a physiological adaptation to a drug.
Depending on the drug, tolerance can develop. Tolerance develops when the
response to the same dose of a drug decreases with repeated use. Heroin and
alcohol are classic examples of a drugs that can bring about a physical dependence,
and gradually a tolerance builds up so that increased amounts of the drug are
needed to achieve the same effect.

Some drugs, such as heroin, alcohol, and barbiturates, have a potential to
promote both psychological and physical dependence. Others, such as marijuana,
are more associated with psychological dependency, though some degree of
physical dependency may be possible. Virtually all of these drugs also involve
withdrawal syndromes, that is, symptoms associated with decreased dosage or
cessation of use. In some instances, these syndromes can be especially severe, such
as in withdrawal from alcohol or heroin.

## Drug Substances

Although common usage of the word *drugs* tends to lump such diverse
substances as tranquilizers, heroin, cocaine, LSD, and marijuana into a single

category, these drugs can be classified into categories according to their effects on the central nervous system: (1) depressants, (2) narcotics, (3) stimulants, and (4) hallucinogens. Although drugs in each category have different effects on the body, these effects are also influenced by the amount of dosage, previous consumption patterns, physical and psychological state of the user, and even by the social environment in which drugs are consumed.

## Depressants

Drugs in this category function to depress the central nervous system and to reduce pain. The most widely used licit drug in this category is alcohol (see discussion in Chapter 5). Other depressants, which also have medicinal uses, include barbiturates (e.g., Seconal, Tuinal), tranquilizers (e.g., Librium, Valium, Miltown), and methaqualone (e.g., Quāālude). Abuse of these substances can result in physical and psychological dependence, a craving for the drug, and physical and psychological withdrawal symptoms. The most common way of ingesting depressant substances is orally, but some can also be administered through injection. Depending on dosage, possible effects of depressants include drunken behavior, slurred speech, and disorientation to the immediate environment. If dosage is excessive, there is definite risk of overdose which can result in death. Signs of possible overdose include shallow respiration, cold, "clammy" skin, weak and rapid pulse, and, in extreme cases, coma. Withdrawal from dependence on depressants can be severe. Symptoms include anxiety, tremors, insomnia and sleeplessness, and convulsions.

## Narcotics

Narcotics, which also have a depressant effect, are highly addictive opiate derivatives, such as morphine and codeine (which have medicinal uses), heroin, and opiatelike drugs, such as methadone (which is used as a substitute for heroin). All of these substances carry the risk of developing psychological and physiological dependence. Typical effects of narcotics are constriction of the eye pupils, a

---

*Panel 6–3*

**Classifications of Commonly Abused Drugs**

All service providers should have a general knowledge of commonly abused drugs. Clients with a history of drug use are especially common in jail and prison populations and among inner-city youths. Most studies of the homeless estimate that from 10 percent to 15 percent have a drug abuse problem other than alcohol, although these rates can run higher among specific subpopulations of the homeless.

Table 5 provides an overview of some of the more commonly abused drugs.

Table 5.   Commonly Abused Drugs

| Substance | Slang term | Effect | Withdrawal |
|---|---|---|---|
| Depressants | | | |
| Benzodiazepines (Valium, Librium) | Downers | Disinhibition | Irritability |
| Barbiturates (Seconal, phenobarbital) | Reds | Sedation | Delusions |
| Quaaludes | Ludes, lemons | Sedation | Hallucinations, paranoia |
| Stimulants | | | |
| Cocaine | Blow, crystal | Euphoria, hyperactivity | Depression, apathy |
| Amphetamine | Meth, crank | Insomnia, anorexia | Lethargy |
| Opiates | | | |
| Morphine | USP | Euphoria | Anxiety |
| Methadone | Juice | Euphoria | Irritability |
| Heroin | Horse, smack | Insomnia | Nausea, vomiting |
| Percodan | Tar | Insomnia | Yawning, lethargy |
| Hallucinogens | | | |
| Marijuana | Pot, grass | Mood change | Depression |
| MDMA | Ecstasy | Hallucinations | Anxiety |
| LSD | Acid | Hallucinations | Sleep disturbance |
| PCP | Angel dust | Hallucinations | Can involve violent dissociative effect |

feeling of euphoria, followed by drowsiness (sometimes called "nodding out"), and respiratory depression, and, at times, a feeling of nausea. Withdrawal symptoms can be severe, which include watery eyes and runny nose, frequent yawning, loss of appetite, irritability, both chills and sweating, tremors, cramps, and nausea. Suffering through these symptoms can bring on a panic attack. Because large doses of narcotics can be lethal, addicts should be considered at risk for overdosing. Methods of ingesting narcotic substances vary. Although heroin can be smoked, it is more commonly administered by intravenous injection. Morphine and methadone can be consumed orally or can be injected.

Opiates suppress the brain center that produces adrenaline, epinephrine, and norepinephrine. These substances are involved with hearing action, bowel action, blood pressure, and other automatic nervous system functions. When opiates are withdrawn, all of these substances are produced in great amounts and they account for all of the symptoms seen in opiate withdrawal. The severity of the withdrawal varies depending on the extent of drug use. High use of a relatively pure substance will lead to more severe symptoms of withdrawal. The intensity of addiction may vary from a mild desire to a craving or to a compulsion to use the drug.

*Appearance.*   The individual in withdrawal symptoms from opiates will show increased fear and anxiety.

*Vital Signs.*   All vital signs, blood pressure, pulse, and temperature of the individual will be elevated.

*Panel 6–4*

## Language and the Drug Subculture

Anyone who has had a brush with the drug subculture knows that there is a unique language—an argot—that heavy drug users share in common, especially those who live on the streets. To New York addicts "black tar," which gets its name for its appearance, is something to get excited about, since it refers to a chunk of heroin that is 50 percent pure. For the pill junkie, "double trouble" is a sedative, known as Tuinal, that is Seventh Heaven!

Argot, of course, is not peculiar to the drug subculture. Indeed, it is a sociological phenomenon that emerges in almost every subculture organized around special activities or lifestyles, lawful or unlawful. Police or prison staff, for example, develop a lingo built around their work; on the opposite side, street people and prison inmates have their own "street language" and "jail talk," much of it focusing on their adversarial relationship with police and correctional officials. In human services agencies, an unofficial nomenclature emerges over time that contains acronyms, abbreviations, or informal terms for services or types of client problems.

Regardless of the subculture, argot becomes second nature for those who live in that lifestyle. At the same time, it also functions sociologically to differentiate "insiders" from "outsiders"—those "in the know" from those who are not. Thus, understanding a special nomenclature is like a badge that gives one entree to an inside perspective, and sometimes even confers privileges in communication. Addicts, for example, use terms like *cokehead* or *crack freak* as a neutral label for their own kind, yet often resent being called these by outsiders.

For case managers or counselors who have clients with drug problems, understanding their language can be important not only from a communications standpoint, but also as a help in establishing trust or rapport in the interview situation. This is not to say that a counselor must use the drug language, yet knowing the argot can be very helpful.

How many of the following terms do you know?

| | |
|---|---|
| Acid head | One who uses LSD. |
| Angel dust | PHP (phencyclidine). |
| Black Beauty | Phenylpropanolamine and caffeine, or "speed," contained in a black capsule. |

*Central Nervous System.*  Watery eyes, yawning, sneezing, sweating, and runny nose will be evident in the individual. In addition, there will be a loss of appetite, tremors, panic, chill and sweating, stomach and bowel symptoms, including nausea. Vomiting and stomach cramps are usually seen 48 hours after the last use of the drug. These symptoms can be severe and, depending on the extent of the habit, can produce extreme discomfort as well as increased fear and anxiety.

*Symptoms of Overdose.*  The individual's slow, shallow breathing is evident along with clammy skin and constricted eye pupils. Coma, or possible death, can occur if not treated.

*Panel 6–4*   (Continued)

| | |
|---|---|
| Chasing the dragon | Smoking cocaine. |
| Cooker | Spoon for heating heroin until it dissolves. |
| Crash | Hard let-down after a drug high. |
| Cut | Substance added to a drug that dilutes the purity. |
| Dynamite | A mixture of cocaine and heroin. |
| Freak out | Psychotic-like experience after a high on drugs. |
| Freebase | Freeing cocaine from an additive base; purifying and smoking cocaine. |
| Fruit salad | Taking different types of pills; often taken with an alcohol chaser. |
| Getting down | Getting high on drugs. |
| Horse | Heroin. |
| Jolly Beans | Pep pills. |
| Lude | A depressant, methaqualone; sometimes called Quālude. |
| Red Devils | Seconal (a barbiturate). |
| Redi-Rock | Small quantity of specially prepared cocaine, sometimes inserted in a cigarette for instant availability. |
| Rig | Syringe/needle. |
| Run | To inject drugs; or "on a run"—using intravenous drugs continuously. |
| Rush | Intense sensation felt after injecting drugs. |
| Scag | Heroin. |
| Score | Make a successful buy of drugs. |
| Shooting gallery | Place where addicts gather to shoot up drugs. |
| Snow | Cocaine. |
| Strung out | Heavily addicted. |
| Tracks | Needle marks on a person's arms or legs from frequent intravenous injection of drugs; collapsed veins. |
| Tweaking | Level of speed intoxication reached after one or two days of continuous use, characterized by obsessive behavior. |

## Stimulants

Stimulants act on the central nervous system to produce feelings of well-being. By far the most widely used stimulants are caffeine and nicotine. Although often referred to as a narcotic, cocaine and its derivative, "crack" cocaine, are the most frequently used illicit drugs in this category, followed by amphetamines (which have limited medical uses), often called "speed" or "uppers." Cocaine can be ingested by snorting, injection, or even smoked. Amphetamines are most often consumed orally, though injection is also possible. Typical effects of stimulants include excitation and euphoria, increased alertness, elevated pulse rate and blood pressure, loss of appetite, and insomnia. With cocaine in particular, there is definite possibilities of overdosing, which can result in extreme agitation, increased body temperature, hallucinations and convulsions, and even death. In fact, considerable publicity has been given to cocaine's potential to precipitate cardiac arrest. The abuse of stimulants can produce psychological dependence, and withdrawal typically entails severely depressed mood, irritability, disorientation and apathy, and especially prolonged sleep.

*Symptoms of Use (Cocaine, Crack).*   Individual shows increased alertness, excitement, euphoria, elevated pulse rate and blood pressure, sense of well-being, insomnia and loss of appetite, rapid speech, and increased physical activity (cannot stop talking, cannot sit still).

*Symptoms of Withdrawal.*   Individual is in a severely depressed mood and displays apathy, irritability, disorientation, and experiences prolonged sleep.

*Symptoms of Overdose.*   Individual shows severe agitation and an increase in body temperature, has hallucinations and convulsions which could result in possible death.
   *Ice, crystal,* and *crank* are street names for forms of methamphetamine, a powerful stimulant of the central nervous system. Although principally confined to Hawaii and West Coast states, smokeable ice is a devastating drug that poses a serious threat both to users and others, especially because its effects induce extreme states of paranoia. Service providers in regions where ice and other forms of amphetamines are prevalent should become familiar with the effects and dangers of this drug.

*Symptoms of Use.*   Individual displays hyper alertness, euphoria, inability to sleep, loss of appetite, rapid speech, dry mouth, increased body temperature, elevated blood pressure, feelings of paranoia, and violent behavior (in extreme cases).

*Symptoms of Withdrawal.*   Individual shows apathy, extreme mood depression, and disorientation.

*Symptoms of Overdose.*   Extreme agitation, elevated body temperature, and nausea are seen in the individual along with amphetamine psychosis (incoherence, hallucinations), and convulsions. Death is possible from stroke or cardiovascular collapse.

## Hallucinogens

Although hallucinogens are less popular today than in previous decades, these substances persist in the drug market. Hallucinogens alter perceptual functions, which can result in visual illusions, hallucinations, and increased or exaggerated emotions. In lay circles, hallucinogens are often referred to as "psychedelic" or "psychoactive" drugs. The most frequently used hallucinogens, both of which are produced artificially, are LSD (lysergic acid diethylamide) and PCP (phencyclidine). Mescaline, a derivative of the peyote cactus, constitutes an organic hallucinogen. Most hallucinogen substances are ingested orally, although PCP can also be smoked. Although no definite withdrawal syndrome is associated with the use of hallucinogens, excessive dosages have produced prolonged episodes of hallucinations that may resemble or simulate psychotic states.

## Cannabis

By far the most widely consumed form of cannabis is *marijuana*. Though less popular in the United States, *hashish* is also a form of cannabis. Both forms are ingested by smoking and typically bring about feelings of euphoria, relaxation of inhibitions, impaired memory and attention span, and oftentimes an increase in appetite. Excessive consumption of cannabis can precipitate "paranoia," that is, unexplained fears, bring on heavy fatigue, and in cases of very high dosage even simulate psychotic-like states. Although there is no definite withdrawal syndrome, insomnia and hyperactivity can be observed in some instances.

---

*Panel 6–5*

### Doing Street Drugs

*Heroin*

Manny makes a life for himself in the back alleys off of New York's Times Square. He described the rush from heroin as like "a giant sexual orgasm that you never want to end. There is instant relief." To get this relief, however, all heroin addicts go through a ritual of preparing the heroin for injection. Powdered heroin, described by Manny as the "white lady," is put into a spoon or bottle cap (called a *cooker*). Then a small amount of water is added, and the mixture is heated with a match or candle until the heroin is dissolved. "I get wild sometimes with excitement," Manny explains, referring to the anticipation of the rush of heroin. This mixture is drawn into a hypodermic needle, then injected into a vein that has been enlarged by using a tourniquet. Oftentimes the addict will draw blood back into the needle so that it mixes with the liquified heroin. Some users also inject heroin just under the skin, a procedure known as *skinpopping*. Because heroin addicts often use "shooting galleries" as places to get high, sharing needles with others is not uncommon, especially if there is a needle shortage.

According to Agar (1973), heroin users can experience four effects.

1. *A Rush*: For most users, this occurs within several seconds, which steadily builds to a feeling of euphoria, a flushing of the face and pleasant visceral sensations.

2. *A High*: A heroin high is a pronounced feeling of well-being that can last up to several hours. In Manny's words, "I

*Continued*

*Panel 6–5*   (Continued)

feel mellow, cooled out, no worries, you might say." Since prolonged use of heroin increases tolerance for the drug, however, greater dosages are required to achieve the same effect.

3. *The Nod*: This third effect is a state of calm in which addicts lose awareness of their surroundings. Oftentimes, eyelids, even the jaw, drop, and for some the nod involves unconsciousness. "You are in another world, your own world," as Manny explains it. "There is nothing like it, no way to really describe it."

4. *Being Straight*: This is the period when addicts are not suffering withdrawal symptoms. The cycle will be repeated when the user ingests more heroin.

*Cocaine and Crack*

Any hardcore "coke user" will tell you that cocaine gives you a "head high"—a feeling of euphoria, of power and confidence, and oftentimes feelings of sexual excitement. In fact, some describe it as the "Cadillac of drug highs." Depending on dosage, its effects will typically last from 5 up to 20 minutes. Many inexperienced coke users report feeling a compulsion to use more of the drug from the onset. As a homeless veteran user explained it, "If I had a half gram, I'd do it. If I had a gram, I'd do a gram. And if I had two grams, I'd do two grams."

Snorting cocaine is the most common form of ingestion. However, some hardcore users prefer "freebasing," which involves mixing cocaine with a flammable product, such as ether or lighter fluid. Although this process is dangerous to carry out, it produces pure cocaine crystals that can be crushed and smoked in a glass pipe or mixed with other substances, such as tobacco or even marijuana. The payoff for coke users is an extraordinary rush and a pleasurable high; the downside comes 20 to 30 minutes later, involving a "crash" or let-down that plunges the user into tension and depression.

Although there is evidence that the number of cocaine users among some age groups has either remained steady or declined in the late 1980s, evidence from the National Institute on Drug Abuse (1986) indicates that the frequency of cocaine use has actually increased among those who are current users. Observable signs that often identify cocaine abusers are: dilated pupils; nervousness, hyperactivity, irritability, and even aggressiveness; "dry mouth" and frequent "licking of the lips"; runny or "stuffed-up" nose, including unexpected nosebleeds; sleeplessness and prolonged lack of appetite (which quite obviously brings about serious weight loss); and if cocaine has been injected intravenously, needle marks (often called *tracks*) on the arms or legs (Winters and Venturelli, 1987).

Although cocaine use can be an expensive habit to maintain, *crack*, a derivative of cocaine, is by comparison a "bargain basement item," costing a fraction of the street market price for cocaine (Goode, 1989). Crack is produced by mixing cocaine powder with sodium bicarbonate (more commonly called, *baking soda*), then heating it to a paste, which is later dried out and chipped into "rock crystals." When a "rock" (which is oftentimes sold on the streets in vials, similar to those used for perfume samples) is smoked (typically in a

*Panel 6–5*   (Continued)

glass pipe mechanism), it produces a "crackling sound" that gives crack its name. Because crack is inhaled, it brings an instant rush, later an intensive high and euphoria lasting from 5 to 10 minutes. Smoking more crack will restore the high; if not the crack user is subjected to an intensive crash, surpassing the let-down experienced after conventional cocaine use.

What makes crack such an extraordinarily devastating drug to users is that "recreational use" rapidly progresses to "compulsive use"—a craving for more crack—within days or a few weeks (Rosecan, Spitz, and Gross, 1987). Crack users are the first to admit this, according to Maria, who abandoned her two children for a life in the crack subculture that flourishes along New York's Eighth Avenue/Midtown District: "It took hold of me. I wanted more the first time I did crack, and look at me now! I am down to 80 pounds, I can't eat, I lost my kids. What's to become of me?"

*Methamphetamine ("Crank," "Ice," "Crystal Meth")*

Methamphetamine, a form of amphetamine, is a synthetic drug that acts as a stimulant on the central nervous system. In fact, it is one of the most powerful stimulants in the amphetamine group. As a street drug, it is called *ice, crystal meth*, or *crank*. In the words of a 23-year-old Seattle man, who first smoked ice in Hawaii, ice gives "a fabulous high like no other dope . . . a feeling of power that goes on and on and on."

Ice gets its name from its appearance—translucent crystals, resembling "chips of ice" or rock candy. Occasionally, it is sold on the street in variously colored capsules or tablets. In white powder form, it resembles baking powder and is called *crank* or *rock*. Hybrid forms of methamphetamines have also surfaced in American cities, such as *croak*, which is a mixture of methamphetamine and cocaine.

In the United States, ice first surfaced in Hawaii, and then surfaced later in the West Coast states, particularly in Southern California. The distribution of ice is thought to be confined principally to these areas. Depending on its form, methamphetamine can be injected, smoked (typically in a stemmed glass bowl), inhaled by snorting it, or taken orally. Smoking ice produces intense feelings of euphoria, tremendous energy, confusion, nausea, and paranoid impulses. Unlike cocaine or crack, the effects of ice can extend from 8 to as long as 24 hours. The use of methamphetamine in any form creates a psychological dependence, and withdrawal can be torturous, involving anxiety and deep depression, even suicidal impulses.

Although consuming ice poses obvious medical dangers, including the risk of overdose, high doses over an extended period can precipitate an "amphetamine psychosis" that resembles paranoid schizophrenia. Thus, ice users also evidence high potential for aggressive and violent behavior. "All I remember is I was crazy," a California man explained in recounting the day he was arrested for assault and possession of drugs. "Anybody who so much as looked at me I would shout at 'em and the day I got busted I hit a guy across the face with a club. I was scared as hell as mean as hell—all at once!"

*Panel 6–6*

**The Life and Death of Hector Torres**

On October 25, Hector Torres got the results of his blood test at a city public health clinic: he had AIDS. "At first it didn't hit me what that really means. I learned about AIDS. I knew that shootin' up can give us AIDS. I knew all that—and still it didn't really hit me until later," he lamented. "I just wanted to get out of there; none of that counseling crap. All I could think about was getting out of there, score some smack and get down!"

Born in New York's South Bronx, Hector was raised in a family with seven children. "We lived in four different places that I remember. The best we ever had was a three-room apartment. My pop—he was killed in an accident at work—died when I was 11." Hector says he and his older brothers "ran wild" after the father's death. "I was gangin' and runnin' the streets. The family sort of fell to pieces. I got two brothers at Riker's Island and another on parole." An uncle and two cousins moved in with his family when Hector was 15. "I done drugs before. That's the way it is where I grew up, but never smack [heroin] until [cousin] Ricky turned me on to skin poppin'." Within a year Hector was mainlining heroin. "Ricky had a good source and scoring dope was never a problem" until his cousin was arrested in a police raid. Life was never the same. He lost his job at a small grocery store when the owner accused him of stealing from the till. "And I was," he confessed. "I got in with a fast crowd. I left home. I just went from one place to another, did some time in the Tombs [jail], but I always scored smack."

For more than six years Hector faced the perils of being homeless in New York City, holing up for short periods in abandoned or unoccupied buildings in the South Bronx, in warehouses along Manhattan's West Side, and in "shooting galleries" where he scored drugs. Prostitution kept him in easy money. "My buddy, Manny—we'd do the porn shops on 42nd, 8th Avenue. I can score a hundred in an hour or two."

"I guess you can say I been my own worst enemy," Hector explained in reflecting back on 27 years of unhappiness. "I been shooting drugs almost half of my life, scorin' smack, gettin' down, dodging the law, doin' time . . . just tryin' to get by, just tryin' to survive. It's no way to live."

On July 13th, Hector's friend, Manny, wrote a letter: "Hector died last week in the hospital and I don't know where to find his mother and sisters so that I can tell them that he is gone. . . . I got it [AIDS]. I don't know what I can do or where I can go."

## Responding to Withdrawal Symptoms

Shelter guests who experience acute withdrawal symptoms requiring emergency medical services must be seen by qualified health care professionals. In instances where symptoms are not severe or life-threatening, shelter personnel should be familiar with the following procedures.

| What to Do (Withdrawal) | Why |
|---|---|
| Urge a drug rehabilitation program. | The person may be more open to treatment at this time. |
| Be firm, but fair. | Be aware that when it is time to use drugs again, the person may act out. This is preexisting drug-seeking behavior and the person will need firm, but fair and consistent limit setting. |
| Determine whether there is a prior history of seizures or other health problems. | Medications at this time should be kept to a minimum. At the same time, the person should not be allowed to go without medication for other clinical problems. |
| Transport the person to the nearest hospital. Consider a direct admission to a drug rehabilitation program. | Most shelters are ill-prepared to care for the person in withdrawal. Treatment in a specialized setting, such as a detoxification center, provides the greatest opportunity for care. |

| What Not to Do | Why |
|---|---|
| Do not give detailed instructions and expect the person to be able to follow them. | The person is unable to concentrate or to think clearly during withdrawal. |
| Do not allow the person to stay in the shelter if the symptoms are acute. | Treatment in a hospital or a detoxification center is necessary. With the right approach, this may be the opportunity for the person to begin treatment. |
| Do not cause additional stress. | The person needs a calm, quiet environment during withdrawal. |

A final word about overdoses—regardless of the drug—should be made clear: any suspected drug overdose requires professional treatment. If you suspect an overdose, transport the person via ambulance, if possible, to the nearest hospital emergency room. While waiting for the ambulance, if the person is unconscious, contact the hospital and follow the instructions provided by the emergency room staff.

## AIDS AND HIV

Like alcoholics, chronic drug users are at risk of developing serious health problems, not the least of which is the danger of overdosing on drug substances. Many of these health problems are also shared by alcoholics, such as hepatitis, tuberculosis, skin diseases and infections, liver and cardiac diseases. In the nationwide Health Care for the Homeless project, Wright and Weber (1987) analyzed the health problems of homeless drug users who made at least two visits to project clinics. Findings revealed that liver disease, cardiac disease, peripheral venous stasis disease, and chronic disorders, such as diabetes, and AIDS were indeed more common among drug abusers.

Yet, for intravenous (IV) drug users, in particular, no threat is more menacing than their risk of contracting Acquired Immune Deficiency Syndrome, more commonly referred to as AIDS. AIDS is a medical condition characterized by a defect in the body's immune system. This defect is caused by the human immunodeficiency virus (HIV), which attacks and destroys white blood cells. This risk is especially acute among those addicts who share needles, since the HIV can be transmitted through exchange of bodily fluids, such as blood. Thus, needle-sharing with another drug user infected with the HIV is a near-certain means of transmitting this disease. Pregnant women who are infected with the AIDS virus can also give this virus to the fetus (intrauterine) or during delivery (peripartum). AIDS is not an airborne disease, and there is no evidence that the HIV can be spread through casual contact with infected persons. At the present time, IV drug users constitute the second largest risk group for AIDS, surpassed only by homosexual and bisexual males. Health statistics on AIDS, however, clearly show that AIDS has claimed lives in virtually every social and demographic group.

Those infected with HIV are vulnerable to opportunistic infections and illnesses which are not normally a threat to those with a properly functioning immune system. The two most common opportunistic diseases associated with AIDS are *Pneumocystis carinii* pneumonia and Kaposi's sarcoma.

HIV can also attack the central nervous system, resulting in progressive dementia, memory loss, impairment of coordination, and even partial paralysis. Although knowledge about the dynamics and patterns of the disease continues to develop, mortality statistics currently indicate that 80 percent of all AIDS patients

---

*Panel 6–7*

### AIDS and Opportunistic Illness

Approximately 8 out of every 10 AIDS patients have had one or both of two diseases: *Pneumocystis carinii* pneumonia (sometimes referred to as PCP), a parasitic infection of the lungs, and Kaposi's sarcoma (KS), a relatively rare form of cancer. PCP manifests symptoms similar to other types of pneumonia, such as fever, cough, and difficulties in breathing. KS involves lesions that can occur on the skin's surface or in the mouth or digestive tract. In their early stages, these lesions resemble a bruise (e.g., blue-violet or brown colored); they grow and eventually spread.

*Source*: Adapted from Runck, 1986:6.

die within 2 years of diagnosis. To date, no AIDS patient is known to have recovered from the disease. Statistics reported by the Centers for Disease Control reveal that 161,073 AIDS cases had been reported in the United States since June 1981, and more than 100,000 people had died from AIDS-related complications by the end of 1990. According to the World Health Organization, there were more than 300,000 cases of AIDS worldwide by 1990 and more than 10 million people were infected with HIV.

Although there are no precise figures on drug use in the United States, experts estimate that there are currently several million drug abusers. About one-half million inject heroin regularly and over one million are occasional IV drug users. There are no reliable estimates on the number of cocaine and amphetamine abusers who inject these drugs (Goode, 1989).

Studies (National Institute on Drug Abuse, 1986) of IV drug users suggest that as many as 95 percent share drug paraphernalia (needles, syringes, cookers) or drugs with other users. To the extent that these can carry small amounts of contaminated blood, the AIDS virus can be transmitted from user to user. In addition, the AIDS virus can be sexually transmitted from drug abuser to individuals who do not use drugs. Many public health experts believe that IV drug users (in addition to bisexual males) are one of the principal ways in which AIDS is transmitted to the heterosexual population. Data from the National Institute on Drug Abuse (1986) are illuminating in this regard:

- Among women who have AIDS, 53 percent are IV drug users.
- 54 percent of pediatric AIDS are traceable to an IV drug-using parent.
- More than two thirds (at present 70 percent) of heterosexually transmitted AIDs cases are traceable to an IV drug user sex partner.

---

*Panel 6–8*

**Reducing the Risk of AIDS Among Active IV Drug Users**

The only certain protection against contracting AIDS through shared drug paraphernalia is to stop using drugs. If drug abusers are unwilling to do this, at the very least they must understand how they can reduce this risk:

- Avoid "shooting galleries" where needle-sharing is common.
- Refrain from sharing drugs and paraphernalia.
- Use only new needles; utilize "needle exchange" programs if they operate in the local area.
- Sterilize used syringes or needles by soaking them in a solution of Clorox (or sodium hypochlorite bleach) and water for at least 10 minutes, then rinse with tap water; or boil them in water for 30 minutes.
- Sexual relations with other high-risk groups should be avoided. If this advice is not followed, the use of condoms can reduce the risk of infection.

Since the time-lapse interval between exposure to HIV and testing positive for HIV is not uniform, ranging from 2 weeks to 6 months or longer, people infected with HIV may feel and appear to be well, yet can transmit the virus. Among people identified as HIV-positive (meaning that one or more blood tests have confirmed that there are antibodies to the HIV disease), active symptoms and opportunistic infections may not appear until months later, even a year or longer.

The Center for AIDS Prevention Studies offers a list of symptoms that warrant immediate medical attention (McKusick, 1990:11–12):

1. Persistent fevers with temperatures above 101° to 102°F lasting 2 or 3 days, and especially if they result in "night sweats."
2. Persistent dry cough associated with a "tight chest" or pressure in the front of the chest or under the breastbone.
3. Shortness of breath, particularly if this occurs while undertaking ordinary activities.
4. Persistent diarrhea (more than several bowel movements daily) extending several days.
5. Increased fatigue after moderate physical activity.
6. Slow healing sores, including mouth sores, whitish patches on the mouth, gums, or tongue; or uncommon appearance of hives or rash or purple-like spots on the skin that do not fade away.
7. Difficulty in swallowing, involving pain or discomfort in the throat (especially when swallowing liquids), or a persistent lump in the throat or beneath the breastbone.
8. Unexplained weight loss, such as 8 to 10 pounds or a pound each week that is not due to dieting.
9. Severe headaches that are worse or unlike headaches in the past.

Although a single symptom may indicate a variety of medical problems, combination or clusters of these symptoms warrant immediate medical attention and referral of the guest or client for HIV testing.

## AIDS and Homelessness

Based on medical data collected at Health Care for the Homeless project sites in 16 cities in the United States, Wright and Weber (1987) estimated the prevalence of AIDS and AIDS-related complex at 185 cases per 100,000 homeless people in those cities. At the time of data-gathering, the rate of AIDS cases in the United States population was 144 per 100,000 (Wright and Weber, 1987).

Recent estimates by the Centers for Disease Control indicate that as many as one in five homeless people are HIV-positive, and there is indirect evidence that this rate can be expected to escalate. For example, Wright and Weber (1987) also reported that homeless youths have higher rates of substance abuse, sexually transmitted diseases, and pregnancies— compared to domiciled youths—which carry obvious risks for transmitting HIV. In addition, studies reviewed earlier in this chapter suggest that an estimated 10 percent to 15 percent (in some studies, higher percentages) of the adult homeless population have histories of drug abuse, placing them at higher risk of contracting the AIDS virus.

Yet the incidence of AIDS cases among the homeless can be expected to increase precisely because the victims of AIDS often lose housing and employment. As the disease progresses, persons with AIDS face increasing difficulties in maintaining financial stability and in coping with everyday responsibilities, which, for some, makes homelessness a near certainty. Thus, the AIDS epidemic has in effect created a "fast track" into homelessness. As this epidemic worsens and as the costs of caring for AIDS patients increase, the prevalence rate of AIDS cases in the homeless population will undoubtedly escalate.

One of the most alarming examples of how AIDS victims are forced into homelessness is cited in an Institute of Medicine (1988) report on homelessness and health. Highlighting findings from a study conducted in New York by the Institute of Public Performance, Inc., their report noted that of the 377 people with AIDS in the metropolitan New York hospitals, 77 (including 7 pediatric cases) were actually homeless at the time of data-gathering in 1985. In fact, 57 percent of the overall 377 AIDS cases indicated that they needed assistance in securing permanent housing (Institute of Medicine, 1988:31–32).

## Helping Homeless Persons with AIDS

Service providers working in shelters and in related settings for homeless people can make major contributions to caring for persons with AIDS (PWAs) and in preventing the spread of HIV. First, shelter personnel should keep informed about the AIDS epidemic and the methods for its prevention. This knowledge contributes to an educational platform that can inform clients about the risks of AIDS and the precautionary measures they must take. Experience gained from AIDS education campaigns in the gay community offers evidence that organized education and prevention programs can be effective in informing at-risk populations and in sharply reducing the number of new cases. Reaching drug abusers, however, is more difficult. Because shelters collect the most diverse cross-section of homeless people, including varying numbers of IV drug users, they offer ideal settings to deliver educational messages about AIDS to hard-to-reach groups. These efforts can range from passive approaches, such as posters and literature on AIDS, to action-oriented programming, such as conducting informal classes or educational sessions which emphasize behaviors that can reduce the risk of HIV infection. Many shelters distribute condoms and offer instructions as to how these can be used to reduce the risk of exposure to HIV from sexual activities.

Second, service providers also play a pivotal role in connecting high-risk groups and PWAs with needed services. Although most shelters are not capable of providing extensive medical services, intake and counseling personnel can make referrals that link homeless guests with AIDS to appropriate services, including entitlements, HIV-testing services, medical attention, housing arrangements, and even support groups that can help in coping with the anxiety caused by AIDS.

Finally, each shelter or agency serving homeless clientele has an obligation to

## Panel 6–9

## AIDS, HIV, and Shelter Policies

Although the actual number of persons with AIDS who are also homeless is not known, it is clear that the crisis of AIDS has taken its toll on the homeless population. For this reason, every shelter and agency serving homeless guests must develop policies that will safeguard the dignity of PWAs, respect their right to confidentiality, and protect the health and well-being of shelter staff and other guests. Although these policies should be written according to the individual organization and its mission of service, they must also be sensitive to legal and ethical considerations.

Because of the complexity of the AIDS problem, however, agencies oftentimes struggle with developing policies on AIDS. It was this realization that in part brought together a team of Boston-area service providers who compiled a manual to serve as a blueprint for developing sound, yet sensitive policies on AIDS. Entitled *AIDS and HIV: A Manual for Shelter and Residential Program Providers* (Bennett et al., 1990), this handbook addresses legal and ethical issues in serving PWAs, psychosocial needs of the person with HIV/AIDS, a summary of medical knowledge about AIDS, information on general infection control, a glossary of AIDS terms, and an addendum on substance abuse. Its section on policies, however, is especially instructive in that it maps out key areas that shelters and similar organizations should include in their policy statements:

- Client, staff, and volunteer confidentiality
- Guests with AIDS or HIV infection
- Staff and volunteers with AIDS or HIV infection
- Discrimination
- Possible accidental exposure to HIV on the job
- Information for pregnant personnel
- Action to be taken should policies be violated

Boston's largest shelter, the Pine Street Inn, offers an illuminating example of how these areas are configured into a policy statement consistent with their service mission.

### Referrals

The Inn will accept referrals of guests with AIDS or ARC [AIDS-related complex]. Pine Street, however, is not an appropriate long-term residence for persons with AIDS because of many other communicable diseases to which persons suffering from AIDS may be susceptible. Therefore, although we will accept referrals, the Inn should be considered only when all other alternatives have been attempted. The referring agency should continue to seek appropriate placements while the person is residing at the Inn.

### Alternative Placements

A guest should not be refused accommodations simply because he or she has

*Panel 6–9*   (Continued)

AIDS. A guest should be encouraged to accept responsibility for finding a more appropriate placement when possible.

*Confidentiality*

State and federal laws protect the confidentiality of people with AIDS, ARC, or who test positive for HIV. Because precautions such as hand washing and wearing gloves are the exception here, there is no legal justification for violating the confidentiality of our guests. If a guest shares this information with us, we can encourage him or her to share it with our staff as it seems appropriate, either for referral work or health care, etc. However, it is up to the guest to decide who should have this information.

*Staff Interactions with Guests with AIDS*

It is the philosophy of Pine Street that our guests have the right to be treated with dignity and respect. While we recognize that there may be some staff persons who are not comfortable working closely with a guest who has AIDS, we believe we have a responsibility to see that this philosophy is conveyed to all guests by our attitude and that we work out among ourselves the division of responsibility for working with a particular guest.

*Precautions*

Staff should assume that any guest is a potential carrier of the AIDS virus, and, therefore, should use gloves when coming in contact with any body fluids (blood, urine, vomit, feces, etc.) from any guest. If accidental contact is made with body fluids, hands should be washed immediately. CPR should always be done with a protective face mask. However, day-to-day contact with guests, including those actually diagnosed with AIDS or ARC, requires no additional precautions. For more information, please contact the clinic.

*Education*

The Inn should initiate a program for informing guests about AIDS. The Inn should also continue to provide in-service training for staff on the topic of AIDS.

*Advocacy*

At the present time, the Inn will not be directly involved with advocacy in this area. However, we will continue to be in contact with other advocacy groups such as the AIDS Action Committee. We will also investigate the possibility of developing resources, such as a hospice, for this segment of our population.

*Staff with AIDS*

Should a staff person contract AIDS, he or she would be covered by all applicable sections of the Inn's Personnel Policies as would any other staff person. The decision whether or not to share information on [his or her] condition would be up to the individual.

*Source*: Panel text adapted and reprinted from Bennett et al., 1990:VII.4–VII.5.

formulate policies concerning PWAs or guests who are HIV-positive than are consistent with their service mission. The formation of sound policies is absolutely essential to safeguarding the health of both personnel and the guests or clients they serve, in protecting the right to privacy of PWAs, and in assuring that discriminatory practices do not intrude upon delivery of needed services. (See pp. 177–180 in Chapter 7 for a discussion of HIV/AIDS and for procedures in providing care to guests who are HIV-positive.)

## CONCLUSIONS

Evidence from a variety of federal government reports suggests that the drug epidemic in the United States may be subsiding in the 1990s. The National Household Survey on Drug Abuse (National Institute on Drug Abuse, 1990), for example, showed that cocaine use has dropped by 72 percent since 1985 and by 45 percent since 1988; the Secretary of Health and Human Services announced that for the first time in 16 years less than half of all teenagers in the United Sates admitted trying illegal drug substances (Gelb, 1991).

Although such evidence is encouraging, these reports are not without critics, who point to steady increases in drug arrests and cocaine-related deaths, as well as to drug abuse rates among all arrestees, which run as high as 75 percent. Moreover, a study from the Senate Judiciary Committee, based on admissions to treatment clinics, prison drug-testing, and conservative estimates of addiction among the homeless, found that the number of addicts grew somewhat in the last half of 1990 (Gelb, 1991). Thus, whatever progress has been made nationwide in combatting America's drug problem, there is no direct evidence that this success extends to the ranks of the homeless. On the contrary, there is every reason to believe that homelessness will continue to collect society's drug abusers, which carries with it the burden of caring for those who are afflicted with AIDS.

For these and other reasons, service providers should feel a special obligation to be informed about the drug problem and to seek an active role in developing education, treatment, and prevention strategies tailored to homeless people. Materials presented in this chapter provide only an overview of basic knowledge that can serve as a point of departure for further training and professional development. Past experience suggests that drug abuse prevention and treatment programs do work, especially when they are sensitive to the special needs and problems of their target population. No one understands the complexity of these needs better than those providing services to America's homeless.

# Health Care and Homeless People

BARBARA A. BLAKENEY

As Minnie, a 63-year-old homeless woman in New York, explained it: "It's not easy for people like me to take care of myself. I'm older and I got no place to go. I don't have a doctor and if I get sick or hurt the best I can hope for is the line is short at the shelter's clinic."

Minnie's concerns are not unlike those of thousands of homeless people nationwide, who face substantially higher risks of injury and physical illness than virtually any other population group in the United States. And the inherent health risks posed by living on the streets and in crowded shelters are multiplied both by homeless persons' lack of economic resources and by the lack of an established health care system for them.

This chapter describes health care problems among the homeless and reviews guidelines for responding effectively to these problems. The chapter begins by describing the prevalence of physical illnesses and injuries among the homeless and the impact of these problems on the rate of homelessness. The symptoms of common illnesses and injuries among homeless persons are then described, and emergency procedures for responding to these problems are identified. The chapter concludes with a discussion of the ways in which shelters and the health care system can improve the delivery of health care to the homeless.

# INTRODUCTION

Health problems interact with homelessness in three principal ways. First, health problems can contribute to the likelihood of becoming homeless. For example, complications that are due to chronic health problems may result in a general decline in coping ability, which in turn disrupts established living patterns. This predicament worsens if there is inadequate insurance coverage to pay for medical expenses, an inability to sustain employment or self-support, and a lack of personal or welfare resources to see the person through the crisis; homelessness may be one result (Institute of Medicine, 1988).

Second, being homeless increases the risk of developing serious health problems. Homeless people face a hazardous environment: many make their way on the streets, sleeping in alleys, parks, abandoned buildings, or makeshift shelters. This lifestyle can take its toll: frostbite, hypothermia, heat stroke, pneumonia, infectious disease from rodent bites, parasitic infestations, skin disorders, and serious injuries that are due to their increased risk of accident, assault, or rape (Institute of Medicine, 1988). Even on occasions when they enjoy the advantages of a shelter bed, homeless persons face increased risks of contracting infectious and communicable diseases compared to domiciled people, since shelter accommodations are almost always under institutional arrangements that include close sleeping quarters, communal showers and toilets, and common dining facilities.

Third, many homeless people have difficulty in accessing traditional health care facilities and in complying with traditional health care regimens. The health care facilities available to homeless persons are usually large hospital emergency departments or ambulatory care centers, which often have long waits and fast, impersonal services. Hospital-based clinicians, unaware of the barriers to compliance faced by homeless people, often prescribe treatments that are not easily followed. Even a simple order—"take two aspirin, go to bed, and get plenty of rest"—is virtually impossible for the homeless patient to obey. Thus, an undomiciled life mitigates against regular use of prescribed medicine or controlling chronic medical conditions, such as high blood pressure, ulcers, or diabetes, through special diets (Institute of Medicine, 1988).

# INTERACTION OF HEALTH PROBLEMS AND HOMELESSNESS

Numerous studies (Brickner, Scharer, Concanan, Elvy, and Savarese, 1985; Brickner, Scharer, Concanan, Savarese, and Scanlan, 1990; Dockett, 1989) document the fact that physical illness or morbidity is high among the homeless population. No work is more definitive in this respect than research conducted in conjunction with the national Health Care for the Homeless (HCH) program (Wright and Weber, 1987). Established by the Robert Wood Johnson Foundation and the Pew Memorial Trust, this 4-year demonstration project was designed to create and test different health care delivery systems for people who are homeless and to suggest various approaches that could reduce the problems of access and continuity of care. Findings from this program are instructive.

According to records on clients visiting Health Care for the Homeless clinics, about two thirds had acute disorders. The most common acute disorders were upper respiratory infections (33 percent) and traumas (23 percent), followed by minor skin ailments (14 percent). Infestational disorders (e.g., scabies or lice) and serious skin disorders were also common (4 percent to 5 percent). Nutritional deficiencies, such as malnutrition and vitamin deficiencies, were present in approximately 2 percent of all HCH clients. Morbidity rates for homeless clients were higher for each of these acute ailments than for a comparable, but domiciled population.

Homeless persons also evidence high rates of chronic physical disorders. The most common chronic diseases among HCH clients were hypertension (14 percent), gastrointestinal disorders (14 percent), peripheral vascular disease (13 percent), poor dentition or dental problems (9 percent), neurological disorders (8 percent), eye disorders (8 percent), cardiac disease (7 percent) and genitourinary disorders (7 percent).

Nearly one third of HCH clients had at least one chronic disorder; among clients seen at a clinic more than once, this figure increased to 41 percent. Men had somewhat higher rates of chronic disorders than women; prevalence was also slightly higher for nonwhites than whites. As expected, chronic disorders were sharply higher among those over the age of 50 (Wright and Weber, 1987:105).

In virtually every disorder category, morbidity rates among the homeless exceeded—in some instances, substantially—those of the study's comparison domiciled population. Some potentially fatal diseases that appear only rarely among the settled population are not uncommon among the homeless: the rate of active TB cases among Boston's homeless in 1988 was 267 per 100,000, compared to 25 per 100,000 for the city as a whole (McAdam et al., 1990); HIV seroprevalence rates may be at least 20 percent among most homeless subgroups, and as high as 60 percent among some (Raba et al., 1990).

## HEALTH CARE EMERGENCIES

Although some larger shelters now have clinics, even with these facilities it is unlikely that there will always be professional health care providers on site. For this reason, shelter workers, such as counselors and case managers, should become familiar with health care emergencies common in the shelter community. This is especially true of those working in smaller shelters, since they are unlikely to have on-site health care personnel.

Whenever possible, it is recommended that at least one person per shift be certified in cardiopulmonary resuscitation (CPR) and basic first aid. Most communities offer such programs through the local chapter of the American Res Cross, the local hospitals, or the American Heart Association. Recertification is usually required every year. Establishing a strong working relationship with the local health department or hospital will provide access to information and consultation services whenever there is a need. Working together to establish a partnership for health care will increase access to care.

The specific medical problems identified in this section are those most frequently seen in shelters. Although the recommendations as to action are correct and complete, they should never be viewed as proper substitutes for qualified health care. *They are intended as safety and first aid measures only.*

## Weather-Related Conditions

### Hypothermia

*Hypothermia* is a condition in which the core body temperature drops below 95°F. Core body temperature refers to the temperature deep within the body and includes the temperature of such vital organs as the heart, lungs, stomach and intestines, and kidneys. The condition is usually brought on by a combination of cold weather and inadequate clothing. However, especially with certain high-risk groups, the weather does not have to be very cold to bring on the problem. Under certain weather conditions and with certain risk factors, such as old age or intoxication, people have been known to die from hypothermia due to exposure at temperatures in the high forties.

High-risk groups include the elderly, infants, alcoholics, severely mentally ill, and people on certain types of medications, such as antidepressants, tranquilizers, and heart medications.

Hypothermia is always an emergency. The person with hypothermia must always be treated immediately by health care professionals.

### Symptoms of Hypothermia

*Skin Appearance.*   The skin of the person with hypothermia is usually cool or cold and pale. The best places to check for this are the abdomen, lower back, and the arms and legs. Skin color, while pale, may also have irregular blue or pink spots.

*Muscles.*   The muscles of the person with hypothermia are usually stiff, especially those of the neck, arms, and legs. The person may be shivering, although the absence of shivering should not be seen as a sign that the person is not cold. On the contrary, the lack of shivering may be an indication that the hypothermia is severe. Many elderly persons, infants, or intoxicated people may not be able to shiver at all.

*Coordination.*   Balance and gait problems are usually present in the person with hypothermia, secondary to stiff muscles and confusion. Watch for jerklike or uneven walking movements.

*Confusion.*   This is often the first sign that there is something wrong. The lower the core body temperature becomes, the more confused the person with hypothermia will become. Because confusion can also be part of the presentation of intoxication, drug use, or mental illness, it is important to get to know the person. A prior knowledge of the person's usual presentation will help to establish a baseline which will assist in the assessment of confusion as it relates to hypothermia.

*Heart and Lungs.* The colder the body becomes, the slower all the vital organs will function. Thus, in the person with hypothermia, the heart and breathing rates will slow as the core body temperature drops, Eventually, the heart and lungs will slow to the point where they stop. Without proper emergency care, the person will die. Even with the rewarming process, cardiac irritability is a serious problem and many people who die of hypothermia do so because the irritability cannot be properly controlled during rewarming. This is especially true for people who have preexisting cardiac problems.

| What to Do | Why |
|---|---|
| Get the person to proper treatment as quickly as possible. | Severe hypothermia must be treated by skilled professionals in order to control complications. |
| Handle the person gently. | Body systems are very fragile when cold. Sudden movement or activity can cause serious complications and even death. |
| Wrap the person in extra clothes and blankets and cover the head and neck. | This helps to conserve body heat. |

| What Not to Do | Why |
|---|---|
| Do not give hot foods, drinks, or alcohol. | Hot foods and drinks will not increase core body temperature that much. The stomach and intestines will not work properly when cold. Thus, the person is at risk of vomiting anything that is given. Reflexes are also dulled in the cold, so the person is also at risk of choking and aspirating. |
| Do not raise the person's feet above the head. | By doing this, blood from the cold legs returns to core areas and further decreases the core body temperatures. |
| Do not rub the arms and legs or place them in warm or hot water, or in any way try to actively rewarm the person. | Rewarming is a complicated process that has many risks of sudden death. It is best done by experienced health professionals who can closely monitor the process and respond to any complications. |

### Frostbite

Frostbite is a local cold-related injury caused by exposure of the body to cold weather or some sort of chemical contact, that is, dry ice. Frostbite causes burnlike damage to the tissues involved which are most often the fingers, toes, ears, nose, or chin. The extent of the damage to the tissue is based on the length of exposure, the extent of the cold, and underlying physical problems which may increase susceptibility to cold, such as malnutrition, anemia, edema, alcohol and drug abuse, decreased circulation to the tissue because of diabetes, peripheral vascular disease, smoking, or previous episodes of frostbite. Another risk factor is decreased awareness of the cold secondary to acute intoxication, drug use, or mental illness.

It is important to remember that a person suffering from frostbite may also be hypothermic as well.

### Symptoms of Frostbite

*First Degree (Mild).* Affected skin in the frostbite area may be red or blue and slightly edematous. Underlying tissue may remain resilient. The person may complain of pain, followed by numbness.

*Second Degree.* The first-degree symptoms are present and, in addition, blisters form 2 to 3 hours after rewarming. The skin will feel hot and dry to the touch. Movement of the affected part may become difficult and painful.

*Third Degree.* The skin takes on a bluish or purplish color, the blisters will fill with a purple-colored fluid and become deeper. The underlying tissue becomes hard and woodlike to the touch. This is a sign that the affected tissue is dying. Movement is very difficult and painful, if possible at all. There will be extreme aching pain which can persist for weeks following exposure. recovery of this degree of injury can take up to 6 months. During this time, the area of frostbite is extremely susceptible to exposure to the cold.

*Fourth Degree.* Dry gangrene is present; the underlying tissue and often the bone is dead. The area of frostbite appears deep red and mottled or cyanotic. The area is completely numb. At this stage, unless the affected area is surgically removed, mummification will occur.

| What to Do | Why |
|---|---|
| (For first-degree frostbite with no indications of hypothermia present) Remove the person from the source of cold. | Prevents further damage and allows for full assessment of the problem. |
| Place the affected part in warm water (90–110°F) for 20 minutes. | Warm water will assist the circulation to the area, provide warmth, and assist in recovery. |
| Elevate the involved part. | Elevation will decrease any edema that may occur. |

For greater than first-degree frostbite) Remove the person from the source of cold.

Prevents further damage to the involved parts.

Support and protect the involved part; seek consultation from a health professional.

Anything beyond first degree frostbite may require further treatment and follow-up. Proper care must be taken to ensure that secondary infection of any blisters is prevented and that any other underlying problems, such as gangrene, are treated.

| What Not to Do | Why |
| --- | --- |
| Do not rub anything on the involved area, such as snow or towels, or in any way cause friction. | Friction will cause further damage to the skin and underlying tissue. Instead of increasing warmth, friction causes more damage. |
| Do not place the involved part in water warmer than 110 degrees. | Temperatures greater than 110 degrees will also cause damage to the skin and tissue, including burns. |

## Heat-Related Conditions

Heat-related problems can occur almost any time. Hot weather combined with high humidity places many people at risk for heat-related problems. This risk is further increased by physical activity, especially if the person is not well conditioned. Other factors that increase risk include (1) some forms of chronic illness, (2) dehydration caused by excessive alcohol consumption, and (3) lack of access to nonalcoholic fluids.

### Heat Edema

*Heat edema* refers to the swelling that occurs in the legs after a person remains standing for prolonged periods in the heat. During hot weather, blood flows through blood vessels that have expanded in an effort to move blood to the skin surface in order to cool it. Blood return, especially from the legs, slows and causes the edema.

| What to Do | Why |
| --- | --- |
| Allow the person to elevate his or her legs. | Elevation assists in removing excess blood from the legs thus decreasing the edema. |
| Provide cool fluids. | Extreme heat and humidity lead to the possibility of dehydration. Providing cool drinks helps to prevent excessive fluid loss and assists in body cooling. |

*Heat Syncope*

*Heat syncope* or *fainting* occurs for much the same reason. Blood flows to the skin surface in an attempt to be cooled, thus pulling blood from the core, especially the brain. When this happens, the person faints.

| What to Do | Why |
|---|---|
| If the person has fallen, allow him or her to remain on the floor. | Keeping the person flat allows the blood to flow to the head. |
| Loosen any tight clothing. | Assists in circulation. |
| Elevate the person's legs to a level above the chest. | Allows the blood to flow from the extremities to the head. |
| Allow the person to remain flat for several minutes before getting up. | Allows time for the body to stabilize. |
| Provide cool fluids and, if possible, a cool environment for as long as possible. | Cool fluids replace lost body fluids and assist in stabilizing the body; cool environment assists in further cooling of the body. |

*Heat Exhaustion*

*Heat exhaustion* is usually the result of exposure to hot humid weather and too little fluid intake. Body temperature will increase to as much as 103 to 106 degrees, resulting in dizziness, headache, nausea, and possibly some minor mental status changes. Usually the skin is warm and moist to the touch.

| What to Do | Why |
|---|---|
| Provide a cool environment where it is possible for the person to rest. | Rest decreases the body's production of heat. A cool environment assists in the body's cooling process. |
| If there is no nausea or vomiting, provide cool fluids. | Cool fluids replace lost body fluids and assist in cooling. |
| If there are no health professionals on site, transport the person to the nearest hospital. | It is sometimes difficult to distinguish between heat exhaustion and heat stroke. It is best if the person is evaluated by professionals. |

| What Not to Do | Why |
|---|---|
| Do not give fluids if the person is nauseated or vomiting. | Under these circumstances, fluids will probably cause vomiting. |

*Heat Stroke*

*Heat stroke* is a condition in which the body temperature goes too high (over 105 degrees). This results in a state of mental confusion and the person no longer sweats. The ability to sweat is critical for normal body cooling. When sweating stops, as in heat stroke, the body temperature can climb very rapidly to extremely high levels. Prolonged exposure to such high temperatures is life threatening. Heat stroke is an emergency which must be responded to at once. Heat stroke is most commonly associated with physical exercise in hot, humid weather. Other factors can increase this risk, such as alcohol consumption, certain heart medications, drugs used in the treatment of mental illness, tranquilizers, diuretics, cocaine, malnutrition, chronic skin disorders, and Parkinson's disease.

| What to Do | Why |
| --- | --- |
| Call an ambulance and get the person to a hospital as quickly as possible. | This is a life-threatening emergency. Quick action is required to prevent death and/or permanent damage to vital organs. |
| If possible, it would be helpful to call the emergency room and seek specific instructions while waiting for the ambulance. | Specific instructions will allow you to safely begin treatment of the person while waiting for the ambulance. |
| While waiting for the ambulance or while in transit, remove all excess clothing from the person and maintain as cool an environment as possible. | It is essential to cool the person's body as quickly as possible. |

| What Not to Do | Why |
| --- | --- |
| Do not delay seeking treatment. When in doubt, always err on the side of treatment. | The longer the person's extremely high temperature continues, the greater the risk of permanent damage or death. |

## Grand Mal Seizures

Seizures are among the most frequently occurring health problems among people who are homeless. All shelter staff should be prepared to provide support and assistance during a seizure. It is only a matter of time before staff will be called upon to respond.

Seizures have a variety of causes, from brain tumors to epilepsy to alcohol. Regardless of the cause, a seizure is brought on by a "misfiring" of electrical impulses in the brain. People who experience seizures because of alcohol usually do so when their alcohol intake is considerably reduced from their "normal" amount (typically, for a 2- to 3-day period).

### Symptoms of Seizures

*Auras.*   Sometimes people know a few minutes before that they are about to have a seizure. An *aura* is an unusual or "out of place" sensation that is almost always followed by a seizure. Auras are often a vague feeling, but can also be a particular smell, sound, taste, or light that is not really present in the environment.

*Severe Muscle Spasms.*   A spasm is usually a severe jerking movement throughout the entire body. The jaw will clamp shut, the head may strike the floor as the person falls, the arms and legs will move in a jerking motion, and the body may arch. All of these movements may be very powerful and difficult or impossible to control. Attempts to hold the person may lead to severe damage to both the person and to the helper.

*Loss of Consciousness.*   Persons having a seizure are unable to respond to other people. They cannot answer questions or talk during the seizure. Their eyes may roll back, and they may lose control of their bladder and bowel and become incontinent. Unconsciousness may continue for several seconds to several minutes. In general, anyone whose seizure lasts for longer than 5 minutes, or who has breathing difficulty, should be transported to the hospital as quickly as possible.

*Postictal Phase.*   This is the time immediately following the seizure during which the person may be confused, sleepy and have a slight fever. During this time, the person may babble and appear incoherent, give nonsense answers to simple questions, or just sleep. The confusion should clear within a few minutes. The sleepiness will disappear after a nap and fever will resolve quickly. If this fails to happen, the person needs to be seen at the nearest hospital or clinic.

In general, people experiencing their first seizure should be evaluated to determine the cause. Usually, this means transporting the person to the hospital as soon as possible. Some shelters prefer to send all people to the hospital following a seizure; others do not. Each shelter should establish a policy to deal with these situations.

| What to Do | Why |
| --- | --- |
| Turn the person on his or her side. If unable to do so, turn the person's head to the side. | Allows saliva and possibly vomitus to drain. Also prevents fluids from getting into the lungs and causing breathing difficulties. |
| Clear surrounding area of potentially dangerous objects, such as furniture or sharp objects. | Provides a safe place for the seizure victim and decreases the possibility of injury during seizure activity. |

Monitor the person's breathing throughout the seizure; time the seizure.

Important for determining best course of action.

After the seizure, allow the person to rest and provide as much privacy as possible.

Allows the person time for privacy and recovery.

Monitor the person to determine that the postictal phase has passed.

Monitoring allows you to determine that the person has returned to the preseizure state. If this fails to occur, the person needs to be evaluated.

### What Not to Do

### Why

Never try to force anything into the person's mouth.

Trying to force something into the mouth can cause severe trauma to the jaw, tongue, and teeth, as well as to surrounding tissue. It is also possible for the helper to get hurt.

Do not try to put anything sharp or breakable into the person's mouth. Never put your fingers into the person's mouth.

During a seizure the tension and strength of all muscles is very great. Anything held between the teeth will be under tremendous pressure. Something that is sharp or that can break may cause severe trauma to the mouth, because the person is not able to control muscle movement.

Do not attempt to hold the person down.

It is almost impossible to subdue the person; the strength of jerking movements can cause bones to break and ligaments to tear, if restrained.

## Infectious Diseases

The world is filled with viruses, bacteria, fungi, and other so-called pathogens, but the human body can ward off literally thousands of such potentially harmful pathogens. Some of the body's ability to manage this feat is internalized and occurs largely without any conscious effort. However, what people do or fail to do can alter greatly their risk for exposure and illness from these pathogens.

Reducing exposure to harmful pathogens obviously can reduce the risk of illness, but such reduction can be difficult. Some infectious illnesses, hepatitis, for example, are most contagious during the time just before a victim shows any symptoms of the illness. For infection spread by body fluids, there is only one way to reduce risk: always assume that there is risk of infection and isolate any substance that is thought to be a body secretion. This concept is known as Body Secretion Isolation or BSI.

The idea is a simple one: if it is a body secretion, no matter what, no matter whose isolate it is, wear gloves. Such activities would include changing soiled linens, cleaning up after a person vomits, cleaning the bathrooms, handling bloody or soiled dressings from wounds, ulcers, or surgical procedures, or "patting" persons down while looking for contraband before admitting them to the shelter. When in doubt, *always* wear gloves!

There is a proper way to use and discard gloves in order to obtain maximum benefit. It is advised that shelters develop a policy on when and how to use gloves. Ask the local Department of Public Health for assistance in the development of such a policy and in the education of the shelter staff in the proper use of the gloves.

The remainder of this section presents some of the more commonly seen illnesses that are contagious. These illnesses can be transferred from one person to another through the air, by sharing contaminated items (utensils, dishes, etc.), or by exposure to infected body secretions.

## *Hepatitis*

There are many different types of hepatitis, both contagious (hepatitis A, hepatitis B, non-A and non-B viral hepatitis) and noncontagious (drug or alcoholic hepatitis, obstructive hepatitis, and hepatitis caused by toxins). This section will focus on the contagious forms of the disease.

Regardless of its cause, hepatitis affects the liver's ability to function properly. During an infection with hepatitis, the liver swells and is unable to function efficiently. This leads to poor digestion and clearance of toxins and waste by-products from the system.

*Hepatitis A*, sometimes called *infectious hepatitis*, is spread from one person to another by the so-called fecal-oral route. Improper hand-washing technique after contact with an infected person, or eating contaminated food or drinking contaminated fluids are the usual methods of transmission. Eating shellfish that has been exposed to inadequately treated sewer waste is a major cause of outbreaks of the illness. The peak periods of contagion is the 2-week period before the infected person becomes sick. Usually, the person stops being contagious about a week after the symptoms appear. The incubation period (the time between the point of exposure and the onset of symptoms) is usually 2 to 6 weeks.

*Hepatitis B*, sometimes called *serum hepatitis*, is spread by contact with a contagious person's body fluids, such as blood, semen, and saliva. A frequent method of transmission is the practice of sharing dirty needles by intravenous drug users (see Chapter 6). Other methods of transmission include unprotected sexual intercourse with an infected person, accidental exposure to needle sticks among health care workers, and childbirth by an infected mother (transmitting the disease to her baby). The sharing of toothbrushes, razors, and face cloths from someone who is infected has also been known to spread the infection. The incubation period for hepatitis B is usually between 2 and 6 months. Most people recover from hepatitis B. However, there is a diseased state during which the individual will become a chronic carrier of the virus. Carriers are capable of spreading the virus long after they apparently recover from the acute symptoms of the virus.

The symptoms of hepatitis, regardless of the type, are variable and can range from no obvious symptoms to sudden onset of severe symptoms leading quite rapidly to death. A frequent presentation may include several days of chills, headache, fatigue, loss of appetite, nausea and vomiting, and diarrhea. Smokers may notice a sudden distaste for cigarettes. There may be some upper right quadrant abdominal pain as the liver begins to swell. During this period, the person is contagious.

## Symptoms of Acute Hepatitis

*Skin and Eyes.*   Both the skin and whites of the eyes of the person with hepatitis may develop a yellow color.

*Lymph Nodes.*   If the person has acute hepatitis there may be swelling of the lymph nodes that are located in the neck.

*Urine and Stool.*   The urine of the person with hepatitis will become darker in color and the stool will become lighter.

*Liver.*   The liver of the person with hepatitis becomes enlarged and sometimes painful, and it is easily felt through the abdomen.

*Fatigue and Appetite.*   These symptoms vary greatly from person to person with some people experiencing profound fatigue for some time and others feeling hardly any fatigue at all. Appetite often returns within a week or two of the onset of acute symptoms.

In the usual course of the illness, all these symptoms gradually diminish and the person feels fairly recovered within 3 to 6 weeks of the onset of the symptoms.

| What to Do | Why |
|---|---|
| If you suspect hepatitis based on risk factors (e.g., needle-sharing, at-risk sexual contact, or other reasons) refer the person for evaluation. | Remember: hepatitis is most contagious during the time just before the onset of symptoms. Early diagnosis can assist in preventing the spread of the illness. |
| Always consider all body fluids or secretions contaminated. (Remember the concept of BSI.) | |
| Wear gloves when in contact with or at risk of being in contact with a person's body secretions. | Body fluid spills can be cleaned with a solution of one part household bleach to nine parts water. Linen that may be contaminated should be properly bagged and not left about the general area. All sheets should be |

stripped and washed each day unless the bed will be used by the same person each night and it is not soiled. Mattresses should be covered with a plastic cover which can be disinfected, as necessary. Use gloves whenever the task at hand may expose you to body fluids. Carry a pair of gloves with you.

Be familiar with and reinforce the health teaching regarding proper hand-washing and other techniques, such as not sharing razors, toothbrushes, etc., with others. Use these techniques yourself.

Following the diagnosis of hepatitis, the person will have been taught about hepatitis and how it is spread. Reinforcement of that education is important in order to ensure that the person follows the precautions as much as possible in order to limit the spread of the illness.

If the person is using drugs, strongly encourage him or her to stop at least during the time of acute symptoms.

During the acute phase, the liver is very limited in what it can do and is very vulnerable. Continuous exposures to drugs and infection from dirty needles and unpure substances can put the liver at great risk for further problems.

| What Not to Do | Why |
|---|---|
| Do not delay in getting the person into treatment. | The sooner the diagnosis is made, the sooner precautions can be taken to prevent the spread of the illness. |
| Do not deny the person shelter. | Although hepatitis is contagious, it can be managed, as has been described above. Casual contact is not a serious problem as long as the person follows the basic precautions described above. |
| Do not ignore indications that the person is not following through on precautions or follow-up appointments. | Most of the time, hepatitis will run a predictable course and will leave the person with little residual effect. There are times, however, when this is not the case. Proper follow-up is thus necessary. |

### Human Immunodeficiency Virus (HIV) and Acquired Immunodeficiency Syndrome (AIDS)

The Human Immunodeficiency Virus (HIV) works by attacking certain cells in the immune system, called *T4 lymphocyte cells*. T4 cells are a major factor in triggering the body's defense mechanisms against infections. Over time, the virus destroys so many T4 cells that the body can no longer mount a defense against infection. Thus, people with AIDS become ill and sometimes die from so-called opportunistic infections, such as *Pneumocystis carninii* pneumonia (PCP), toxoplasmosis, meningitis, tuberculosis, Hodgkin's disease, Karposi's sarcoma, and many others. Other problems, while not necessarily life-threatening, may cause difficulty in living from day to day, and include: dementia, fungus infections (candida) of the mouth, which makes it impossible to eat or swallow without pain; herpes; cryptosporidiosis, which causes diarrhea; cytomegalovirus (CVM), which almost half of the general population carries without symptoms, but which becomes active in people who are immunocompromised, resulting in fevers, weight loss, profound fatigue, and blindness; and a host of other infections.

Being infected with HIV does not mean that the person has AIDS. Many people who test positive for the virus remain healthy and without symptoms for years. Although it is necessary to have the virus in the body to contract AIDS, it does not necessarily mean that the person will progress rapidly to AIDS. The incubation period (the time between the establishment of the virus in the body and the onset of symptoms) can vary and may be as long as 10 years. Throughout that time, the person is able to pass the virus on to others through blood-to-blood contact, such as sharing dirty needles, as well as unprotected sexual intercourse, both heterosexual and homosexual. Children born to infected women are also at risk.

Because the incubation period can be so long, and people who are infected feel perfectly well, the numbers of people who are infected and do not know it may be very high. The Centers for Disease Control estimates that for every person who is infected and knows it there are between 6 and 7 people who are infected and do not yet know it. For this reason, it is crucial that service providers and health care workers make the assumption that all body secretions carry the potential of causing infection. It is not the person who tells you that he or she is infected who is the risk factor; instead, it is the person who does not know or has not told you and whom you do not suspect who places you at risk.

People with AIDS face a variety of problems that are due to exposure to everyday organisms that a healthy person can fight off. Homeless people who also have HIV infection or AIDS are especially vulnerable and are also without resources. Dealing with such problems as profound as fatigue, diarrhea, vision impairment, and dementia is simply not possible on the streets. Yet, because so many drug abusers are homeless and infected, this is exactly what they must try and do each day. (See Chapter 6, pp. 155–162, for a discussion of HIV/AIDS and drug abuse.)

Efforts are currently underway from a variety of agencies to offer health education programs about HIV infection. Because intravenous drug abuse is a major risk factor among homeless people, education programs have focused on preventing the spread of the virus through sharing of contaminated needles and safe sex practices. In a few cities, a clean needle exchange program for drug addicts has been implemented. Because this is a politically controversial subject, it is not a widespread practice in the United States. Other programs have provided addicts with information about cleaning their needles with bleach and water before sharing.

Providing people with free condoms, teaching safe sex practices, and providing bleach and small bottles for cleaning needles have become the mainstays of many programs serving homeless people. Missing from this effort is support at the public-policy level for treatment on demand and the funds and other resources to support it.

Because intensive research efforts on the AIDS epidemic are in progress worldwide, shelters and other programs serving homeless clients should establish close working relationships with their local board of health and their local hospitals so as to keep abreast of current developments. In any case, anyone who works with homeless clients should understand the basics of infection control.

| **What to Do** | **Why** |
| --- | --- |
| Isolate body secretions. | Isolating secretions prevents anyone else from accidental exposure. If it is a body secretion, isolate it. This should be an automatic response. Remember the concept of Body Secretion Isolation (BSI). |
| Wear gloves | Wear gloves at all times when at risk for exposure to body fluids. Not all body fluids carry HIV, but any body fluid which has blood in it can. Because it is impossible to predict when blood may be present, assume that it is and wear gloves. Ask the local board of health, hospital infection control nurse, or community health nurse for help in teaching the proper use of gloves. |
| Clean areas soiled with body secretion with a solution of bleach and water (1:9 ratio). Then clean the mop or other implement used with fresh bleach and water. | Bleach will kill the virus. A one-part bleach to nine-parts water solution is adequate. |
| Soiled dressings and linen should be properly disposed of and clearly marked for disposal. Soiled linen should be handled as little as possible. It should be placed directly in the proper receptacle and not left on the floor, chair, or bed. All bed linen should be cleaned so as to sterilize it. Use mattresses with plastic covers or with covers that can be washed with a bleach-water solution. | Linen or dressings from wounds soiled with body secretions can carry HIV. Proper handling of material prevents possible exposure. Linen or dressings placed on any surface before placement in a proper container can deposit secretions on that surface. Although it is unlikely that this is a route of contamination, caution should be used. Areas that may have been exposed can be cleaned with a bleach and water solution (1:9 ratio). |

| **What Not to Do** | **Why** |
|---|---|
| Do not assume that because a person does not seem to have any of the risk factors, you do not need to use precautions. | The CDC estimates that for every person who knows that they are infected, six to seven are and do not know it. Assume every body secretion is capable of spreading any number of infections from HIV to hepatitis and many others. Make no exceptions to this rule. |
| Do not isolate the person who is known to have HIV. | One has to work hard to contract HIV. It is not spread by casual contact between people. People with HIV infection have enough to deal with; they do not have to be needlessly isolated or shunned. Casual contact will not spread the virus. Using gloves when there is risk of exposure to body secretions is necessary and strongly encouraged. Using gloves otherwise is not going to make a difference in the spread of the virus and will make people feel unnecessarily isolated. |

*Tuberculosis*

Until the late 1940s and early 1950s, when the drugs isoniazid, streptomycin, and para-aminosalicylic were discovered there was no way outside of the body's normal defense mechanisms to treat tuberculosis (TB). With the advent of these drugs, however, TB could not only be treated, but could also be cured. As a result, the incidence of TB declined in the following decades.

In spite of pharmaceutical breakthroughs, TB remains active in certain subgroups of the population: the elderly, who were infected as children, but did not become active until later in life; immigrants from global areas where the disease is still a significant problem; substance abusers, initially alcoholics and later intravenous drug users, because of HIV infection; and the homeless. The homeless are included because of the number of substance abusers among them, their poor state of general health, and because of the often crowded conditions found in homeless shelters. Under normal living conditions, TB is only minimally contagious. Yet street living, crowded living quarters, poor nutrition, and the practice of sharing bottles among alcoholics are major factors that help to sustain TB among the homeless population. In addition, HIV-infected people are extremely susceptible to infection by TB, because their immune system cannot fight it off. TB is considered an opportunistic infection; as such, it is an emerging health problem for people with HIV infection. In some areas of the United States, as many as 25 percent of the new cases of active TB are found among people with HIV infection.

TB is spread by inhaling the tubercle bacillus (*mycobacterium tuberculosis*). The mere fact of breathing in the bacteria does not in itself mean that the person has TB. Most people who are exposed to TB never progress to developing the disease. Those who develop TB usually develop the problem in their lungs. Other places in the body where TB can become active include the lymph system, spleen, kidneys, and bone. Pulmonary TB is the form of the disease which can become contagious. Not everyone who develops TB is contagious and those who are can be successfully treated, thus stopping the spread of the bacteria. Once a person has been properly diagnosed and treatment has been under way for a sufficient period of time, he or she can return to the community without fear of contagion as long as medication and follow up treatment are continued. Treatment for TB is still a somewhat prolonged process, but the outcome for most people is successful recovery. A resistant strain of TB has recently appeared and may alter the rate of recovery.

TB testing is an effective and efficient way of identifying those who are in need of further assessment. It is imperative that a follow-up process be established prior to testing in order to assure adequate assessment and, if necessary, treatment for those who are found to have a positive test result.

Resources to assist with testing include the local board of health, the Visiting Nurse Association, area hospitals, schools of nursing and medicine, and local chapters of professional organizations, such as the Nurses' Association and the Medical Society.

Some shelters have installed ultraviolet (UV) lighting in areas of high use. There is some evidence suggesting that UV lighting kills the TB bacterium. However, these data are inconclusive. UV lights are expensive and need to be changed once a year. In addition, they must remain on all night, even in the sleeping areas. A check with the Board of Health or the infection control department of the local hospital should be made for recommendations.

### Symptoms of Tuberculosis

The classic symptoms of pulmonary TB include persistent cough, sometimes blood-tinged, sometimes shortness of breath, night sweats, weight loss, and fatigue. Any person with one or more of these symptoms should be seen and tested.

| What to Do | Why |
| --- | --- |
| Because TB is sometimes a quiet illness with subtle symptoms, routine monitoring and testing is a must. Staff and volunteers (if possible) should be tested prior to beginning work and every 3 to 6 months thereafter. | Testing new employees and volunteers as they begin their work establishes a baseline for further testing, and determines current TB status. Periodic testing provides a mechanism for ongoing and case finding and follow-up, as well as protecting those working in the shelter. |

Guests should be tested on a regular basis. Check the local board of health for recommendations specific to the community.

The population in the shelter should be tested on a regular basis. Shelters with established clinics may test on an ongoing basis, as guests come into the clinic, or they may choose to run TB clinics and systematically test everyone at once. Shelters without such clinical services can enlist the help of a variety of health professionals.

Provide adequate space between beds in the sleeping areas of shelters. Check with the local board of health for recommendations. Consider 3 feet a minimum requirement.

Because TB is spread by airborne droplets, the greater the distance between people, the less likely the infection will spread.

Ensure good ventilation in common areas and other areas where people congregate over time.

Good ventilation increases the flow of air out of the room and decreases the possibility that airborne bacteria will cause infection.

## Infestations

Such infestations as scabies and pediculosis (often called *bugs*) are widespread among people who are homeless. As anyone with school-aged children knows, these problems are not a result of poor hygiene, as much as they are problems of contact with infested skin, clothes, or hair.

### Scabies

*Scabies* is a common contagious disease of the skin that is caused by a mite. These mites burrow into the skin and leave pimplelike irritations or burrows as they go. The mite transfers from one person to another by direct skin-to-skin contact. Fortunately, the mite is not able to live long away from human contact, so transmission from clothes, bedding, or other surfaces occurs only if contact by an uninfested person is made immediately following contact by an infested person.

### Symptoms of Scabies Infestations

*Skin.*   Intense itching, which is most noticeable at night, is the first sign of scabies infestation. The areas most affected include the webbing between the fingers, and around the wrists, elbows, waist, thighs, genitals, breasts, lower buttocks, and under the arms.

*Incubation Period.*   Without previous exposure, it can take between 2 and 6 weeks to develop symptoms of scabies infestation. After the first exposure, symptoms may appear within 4 days. The period of contagion will continue until the person is adequately treated.

*Treatment.* Skin lotions for scabies infestation contain lindane or crotamiton and are obtained only by prescription. The lotion should be applied to the entire body except the head and neck and left on for 8 hours. After that, the person should take a shower or bath, being sure to remove all traces of the lotion. If symptoms persist, the treatment can be repeated in a week. It is not unusual for some amount of itching to continue for a time following treatment. Care should be taken not to confuse normal posttreatment itching with reinfestation.

| What to Do | Why |
|---|---|
| Observe the person for indications of infestations, such as scratching, burrows, or tracks of pimplelike eruptions between the fingers, elbows, wrists, etc. | Quick identification and treatment are vital in order to avoid infestation of others and minimize symptoms for the person involved. |
| Refer the infected person for assessment and treatment. | The diagnosis and treatment of scabies must be done by professionals because the treatments can cause serious side effects if not prescribed properly. Indiscriminate distribution of these medications can cause serious consequences which cannot be reversed. |
| Wear gloves if handling the clothes and personal belongings of a person with an infestation. | Spread of scabies is caused by direct skin-to-skin contact or by contact with mites in clothing. |
| All clothing and linen of the infested person should be removed and replaced following treatment. | Reusing infested linen or clothing will only reinfest the person. |
| The bed should be washed down with a disinfectant and not used for at least 2 days. | Washing the bed with a disinfectant will clean the bed, but may not kill the mites. Denying the mites access to a body for 2 days will kill them. Isolate the bed. |

| What Not to Do | Why |
|---|---|
| Do not use treatments without proper approval and instruction. | Treatment for scabies can cause dangerous side effects if not used properly and under the right circumstances. |
| Do not re-treat the person without clear evidence that the infestation has failed to clear. | Unnecessary retreatment can be harmful. |

## Pediculosis

*Pediculosis* is an infestation of lice in the hairy parts of the body or in clothing. There are different types of lice: *head lice* are located on the scalp; *crab lice* in the pubic area; and *body lice* along the seams of clothing next to the skin.

With the exception of body lice, infestations of pediculosis are not an indication of poor hygiene, but rather are the result of direct contact with an already infested person. Body lice can be attributed in part to crowded living conditions with infrequent opportunities to wash clothes or to get clean clothes.

Transmission of lice from one person to another is by direct contact. Head lice can be transmitted by sharing combs and brushes, as well as by sharing a pillow or other close contact. Body lice can be acquired by sharing clothing. Crab lice are most often transmitted during sexual contact.

## Symptoms of Lice Infestation

*Skin.*    Itching is the hallmark of pediculosis. Persistent itching should result in an examination which will reveal the presence of louse eggs or nits attached to individual hairs. Body lice can be spotted in the seams of clothing. Itching can get so intense that the skin breaks down, sometimes causing severe secondary bacterial infections which must also be treated.

*Incubation Period.*    It can sometimes take as long as 2 weeks for the infestation to develop to the point where it is noticeable. The person will remain contagious as long as the lice or eggs are alive.

*Treatment.*    Treatment of lice infestation consists of the application of medicated shampoos and creams. Some of the treatments can be purchased over the counter, but those containing lindane require a prescription. Lindane is not recommended for infants and young children; neither is it recommended for pregnant or nursing mothers. A repeat treatment should occur 7 to 10 days after the first to assure that no eggs have survived. The hair can be combed with a fine-tooth comb to remove any remaining nits.

| What to Do | Why |
|---|---|
| Observe the person for persistent itching and refer him or her for assessment and treatment. | Early detection will prevent the spread of infestations and assist the person in getting early treatment. |
| Wash all linen and, if possible, any clothing in hot water (130 degrees for 20 minutes). Clothes that cannot be washed can be heated in a dryer for 20 minutes. | Heat will kill the lice. |

| | |
|---|---|
| The bed should be disinfected and isolated for several days. | Lice cannot live for long without a host. A bed that is used again the same night may contribute to the spread of infestation. |

| **What Not to Do** | **Why** |
|---|---|
| Do not retreat without reassessing the person for continued infestations. | Treatments for lice contain substances that can be harmful if not used correctly. The side effects are potentially dangerous and some are not reversible. |

## SHELTERS AS SITES FOR DELIVERING HEALTH CARE SERVICES

Historically, shelters were not designed, funded, or identified as health care institutions. Nonetheless, the shortage of health care facilities serving indigent persons and the special difficulties that homeless persons encounter when using traditional health care services have led many shelters to enter the health care business. Most shelters offer basic first aid and some health screening; others offer substantially more.

Because their guests are exposed daily to conditions associated with illness and injury, shelter health clinics that offer routine health care services are invaluable. Shelter-based clinics range in structure from a nursing station in one corner of a shelter to fully equipped clinics staffed by full-time health care professionals. A nurse on-site, a clinic with basic supplies, and a visiting physician are reasonable goals for some shelters. In the absence of such a clinic, close relations are needed with a local hospital or visiting health care team. Provision should be made for staff to help guests maintain a schedule for taking prescribed medication and ensure that clinical evaluations occur when shelter guests appear to need them.

An ounce of prevention is worth every bit as much with homeless persons as it is with those who are housed. Health care crises disrupt shelter functioning and require inordinate amounts of resources. Providing routine checkups and maintaining patient records will help to reduce the incidence of such crises. Accompanying shelter guests on visits to hospitals or other off-site health care facilities should help to ensure that the care needed is obtained. Preventive care is even more important with expectant mothers; a connection with a prenatal clinic is essential (Brickner and Scanlan, 1990).

The catalyst for many shelter-based clinics has been the Health Care for the Homeless project established by the Robert Wood Johnson Foundation and the Pew Memorial Trust. Health Care for the Homeless became one of the most innovative and effective programs targeted for homeless persons on a national basis (Brickner et al., 1990). The two foundations designed the program to address directly the impediments to provision of health care to the homeless. Each local program was required to use locations for health care delivery where as many homeless persons could be served as possible; service teams were expected to include physicians,

---

*Panel 7–1*

**Nashville's Health Care for the Homeless Program**

Nashville's Health Care for the Homeless Program established the Downtown Clinic between two large shelters in the city's skid row district. Clinic staff included a medical director, a physician's assistant, family nurse clinicians, case managers, and mental health specialists. In addition to referrals from other service providers and by word of mouth, cases were to be garnered through outreach workers in other locations. Services were to include physical examinations, medical consultation for a runaway youth shelter, mental health and social services (Somers, Rimel, Shmavonian, Waxman, Reyes, Webido, and Brickner, 1990).

---

nurses, and social workers; service coordinators and mechanisms for making service referrals were encouraged; and welfare and housing agency representatives had to be included among the program sponsors.

Perhaps most importantly, cities were limited to only one application. All potential applicants within a city had to collaborate as part of a local coalition, including the mayor and representatives of religious groups, as well as representatives of public and private nonprofit groups. Nineteen cities were chosen after a competitive review.

Boston's Stabilization Services for Homeless Substance Abusers project, funded by the National Institute of Alcohol Abuse and Alcoholism Community Demonstration Program, also showed that it is possible to deliver effective health services to guests who are in residence at shelters. The project provided extensive recovery services for randomly selected shelter guests, all of whom had histories of alcohol and/or other drug problems. The project demonstrated that despite histories of multiple addictions and prior treatment, lack of social and economic supports, and psychiatric problems, many homeless clients can be stabilized by providing intensive services in shelter settings (McCarty et al., 1990).

*Respite beds* are an important component of a comprehensive clinical services program and can be used to enhance health care in many shelters. Essentially, respite beds are set aside in the shelter for persons recovering from some type of illness. Usually, these beds are in one area within the shelter. Persons allotted a respite bed typically are allowed to keep the same bed as long as they are ill and can remain in the shelter during the day. In addition, they receive more comprehensive care, including nurse practitioner and physician visits. Providing this modicum of stability in the otherwise chaotic life of homeless persons can substantially improve the recovery process, but because of the illnesses involved, more support also is needed (Goetcheus, Gleason, Sarson, Bennett, and Wolfe, 1990).

The necessary support arrangements for persons in shelter respite beds include help with obtaining and taking prescribed medications and regular visits from clinical personnel. A shelter-based respite unit also must develop clear policies concerning admission and discharge. There should be a clear understanding with local hospitals about the type of patients who are appropriate for the respite unit so as not to tax unreasonably the shelter's resources and to discourage hospitals from rushing their indigent patients too quickly to the shelter. Support services also must be planned to facilitate the discharge process and to aid discharged respite guests to adjust to a new schedule and to new surroundings (Goetcheus et al., 1990).

While making health care and ancillary services available in shelters is critical, it is not enough. Too many homeless persons neglect basic health care needs because of overriding problems with substance abuse, mental illness, or immediate survival. Aggressive outreach may be required to make homeless persons, even shelter users, aware of health care facilities and convince them of the benevolence of those who provide the health care. It was the commitment of Health Care for the Homeless teams to set up clinics within shelters, rather than waiting for homeless persons to come to off-site hospitals or clinics, that made the HCH approach so successful. Within shelters, an outreach-oriented approach also is necessary to maximize success.

An outreach mentality should pervade the approach of those staff members who provide health care for persons with physical as well as mental problems (see Chapter 4) who are in shelters (Wobido et al., 1990). Health care workers should be prepared to offer services in different ways to different guests, respecting a desire to withhold information or to refuse care entirely, except in emergencies, and yet continuing to build a relationship through low-demand contacts—saying hello, checking on how people are doing, asking about the quality of the food.

## CONCLUSIONS

Many basic issues of health care need to be addressed by the shelter community. Infectious diseases, such as tuberculosis, hepatitis, lice and other infestations, herpes and the so-called childhood illnesses, such as measles, mumps, and chicken pox are public health issues that every shelter, both adult and family, will face. In addition, health issues secondary to drug abuse and alcoholism will be prevalent.

HIV infection is rapidly becoming a major health issue for the homeless population. In fact, some reports estimate that as many as one third of the homeless population are HIV-positive. Therefore, it is important that the shelter community be aware of these issues and be prepared to address them within their own facility. The first step in addressing these issues is a sound knowledge base.

Health problems function as both antecedents and consequences of homelessness. Evidence from health care studies and clinical observations point to substantially higher morbidity rates among homeless people, compared to other populations. Thus, responding to the health care needs of the homeless should be seen as a cornerstone of policy and human service solutions to the crisis of homelessness. Yet, while homeless persons' health care needs are acute, it is not easy to separate health care from other urgent survival needs—income, employment, and housing, in particular. For this reason, it is vital that health care and treatment providers integrate as closely as possible the provision of health services with the other segments of the local service network—the Health Care for the Homeless approach. Shelters can play a critical role in linking homeless people with health care opportunities and in providing directly essential emergency services.

---

*Panel 7–2*

## The Case of Dwayne

When Dwayne was 12 years old, he saw his father gunned down as he stood beside him. The victim of a robbery, the father died while cradled in his son's arms. Because he believed that men don't cry, Dwayne stuffed his feelings of anger, fear, and grief. Not until many years later did Dwayne admit to crying. Dwayne described his father as a self-made success. A retired merchant marine, who had built a successful business for himself and his family after his retirement, he was everything young Dwayne wanted to be. Dwayne missed him terribly. It was shortly after his father's murder that Dwayne began to drink. He found that the effect of alcohol helped him to deal with his pain. Because he continued to deny his emotions over his father's death, he never had the opportunity to get out the anger, pain, and grief that was eating at him inside.

By the time he was 15, Dwayne had added marijuana to his alcohol use. During his junior year in high school, he discovered cocaine and was soon totally overcome by his addiction. He was expelled from school before Thanksgiving of his junior year, later to be arrested for possession and driving under the influence. Because it was his first offense, he was released with a sentence of supervised community service. In the months and years that followed, Dwayne was arrested several more times, and later sent to prison. Prior to incarceration, he survived being shot at because of money he owed a drug dealer, underwent multiple hospitalizations for several drug overdoses, and ended up living on the streets. In spite of all of this, his life did not collapse until the day he was told he was no longer welcome at his mother's home. That day was the turning

---

*Panel 7–2*   (Continued)

point. As he stood on the porch that afternoon, Dwayne realized that he had nothing and no one left in his life. He had to get his life under control.

Although he had been in several detoxification programs, Dwayne had not been ready to get straight. Admission to detox centers were little more than efforts to bring his habit under control and to decrease the amount of drug he needed each day. But this time, things were different; he had nowhere else to go.

Dwayne went through a public detox program. On the next to the last day, he was asked if he wanted to participate in an experimental project, called the Stabilization Services Program. Dwayne agreed. He arrived at Boston's Long Island Shelter for the Homeless the next day. Tall at 6 feet 5 inches and thin at 135 pounds, Dwayne showed the physical results of years of drug abuse and living on the streets. He was apprehensive and nervous, especially when he realized that the shelter was not "dry," that is, shelter guests were often under the influence of one or more substances. On the other hand, Dwayne was desperate—he'd try anything to get his life back. His entry into the program was tenuous at first, but he soon found himself speaking out at the meetings and sharing things about his life as a drug abuser that he had never told anyone before. To his surprise, no one was judgmental about his self-disclosures; this gave him the courage to become more open. For the first time, Dwayne shared his hurt and grief about his father, crying openly; when he looked up at the others in the group, he saw many of them were also crying. When the meeting was over, the entire group gathered around him and just held him for several minutes. It was like a huge weight had been lifted from him. Following this emotional meeting, Dwayne began to seriously address his addiction. He stayed with the program for about 8 weeks, then moved on to a 6-month halfway house where he continued to do well.

Dwayne got a job working with disadvantaged youth in some of the toughest housing projects in the city. He frequently returns to the shelter to put on meetings with the current residents of the program. On occasion, he brings a group of "his kids" to the shelter so that they can talk to the program residents. Many of the kids actually know some of the residents. It is a powerful experience watching struggling addicts and alcoholics tell these kids their stories. Invariably, they describe the experience as being among the toughest but most rewarding experiences at the shelter.

Most recently, Dwayne became engaged. The wedding will be just before Thanksgiving. This year Thanksgiving for the whole family will be at Dwayne's.

*Panel 7–3*

## A Shelter Report on Jane

She was one of those people who easily disappeared into a crowd. Quiet and nondescript, she came and went in the shelter without too much notice being paid to her. If approached, she would say a few words, but beyond that she would pull back. If pushed to interact with others, she would become anxious and hostile. Most of the other guests, as well as the staff, soon learned to keep their distance. On a few occasions, a psychiatric clinical nurse specialist attempted to establish a relationship, but Jane would not allow it. Rather than make it too uncomfortable for her and because there did not seem to be any acute problems, Jane was left to herself.

One day the triage nurse noticed a small amount of discharge coming from Jane's right eye. From a distance it appeared that she may have had a common problem known as conjunctivitis. Jane would not allow any close-up examination, however, so the assessment was literally done from 10 feet away. For 4 days, the staff gently suggested that Jane allow an examination. Each day she refused. By the fourth day when the eye had not im-

proved, the staff approached her with greater urgency. Jane would not allow any close examination and denied that there was any problem, pain, or loss of vision. She threatened to leave "for good" if the staff persisted in trying to examine her. It was noted, however, that she was not able to open the eye. On the fifth day, discharge from the eye was much worse and had changed in character. It was clear that the situation was deteriorating. The decision was made to seek care for Jane and the plan was to transport Jane against her wishes for both physical and psychiatric examination.

Physical examination revealed that Jane had developed a corneal abrasion (a scratch or small cut on the cornea of the eye), which developed into an ulcer. Because there had not been any treatment, the ulcer had continued to develop until it finally got so deep that it went all the way through the inside part of her eye. The change in the character of the discharge occurred because the fluid from the inside of the eye (the aqueous humor) had begun to leak out. Jane was immediately admitted to the hospital against her will. Ini-

*Panel 7–3*   (Continued)

tially, Jane refused all treatment, fought and threatened the nursing and medical staffs, and even tried to leave the hospital. She was evaluated by a psychiatrist who deemed her incompetent to care for herself and treated her with Haldol and Cogentin in order to manager her behavior. She was treated for her eye infection with intravenous antibiotics and a variety of eye drops. Her vision could not be saved because of the extent of the ulcer. The goal of the treatment was to save the eye itself.

Following several days of treatment during which Jane's eye and her behavior improved, she was discharged back to the shelter. One of the shelter nurses had visited Jane during her hospitalization and had participated in her treatment plan so that the shelter nursing staff felt prepared to provide her care. In addition, Jane began to respond to the nurse, seeing her as a friend and protector. Jane agreed to continue her treatments at the shelter and to the schedule of follow-up appointments that had been arranged.

Upon her return to the shelter, Jane settled into a routine that revolved around her eye treatments. In order to positively reinforce her behavior, the nurses would immediately respond to her even if it meant asking the other guests to wait a little longer. Jane also continued to take her Haldol and Cogentin. The difference in her ability to interact was profound. We were at last able to get to know her and what we found was an intelligent, thoughtful, humorous woman.

Follow-up with the hospital soon revealed that Jane had progressed well. The eye would be saved and she would be a candidate for a corneal transplant. Although she is apprehensive about the surgery, Jane is excited about the possibility of once again seeing with that eye. If all goes well and Jane agrees to continue with the Haldol and Cogentin following surgery, it is our belief that we may be able to help her get off the streets. We realize, however, that this part of the plan must proceed slowly. We have helped Jane to establish a place where she feels safe and secure. We must now work carefully to transfer those feelings to another place where she can be off the streets, supported and integrated into some type of community that will care for her.

# Housing: From Street, to Shelter, to _____?

Friedner D. Wittman

The problem of homelessness begins with an insufficient supply of accessible housing. Obvious as this fact may seem to those working in the shelter system, policy-makers and service providers often do not pay enough attention to housing issues. As a result, shelter workers often are unable to do as much as they would like to meet homeless persons' housing needs. But there are many steps that shelters can take to help improve homeless persons' housing opportunities.

## INTRODUCTION

Improving homeless persons' housing opportunities also requires some understanding of the housing types that different homeless persons may need. Persons who suffer from mental illness, alcohol, and other drug problems may require social and medical services in their residence, whereas others need only affordable independent housing; institutional care may be required by a small proportion. So this chapter will begin with a review of these housing types.

None of these housing types represents a new approach to housing the poor; each has a long history of application. Rather, what was different in the 1980s was the decline in availability of these housing types. Since restoring the affordable housing stock ultimately is the focus of efforts to house the homeless, we will review in some detail the historical factors that seemed to result in the current housing deficit.

Of course, in the final analysis, it is neither knowledge of housing alternatives nor of historical vagaries that improves housing for homeless persons; it is actions by shelters, their staff, and other advocates to develop new housing and to place their guests in available housing. Some shelters have begun to develop housing for their guests, some employ special staff to help their guests locate housing, and many advocate vigorously in their local communities for more affordable housing programs. The last section of this chapter will examine such techniques.

## DIFFERENT HOUSING TYPES

More housing at an affordable price must be the first concern of those who seek to improve housing opportunities for homeless persons. But among the homeless population are some who need a more supported form of housing, and a small proportion who cannot always manage outside of institutions.

### Conventional Housing

Conventional housing consists of apartments and family dwellings for people living independently. Conventional housing has self-contained living units for each occupant (or group of occupants): bedroom(s), bathroom, kitchen, living/dining area (which may include sleeping areas for studio apartments).

Thus, low-income housing can occur in all types of residential buildings—apartment houses, duplexes or other multifamily units, and single-family homes. According to the Fair Housing Act Amendments of 1988, low-income people, mentally ill people, and people recovering from alcohol or drug abuse problems can occupy such housing in any residentially zoned neighborhood in any community.

There is nothing "special" about this housing in its use by low-income people. As Tucker (1990) pointed out, "low-income" housing in most communities began life as middle-class housing and then has been redistributed when the original residents moved to new neighborhoods and the housing stock aged. Generally speaking, more than half of the homeless people in shelters need only such conventional housing, with adequate space, building systems that work properly, and a safe location that is well served by public transportation. Even most persons with physical or mental health problems, including those with alcohol and other drug problems, can live normally in conventional housing while receiving services from off-site sources.

### Single-Room Occupancy and Specialty Housing

Single-room occupancy (SRO) housing is designed specifically to accommodate single individuals as efficiently as possible. Specialty housing is designed to accommodate groups that do not fit readily into conventional housing, such as mothers with children who wish to share a residence, or group homes for people who are mentally ill. SRO and specialty housing achieve their efficiency by providing social, kitchen, bathroom, and utility areas that are shared among all residents. Lobbies, parlors, and management offices located near the main entrance provide for common use and ease of supervision.

### Physical Configuration

The SRO comes in two architectural varieties: the SRO hotel and the boarding house. Both configurations provide units (bedrooms) for a large number of people; as a result, special on-site management is required.

*The SRO Hotel.*   An SRO hotel contains many identical rooms, usually located along a corridor with the rooms on either side. Larger buildings have a number of wings, perhaps with several stories each. Usually, the bedrooms measure about 100 square feet in size, and the SRO hotel can range in size from a few rooms to several hundred. Rooms are almost always suitable only for single occupants, though management in some SROs may allow exceptions.

None of the bedrooms has its own kitchen, and usually the bedrooms do not have their own bathrooms (some SRO hotels may provide sinks in the room; others may provide a small bathroom). Residents obtain meals from nearby restaurants, or board is provided from a kitchen on the premises (with meals prepared by a cook or sometimes by the tenants themselves).

Usually, SRO hotels emphasize individual rather than communal living, and those who live successfully in SRO hotels are more likely to be working or to have a stable income, and less likely to have extensive health and social problems. But recent experiments with the use of SRO housing for people recovering from alcohol and other drug problems have led to innovations in the use of traditional SROs as facilities that support recovery.

*The Boarding House.*   The boarding house is usually a converted single-family residence in which bedrooms are leased to individual tenants. The organization and operation of the boarding house are the same as the SRO, but at a reduced scale. The architecture of the boarding house places greater emphasis on communal living, with a shared living room, dining room, kitchen, and utility areas. Usually, boarding houses accommodate from 3 or 4 to a maximum of about 20 residents.

Design changes are required in some cases when large traditional single-family homes are converted for shared use by unrelated individuals. Congregate living facilities, for example, generally require more social space and dining-room area than in a single-family home. Women with children will require large bedroom suites and special areas in which children can play. These design changes may seem of minor significance physically, but they are extremely important for the social and psychological well-being of the residents.

## Institutional Housing

Institutional housing is provided by the health care system—hospitals, mental hospitals, nursing homes—and, in a sense, by the correctional system—jails, prisons, prerelease halfway houses. The residents' day is managed by a formal

## Panel 8–1

## Arlington Hotel

The Arlington Hotel, an SRO with nearly 200 rooms, is a four-story building located in an area of downtown San Francisco that has long served transients. In May, 1985, the Arlington converted to an alcohol- and drug-free (ADF) residence. Since then, the Arlington has thrived both as a social community and as an economically viable hotel operation.

The need for an alcohol- and drug-free SRO emerged from deliberations in 1981 by a Mayor's Task Force on Public Inebriates for those living in San Francisco's Tenderloin and South-of-Market areas. The Task Force sought alternatives to the expensive and futile "revolving-door" system of shuttling alcoholics from the street, to the hospital detox ward, or to the jail drunk-tank, and then back to the street. The Task Force proposed ten SRO hotels be established as "islands of sobriety" for 1,000 public inebriates. The Arlington was the first such "island."

Several aspects of the Arlington's development were critical to its establishment as an alcohol- and drug-free SRO.

1. From the beginning, an agency capable of managing an ADF program in the Arlington was included on the development team. The development team for this financially complex and technically difficult remodeling project remained responsive throughout the development process to program concerns of the Arlington's operator, the St. Vincent de Paul Society of San Francisco. Accordingly, the development team never lost sight of the development objective to create effective ADF housing.

2. Architectural remodeling at the Arlington placed heavy emphasis on design to promote recovery from alcohol and other drug problems. Architectural design emphasized physical and psychological comfort (including generously sized bedrooms) and social arrangements to encourage mutual help among recovering residents. Seven living units of approximately 25 beds each were created by providing community kitchens and sitting areas. The design also emphasized security of the premises (controlled entrances to protect against theft and intrusions by nontenants) and dignity (high-quality fixtures and furnishings that would stand up to heavy use and would be easy to maintain and repair).

3. The Arlington was planned to be economically accessible to the tenants. Rent for each room varies between $232 and $275 per month. This compares favorably with the average San Francisco rental of $406 per month (1990 dollars).

4. The Arlington's management policy is explicit about alcohol and other drug use. Tenants, who must have 6 months sobriety to be admitted, sign a tenant agreement not to drink alcohol or to use other nonprescribed drugs either on or off the premises. Tenants also agree that they may be evicted if they violate the agreement. The architectural design for frequent contact among residents in the course of daily living and the operation of an active tenants' council both are critical to the agreement's effectiveness. Because it has resident support, the tenant agreement has been successful in a city that is noted nationally for its tenant protections.

5. It is a home for as long as one wants: with no fixed length of stay, the Arlington supports residents' recovery for as long as the resident wishes. Recovering tenants get along well with its "regular" apartment dwellers (many of whom lived at the Arlington prior to its conversion as an ADF residence).

(For a complete discussion of the Arlington, see Curtiss et al., 1991:85–94.)

*Panel 8–2*

## Hutchinson Place

Hutchinson Place provides one example of how the specialized needs of current subgroups of the homeless can challenge traditional thinking about "boarding house" facilities. Hutchinson Place is home for up to 20 women with babies and young children under 6 years of age. The women (and sometimes their children) are recovering from dependence on alcohol and other drugs, especially crack cocaine. All of the women have come to the program from the street, from crack houses, or from abusive settings. Most of them have never known a stable home. Their recovery from alcohol and other drug use is intimately connected to learning how to live an ordinary life free of drinking and drug use.

Hutchinson Place provides a recovery environment that includes architectural, interpersonal, and clinical settings within a single program. Hutchinson Place provides a 6- to 9-month residential setting where women can learn parenting skills, complete their basic education, receive counseling for interpersonal and alcohol/drug use problems, and learn basic household skills. The program, operated by the Philadelphia Diagnostic and Rehabilitation Center (DRC), received demonstration grant funding from the National Institute on Alcohol Abuse and Alcoholism (NIAAA) to create the program. NIAAA funding was provided from 1988 to 1991. A combination of local and state resources is expected to maintain the program after federal funding expires.

Architectural aspects of the Hutchinson Place program emphasize daily householding and parenting skills. Space for the residential facility, a converted warehouse, provides a warm, homelike atmosphere in ways that defy conventional thinking about family housing. The facility provides a private sleeping and dressing cubicle for each mother/child. All other spaces are shared, including utilities (bathrooms, laundry, kitchen) and three high-ceilinged social areas of about 2,500 square feet each (living area, dining area, children's play area). Oversized by conventional standards, the social areas work extremely well for up to 60 women and children participating in the program.

DRC views linkage of on-site support and off-site therapy as a critical part of the recovery process. Design of the Hutchinson Place setting provides ample opportunity for the women to develop personal and interpersonal skills, and to help each other work out their problems. Each woman has both a case manager at Hutchinson Place and a therapist at DRC's Women's Program at another location. Women work on their recovery through a combination of contacts with each other, attendance at AA, counseling, and participation in therapy at the Women's Program.

Hutchinson Place hums with activity during the day. Children are everywhere, cheerfully underfoot in the cavernous rooms, brightly skylit to make an indoor park. Activity swirls especially in the children's play area, where mothers, many of them just past childhood themselves, play with their children, chat with each other, or talk with their case managers. The smell of dinner cooking rises in the air, and the light changes as daylight plays between sun and shadow overhead. Sounds of laughter, excitement, and tears mix with the humid air of late summer. Children's posters for a house party seem at home on a warm, red, brick wall. Expressions are animated, eyes glisten. Everyone is safe here, getting on with life. It really does beat doing drugs.

(For a complete discussion of Hutchinson Place, see Curtiss et al., 1991:110–117. See also Comfort, Shipley, White, Griffith, Shandler, 1190:129–148.)

program and operated by certified staff who work in a licensed facility. This "housing" is not residential in character, and is not considered to be a residence under the usual residential land-use classifications of local zoning ordinances. Nevertheless, this housing represents part of the continuum of domiciliary facilities used by homeless people entering the shelter system, and so should be discussed here.

Only a small fraction of the homeless who are mentally ill or who have alcohol and other drug problems need to be institutionalized. Federally sponsored research by the National Institute of Mental Health (NIMH) and the NIAAA has found that most people with alcohol/other drug and mental health problems can live successfully in both conventional and SRO/specialty housing, *provided* the housing is appropriately managed and the resident is involved in off- or on-site treatment and recovery programs. If these provisos can be met, only those people need be institutionalized who are a danger to themselves or others, or who are so debilitated that they are incapable of taking care of their own daily needs— probably no more than 10 percent to 15 percent of the homeless population.

Theoretically, those homeless persons who can benefit from institutional care facilities are also those who are a danger to themselves or others, or who are so debilitated they cannot care for their own daily needs. Groups who are included in this definition are the brain-damaged or debilitated chronic public inebriate; the actively psychotic mentally ill; those with life-threatening injuries or physical ailments; and persons greatly at risk for such health or mental health problems, such as babies born to mothers who used drugs during pregnancy.

## PROBLEMS IN ACCESS TO HOUSING FOR LOW-INCOME PEOPLE

The accessibility of all types of housing for low-income people in the United States has eroded steadily for more than 30 years. Three interrelated forces have contributed to this housing shortfall.

### Decrease in the Supply of Affordable Housing

The supply of housing for low-income people has been shrinking since the early 1970s. Today the United States faces a shortfall of low-income housing estimated to be as high as 5 million units. Currently, two of every five very low-income households have no access to low-rent housing. In the next 15 years, up to one million more low-rent units could be lost as privately owned, publicly subsidized units are returned to the general housing market (Barbieri and Fricke, 1989).

The National Housing Act of 1949 promised to provide decent housing for all Americans, but it was clear by the 1960s that this promise had not been met; at that time, 12 million American families were living in substandard units (Hartman, 1967). An outpouring of studies, recommendations, and pilot programs stimulated the urban renewal programs, but this may have done little good for low-income people. Too often, viable low-income communities and residences have been destroyed rather than protected (Fried, 1963; Jacobs, 1961) or funding levels and public support have been insufficient to meet demonstrated levels of need (Hartman, 1983). Low-income housing was torn down or refurbished for other purposes, was not rebuilt, or was replaced with other low-income units. Even federal urban renewal funds designated specifically for low-income housing were often used inappropriately (Bauman, 1987).

## Problems with Public Housing

Public housing is housing which is constructed with public financing and is operated by public housing authorities. Generally, the creation of special (segregated) public housing projects has been neither a social nor an economic success. Where public housing has been provided for low-income people, critics have long observed that the housing's utility can be sharply reduced by insensitivity to the needs of low-income, ethnically distinct, and special-needs populations (Rainwater, 1973).

Over the years, large public housing projects have tended to perpetuate poverty, and some have been so difficult to live in that they have been destroyed (e.g., the infamous Pruitt-Igoe public housing project in St. Louis was eventually dynamited; see Rainwater, 1967). No large-scale public housing projects have been built in the past 15 years, and some communities have even stopped using the term *public housing project*. In recent years, public housing has been particularly hard-hit by drug-dealing and by the onslaught of a crime-oriented drug culture based on cocaine and heroine. Difficulties that are due to drugs are compounded by alcohol abuse, by inadequate social and health services, and by inadequate funds for maintenance and security.

In spite of these difficulties, large cities continue to operate considerable stocks of public housing built 20 and 30 years ago, and public housing authorities are struggling to make them better places to live. Some authorities have developed partnerships between public service agencies and tenants in order to reduce social and health problems (Ille, Lynn, and Wetzel, 1991). Even so, high levels of effort are required to create viable communities in the framework of these large-scale projects.

Dissatisfaction with large-scale public housing projects has influenced efforts to house homeless persons. In situations similar to those leading to the demolition of Pruitt-Igoe, the cities of New York and San Francisco in 1989–1990 stopped purchasing rooms from large "welfare hotels" that had been contracted to provide housing for homeless people who had nowhere else to go. The large old hotels, like the large public housing projects, proved too difficult to manage.

In spite of these problems with large-scale projects, many smaller public housing complexes are well designed and well maintained. Some private organizations that specialize in the management of housing for low-income people (such as Phipps Houses in New York City) have been able to limit the severity of alcohol and other drug problems and to provide some of the necessary social, educational, and health services. Usually, these organizations welcome strong referral relationships with shelters. The problem is that few such units are available and waiting lists often stretch for months or years.

## Community Resistance

Another major factor limiting low-income people's access to housing is resistance from neighbors and community groups who do not want low-income people or people with disabilities living near them. The NIMBY ("not in my backyard") syndrome expresses itself through denial of zoning-use permits and demonstrations against alcohol, drug, and mental health (ADM) service programs that seek to provide supportive housing. Despite federal polices that protect against discrimination and require that access be provided for the handicapped, many localities and states still impose restrictions that reduce access.

These experiences with housing make clear that homelessness is not due only to personal disabilities: our national housing system has failed its low-income citizens. The failure is a historical one that has ebbed and flowed since the nineteenth century (Bauman, 1987), and the 1980s were a particularly painful "ebb" period.

## Loss and Reemergence of SRO and Specialty Housing

The loss of SRO and specialty housing has been due in part to these general factors, but the history of SROs also reveals some unique influences.

### Early History of SROs

From the 1880s through the 1920s, SRO housing was respected as economically viable housing for blue-collar workers and laborers. Dozens of SROs often were located near transportation and manufacturing centers that needed unskilled and semiskilled laborers for work that varied seasonally and with economic cycles. SRO tenants, mostly single men, could come and go easily, and could live comfortably between jobs in the inexpensive housing. Other services (education, health care, recreation, and cultural activities) were readily available in the nearby city center.

Unemployment and labor unrest during the Great Depression of the 1930s eroded the economic base of the SRO, although the enormous housing dislocations during World War II produced a brief SRO resurgence. By the end of the war, new patterns of social and geographic mobility changed fundamentally the market for SRO housing. Poor people's movements from the south to the north and from the country to the city, stimulated by World War II's labor shortages, continued to increase. Increasingly, middle- and working-class families moved from the cities to the suburbs, aided by benefits available to returning war veterans.

SROs (and the central cities in which they were located) increasingly housed only poor (usually minority) populations. By the mid-1950s, SRO housing was associated in the public mind with multiple social ills: poverty, race problems, crime, prostitution, and alcohol and drug use. In some large SROs, hundreds of cubicles were packed in large rooms; topped by chicken wire, the cubicles frequently contained no more than a desk, mirror, and old bed. The worst were redolent with filth, noise, and vermin and were plagued by crime; urban renewers

---

*Panel 8–3*

**SRO Accommodations: The Best and the Worst**

In New York's Greenwich Hotel, 1,400 cubicles became a haven for chronic alcoholics, the impoverished elderly, and heroin addicts. "At night the hotel became a jungle in which the aged and disabled barricaded themselves in their rooms or were subject to assault" (Brickner et al., 1985:12). Unable to remain in the hotel during the day, its residents loitered outside, hustled passersby and wandered in the park.

On the other hand, New York's Dakota Hotel was quiet and clean; customers were recruited by the owner; staff developed personal relations with the guests while strictly enforcing behavioral rules. Long-term lodgers lived in the same cubicle for years; they drank, gambled, talked, and watched TV together (Bahr, 1973).

---

achieved widespread support for their elimination (Bahr, 1973:112–116). Other SROs, however, functioned as mini-agencies for social service.

Urban renewal plans in all major cities, which were drafted to meet funding requirements of new federal urban renewal and housing programs, identified the SRO and its neighborhood as substandard "blighted" areas to be demolished and rebuilt with conventional housing for family-oriented living. The Department of Housing and Urban Development's minimum property standards, set in 1973, exceeded the standards to which nearly all SROs had been built.

### Collapse of SROs as Viable Living Units

By 1962, transformation of the SRO population had become complete. Poor (largely African American) people now lived in inner-city areas and SROs housed increasing numbers of destitute families. Many psychiatric patients discharged from hospitals during the 1960s ended up in SROs instead of supervised living facilities. Older people, economically unable to move, stayed behind in retirement hotels that gradually filled up with younger, more aggressive, and sicker people.

By the 1970s, developers began looking to inner-city areas for growth possibilities as suburban expansion slowed and energy costs rose. The neighborhoods in which SROs were located became increasingly popular for redevelopment, or "gentrification," and pressure to remove SROs increased accordingly. Urban renewal authorities and developers discredited SRO residents as problematic and undesirable groups (often pointing to alcohol and drug use in cheap flophouses as exemplary of the whole class of facilities). Ownership turned over, management services declined, city/county programs for social, health, and mental health services retreated, and problems further magnified. SRO facilities became ripe for the picking—either for destruction for new projects, or for rehabilitation as apartments for new tenants who were able to afford rents in newly refurbished neighborhoods.

These pressures resulted in the virtual destruction of the low-income SRO housing stock between about 1960 and 1985. Very little replacement housing for low-income people was built in its place; housing that was built was generally economically and socially inaccessible to the former residents. New York City saw the number of SRO living units decrease from 127,000 in 1970 to 14,000 in 1983 (a decline of 89 percent); San Francisco lost one third of its SRO stock during the 1980s alone; 18 percent of Detroit's SROs were lost in just 2 years (Caton, 1990:14; Coalition for the Homeless, 1985). In Philadelphia, new housing built at Society Hill Towers was far out of reach economically for those who had been displaced to make way for it.

## The Supportive Residence: Reemergence of the SRO

In the early 1980s, as the homeless population rapidly grew, city planners and human service program providers began looking afresh at the now-maligned SRO, realizing that with strong management, it could efficiently be returned to service for its original purposes (Church, Galbreath, and Raubeson, 1985; Heckler, 1984; Heskin, 1987; Reyes, 1987). Some cities have begun to rebuild SROs as "service-enriched" or "assisted-living" facilities, in which local public health and welfare authorities create formal agreements with owner-operators of SROs to make sure that necessary human services and supports are provided (Curtiss et al., 1991). Slowly, the damage caused by the last 30 years of housing policies is being repaired.

The fate of boarding houses and women's residences has paralleled that of the SRO. For example, private rooming houses in Boston declined from over 1,000 to 37 from 1975 to 1985 (Fodor, 1985), and women's hotels virtually have disappeared. But in recent years, shared occupancy of residences by people recovering from alcohol and drug problems has increased, and numerous specialized residences for formerly homeless women have been opened. After nearly becoming extinct, these facilities have gained a new lease on life.

The growth of "Oxford Houses" provides one example of the renewed appeal of boarding houses. Oxford Houses are large, single-family residences rented by individuals who are recovering from alcohol and drug problems. Operating under a standard charter with a few rules, they provide a stable living environment for a wide variety of people who wish to live alcohol- and drug-free lives. Because all residents share rent payments, low-income people can live affordably in well-located, attractive, middle-class housing (Oxford House Service Board, 1988).

Originally begun by a group of tenants sharing a halfway house, over 100 Oxford Houses are now in operation in 23 states. The self-help principles of the Oxford House are being further explored and expanded to reach new groups who have alcohol and drug problems, such as the mentally ill and women with children. An Oxford House organization is now available to assist in the start-up of the houses, and federally financed state-level revolving loan programs are available to provide start-up funding to open an Oxford House (Oxford House Service Board, 1988). Additionally, a number of alcohol and other drug recovery programs are

## Panel 8–4

## Oxford House

Oxford House began in 1975, when recovering residents of a halfway house were informed that the county alcohol treatment program that had leased the house could no longer pay the rent. The residents decided among themselves to take over the lease. Over the next several months, they established a straightforward set of rules and selected officers to manager the house: pay your share of expenses and no drinking or drug use on or off the premises. Commonsense rules for living among others were also developed: help out with household chores and abide by common agreements about living in the house; and no violence or threats of violence. The founders also developed a democratic governance system in which the positions of house president, treasurer, and comptroller rotate among the residents at intervals no longer than 6 months.

This simple approach to operations has endured remarkably well over the past 15 years. Various experiments have been tried, with mixed results: mixed-sex occupancies do not seem to work, although single-sex residences of either sex work well; no-relapse policies work best; selection of new tenants should be controlled by an admissions committee composed of current tenants; and new Oxford Houses should include a veteran of another Oxford House for at least the first several weeks of the new house.

Because the residential housing stock that is needed is simply existing family housing (preferably large housing with several bedrooms, located in good neighborhoods), and because sharing of rental expenses makes many houses accessible that would otherwise be out of reach, the only real barriers to new Oxford Houses involve possible neighborhood resistance. Here the federal Fair Housing Act Amendments of 1988 provide protection against discrimination. The best strategy to avoid such resistance seems to be simply to move in, as any family would do, and take pains to be a good neighbor. Neighbors quickly realize that the Oxford House is a conventional setting for ordinary daily living.

Perhaps the most remarkable features of Oxford Houses are their ordinariness and their simplicity of operation. One Oxford House has been operating in Washington, D.C., for the past 14 years. The person who signed the lease 14 years ago has renewed it 7 times. Payments have always been on time, and the house members have never asked for help in taking care of their problems. The landlord has never had problems with the tenants, the neighbors, or the upkeep of the house. Yet this residence has taken in a wide variety of residents, ranging from inner-city youth to itinerant chronic drinkers, many of them straight from detoxification facilities or from the street. The house does have to deal with problem residents from time to time; members of the house have learned to take prompt action without fuss, according to the Oxford House's operating principles. (Argeriou et al., 1989; Oxford House Service Board, 1988; Ridlen et al., 1990).

exploring sponsorship and other forms of linkage between treatment/recovery services and long-term residence in alcohol- and drug-free settings (Argeriou, McCarty, and MacDonald, 1989; Ridlen, Asamoah, Edwards, and Zimmer, 1990).

SROs and other specialized facilities are in a period of resurgence because they fill an important niche in providing accommodation for groups of homeless people who require on-site security and facility management where they live. These groups include the elderly, women and children, and people with treatable alcohol, other drug, and mental health problems. People in these groups are able to do a great deal to care for themselves, but cannot live completely independently because of a combination of economic, health, and social problems.

Human service programs and housing developers working together have realized over the past decade that the best response to problems of the homeless is often a mixture of professional help and opportunity for people to take care of themselves. Safe housing managed by on-site managers, by peer-based approaches, or by some combination of the two, provides vital opportunities for homeless people to relearn the skills of independent living.

## Changes in Commitment Policies

Homeless people's access to institutional housing in the health care system also has been reduced in recent years. Since the early 1970s, access to hospitals has been limited by increasing demands on emergency and trauma facilities, by programs to divert people with drinking and other drug problems to detoxification and sobering facilities, and by the deinstitutionalization of care for public psychiatric patients.

Legislation to decriminalize drunkenness and to provide safeguards in commitment procedures of the mentally ill has sharply reduced the use of legal measures to put people with alcohol/drug problems or mental health problems involuntarily into secure facilities. Communities now routinely limit involuntary holds on people to a few hours or a few days; expensive and time-consuming hearings must be held to keep people for longer periods.

Reducing the use of hospitals has long been a goal of the health field, as has been a shift from mandatory commitment to voluntary treatment whenever possible for people with alcohol, other drug, and mental health problems. Early planning for these reductions and shifts was based on the presumption that community-based care would be available through outpatient, day-care, and sheltered housing programs. The hospitals and state institutions discharged patients, but, as described in Chapter 4, many of these patients were overlooked or turned away by the community care system.

Although opportunities for care of homeless persons in health care institutions have declined, opportunities for institutional "care" in prisons have increased dramatically—the number of incarcerated people in the United States rose from 344,000 to 674,000 between 1980 and 1989 (*New York Times*, September 11, 1989, A-2). Many homeless persons, including those who are mentally ill, spend time in correctional institutions. Nonetheless, decriminalization of simple drunkenness and low manpower levels in many police forces have reduced the frequency of incarceration for some portions of the homeless population.

## HELPING HOMELESS PEOPLE GAIN ACCESS TO HOUSING

Shelter workers can provide a great deal of help to homeless people who are seeking housing. Help can be given in three forms: by identifying the availability of low-income housing in the community, assisting shelter guests to seek housing, and advocating expanded availability of housing to meet the needs of the homeless.

### Identifying the Availability of Low-Income Housing

Shelters that know a great deal about their guests are in a unique position to link available housing to those homeless people who can most benefit from it. Shelters can inventory the housing available to low-income people in the community and can then match shelter guests to that housing.

Creation of the linkage begins by conducting an inventory of housing accessible to low-income people in the community. What housing resources does the community have to offer? Shelter workers may be surprised to find that this question has not been asked very thoroughly, and that a number of resources are available that have been overlooked or that have not been linked to the shelter system.

A *systematic* inventory will be needed. To be most useful, this inventory should be updated every day or so in order to identify the availability of a room at the time a shelter guest needs one. The job is a big one, and requires formal assignment of staff time to the various tasks.

*What kinds of housing and how many units of each are available from the following sources*? The first step is to learn about the full range of institutional resources that are available to provide housing. These resources include:

- Public housing authorities
- HUD-financed housing for low-income people
- Human service programs that operate housing by themselves or in conjunction with housing developers and managers
- Low-income housing units enrolled in the HUD Section 8 program (project-based certificates) or that accept HUD Section 8 payments (tenant-based certificates)
- Housing providers in the community affiliated with charitable activities, such as churches or local charities
- Housing providers that are free-standing but dedicated to low-income units.

Each of these agencies or organizations should be contacted directly, and working relationships should be established with each of them, so that continuous updating can be maintained to respond to guests' housing needs.

What does the private housing market have to offer? The first step should include a thorough review of the private market to help establish reasonable housing prices and rents for the area. Ask the following questions (real estate brokers, local planning commission members, board members of human service agencies and charitable organizations, and local landlords are good sources of information):

- Where in the community are the low-rent units located?
- Which units are located in neighborhoods that are relatively quiet, free of crime, with public transportation located nearby?
- Which public agencies and landlords are looking to sell or rent?

Many property owners are interested in turning over their property either in ownership or in management. Looking for these owners may lead either the property owner or the shelter itself to become interested in developing housing for shelter guests—you will be surprised; it happens naturally! For example, as it investigated the need for housing for its program participants, a Boston-based, federally financed demonstration grant program to stabilize homeless alcoholics and drug addicts ended up taking action on its own to create separate alcohol-free living areas in shelters and to stimulate development of Oxford House-type residential facilities.

*Evaluate the quality of the identified housing stock.* As the housing resources are identified, the following questions need to be asked about the facilities themselves:

1. *Facility configuration.* Is the facility configured for independent apartment (regular) living or for congregate (SRO/specialty) living? How much space and privacy is provided for residents? How secure is the perimeter? How safe for fire protection and exiting requirements? How clean is the facility? How serviceable are the utilities? How well is the building maintained?

2. *Policies on accepting residents.* What are the facility's requirements to accept shelter guests? Who is welcome, and how are they expected to behave? How much diversity/homogeneity is present among the residents? How much of the operation of the facility is left to the residents themselves? How much of the operation is left to the management?

3. *House rules.* Are house rules simple and straightforward (no fighting, no threats, pay rent on time, participate in the house's activities) or are they intricate and demanding? If the latter, to what purpose? Do rules emphasize peer-operated housing, or professionally managed housing? If the former, how is supervision of the premises managed and by whom? If the latter, what are the characteristics of the manager? How well are the rules administered and enforced?

4. *House policy on use of alcohol and other drugs.* Is the facility operated as an alcohol- and other drug-free (ADF) house? Would the landlord be willing to convert to this kind of use? What are the policies on the administration and use of psychotropic medication? Would the landlord be willing to negotiate a new policy if the current policy is not appropriate?

5. *On-site house management.* What is on-site house management like? What are the working relationships with other human services agencies? With public safety agencies such as the police and fire department? With neighbors?

House managers shape the character of the residence—its ability to minimize conflicts among residents and to maximize participation in maintaining the house. In the increasingly popular forms of alcohol- and drug-free housing, house managers provide a critical linkage to treatment programs and other services.

Thus, the SRO manager is far more than a neutral, faceless individual. Effective house managers keep tabs on their tenants, usually to make sure they are all right, to provide help as needed, and to enforce house rules. The most important characteristics of the "good manager" are that they are people of strong personal integrity, they are fair, they like people as individuals, and they have some wisdom and experience in dealing with people. Finding a good SRO means finding a good SRO operator. "Mrs. McGillicuddy's Boarding House" is likely to be known first for Mrs. McGillicuddy, second for the meals and upkeep, and third for the comfort of the rooms that are let.

## Assisting Shelter Guests to Gain and Maintain Housing

Assisting shelter guests to gain access to housing is primarily a matter of matching individual's needs to available housing resources. As the foregoing discussion suggests, this "matching" involves linking a wide variety of individuals to a broad range of housing types. Ideally, the matching process is something that occurs naturally, through the marketplace juxtaposition of the individual's desires for housing with the housing that is available to match the individual's desire. In the marketplace system, the individual knows what housing he or she wants or needs. The individual has the resources to gain access to the housing. A housing stock is available to satisfy that desire at a price the individual can afford. Ideally, our free-market, individual-enterprise system should work for the homeless as it is supposed to work for everyone.

This free-market system does not magically work all by itself and it has not worked well for the homeless. First, the housing is not sufficiently available in the first place. Second, many homeless individuals who are poorly equipped to make their choices independently are not given the support they need to make choices. These individuals are in an extremely difficult position: they are ill or disabled; they are poorly educated about the choices available to them; or they have little or no money even if they do not have overwhelming personal problems.

Shelter workers are in a position to help provide the supports that are missing in the housing market. Many of the homeless persons' difficulties in gaining access to housing are "structural" in nature—that is, they are based on regulations, policies, and large-scale trends that can be influenced only by organizing and advocacy. Other difficulties occur at the individual level and can be reduced through case management, personal support, and referrals to alcohol, drug, or mental health services. Shelter workers can provide assistance at both levels.

### Keep in Touch

Program supports are likely to be needed after the person has relocated to appropriate housing. The shelter program and its workers should anticipate a continuing relationship with the homeless person and his or her landlord for an indefinite period to make sure that the person successfully is settled in the new lodging. One of three results will be observed:

1. Residents who are not able to follow the few rules required in the supportive housing environment will leave. Many will clearly need institutionalization in more secure environments, and their stay in the house may facilitate their institu-

---

*Panel 8–5*

**The Shelter Housing Specialist: A New Occupational Role**

Looking for housing is *very* labor intensive; housing specialists must travel throughout the local area looking for housing and then negotiate with clients to identify acceptable placements. The specialist has to have a background in the community and be able to cope with clients (and their problems). In order to preserve their opportunities, housing specialists should be prepared to help landlords resolve problems with clients who are placed with them. Successful housing specialists tend to be persistent and to have a "politician's personality," prizing ambiguity and negotiation.

The following are some occupational "tricks of the trade."

1. Know about Social Security, Veterans' Benefits, welfare (GR), and the AFDC system. You need to be able to help the shelter guest get benefits, veterans' pensions, SSI, and to check on their continuation.

2. Learn what kind of housing subsidies are available.

3. In order to find apartments, walk the streets, talk to those with experience, get to know landlords. Get lists of rooming houses; be sure to visit sites before referring guests.

4. Maintain good relations with landlords. A housing coordinator simply will not be able to find housing for shelter guests if he or she does not know landlords and is not trusted by them.

5. Be prepared for stress and learn to relax.

6. Be able to identify clients who are adequately stabilized. For most, you will need to find a structured program. It is important to accumulate knowledge about service agencies that provide such programs.

7. Provide only the help that is needed. For most clients, this means helping the client to make an informed choice about housing options and helping them to secure economic resources. Shelter guests may be put off if they feel that they are being patronized, that they are not being listened to, or that they are being offered something that is not appropriate for them.

---

tionalization (see below). Some of these residents may cycle through the supportive residence several times before moving on to the next stage.

2. Some residents will eventually become capable of more independent living, though they will not become completely self-sufficient and will not move out of the house. These residents will stay indefinitely, needing fewer social, health, and psychological services. However, they continue to benefit greatly from the supportive structure of the residence.

---

*Panel 8–5* (Continued)

On the other hand, guests are likely to be grateful if they are given the resources they need to accomplish their own ends.

8. Listen carefully and be responsive.

9. The shelter worker must make a determination: What housing does the guest need? What can the guest do for him- or herself? What can I do to help that happen?

Much of what is needed is simply practical assistance, such as freeing up the guest's time and providing transportation. Examples of such supports include:

- Child-care and baby-sitting while house-hunting
- Shower and clean clothes
- Protection for personal belongings
- Telephone answering/messages to follow-up housing leads
- Rental listings and other leads
- Transportation (subway/bus tokens)

Sometimes more personal attention is needed, both to provide support directly and to put the guest in touch with others who also are looking:

- Help the guest review listings and learn to house-hunt.
- Introduce the guest to potential roommates or to others who know of accessible housing units.

- Accompany the guest to provide practical and moral support.

Sometimes the guest needs assistance in qualifying for benefits (VA, welfare, SSI) that can help pay the rent; or the person may be capable of working. If the shelter guest has great difficulty obtaining these benefits, you may need to work with a case manager who specializes in benefit acquisition. Try to (1) assist with the benefits qualification process; (2) identify spot jobs or enlist the guest in a work program to which the shelter has access; and (3) secure a representative payee for benefits to assure that benefits are spent on housing.

Sometimes (often) the guest needs treatment for health, mental health, alcohol, and other drug problems prior to or simultaneously while seeking housing:

- Assist the entry of the guest into a treatment or recovery program.
- Direct the guest to a separate area in the shelter for people who are waiting to be admitted to a treatment/recovery program.
- Assist the entry of the guest into alcohol- and drug-free housing or into a sheltered living facility for the mentally ill.

*Note*: We are grateful for the comments of Paul McGerigle.

---

3. Some residents, hopefully most, will move to conventional housing and will live conventional lives as independent individuals or as participants in families and other committed relationships.

In any case, the need for careful evaluation and matching of shelter guests to housing opportunities should not be used as an excuse for delay. Many of the personal problems that impair independent living should be lessened immensely by a move to safe, secure, and comfortable housing. Although the process may have to be repeated several times, the best way to orient homeless persons to living outside of the shelter system is to make it happen!

## Advocating for More and Better Housing for Homeless People

Some shelter workers may be more interested in working on the housing shortfall at a structural level than at a personal level. Housing advocacy offers an outlet for these workers' energies. In every community, an enormous amount of work needs to be done in several areas to increase the supply of housing available to homeless people:

*Work to create alcohol- and drug-free (ADF) long-term housing for homeless people who are recovering from alcohol and drug problems.* Alcohol and other drug recovery programs are rapidly discovering that long-term ADF housing is an essential program element for services to homeless people with alcohol and drug problems, and the effectiveness of the housing for recovery speaks for itself (Curtiss et al., 1991). Development of ADF housing according to the Oxford House concept is inexpensive and simple, since it is based on rental of regular family homes. Such support as modest financial sponsorship or making housing available for Oxford Homes are strategies for the creation of ADF housing. Participating in formal housing development projects dedicated to ADF uses is another.

*Encourage partnerships between housing providers and service providers to establish specialized housing for low-income people.* A variety of special needs must be met among the homeless—women with children, adolescents, various ethnic groups, older people, mentally ill people, people with alcohol and drug problems, and others. Service programs and housing advocates working together can create partnerships, joint ventures, turnkey projects, mixed-use projects, and other arrangements to create stable, long-term housing opportunities. Shelter programs can provide meeting grounds for bringing these groups together.

*Undertake fund-raising and grant-writing to develop housing projects.* HUD, many states, and an increasing number of foundations have capital programs to support the acquisition, remodeling, and new construction of residences for homeless people. Help is needed in identifying sources of funds, conducting background research, working on the proposal design, and writing proposals.

*Lobby for increased housing benefits for homeless people.* The "marketplace" solution to housing for low-income people is to bring housing within low-income people's financial reach. This can be accomplished through a combination of subsidies for the housing and cash payments (or other income-providing help) to the individual. To those who complain that this kind of policy encourages homelessness or poverty, one may point out that the great bulk of America's middle-class home-owners are given large subsidies every year by the Internal Revenue Service for the deduction of mortgage interest payments.

*Obtain donations of housing and related items for programs serving low-income people.* Housing may be available almost for the asking in some economically depressed communities. Estates may give houses to local philanthropies dedicated to moving homeless people into safe, indefinite-stay housing. Programs can be developed that donate furniture and other household items (e.g., Shelter Partnership, Los

---

*Panel 8–6*

## The McNay House: An Alcohol-Free Living Center

Programs for homeless alcoholics often rely on self-help efforts by guests themselves. McNay House in Los Angeles is an Alcohol-Free Living Center managed by a nonprofit agency (People in Progress [P.I.P.]) (Homelessness Information Exchange [HIE], 1988). It provides a supportive environment for homeless alcoholic men who have been sober for at least 3 months, display motivation for improvement, have only a low income, and are compliant with the rules. A house resident manages the program, coordinating activities, orienting new residents, and reporting any problems to P.I.P. P.I.P. staff visit the AFLCs weekly to check on program operations. Since the rent is relatively high, regular employment is needed to remain in the program.

### McNay House Rules (Grounds for Immediate Eviction)

1. Abstinence from alcohol and mind-altering chemicals will be maintained at all times, both on and off the premises.

2. Guests of residents are prohibited from bringing and/or consuming alcohol and/or mind-altering chemicals.

3. Each resident is responsible for his or her payment of rent on a timely basis. If rent becomes two weeks delinquent, it is grounds for eviction.

4. Residents are responsible for their own purchase and preparation of food, cleanup duties, and personal hygiene.

5. Residents will participate in shared household duties as determined by the resident group and/or the house manager.

6. Fighting and/or verbal abuse between residents, residents and neighbors, guests, and/or staff is prohibited.

7. Theft and/or willful destruction of the property of others are grounds for eviction.

---

Angeles). Local philanthropies may be interested in helping to support these projects. Pine Street Inn in Boston found that after circulating in the community for some time, the word will begin to spread and donations will begin to come in.

*Work to overcome community barriers to location of housing for very low-income people in residentially zoned areas.* The Fair Housing Act Amendments of 1988 make it absolutely clear that low-income people may live in any part of the community-zoned as a "residential" area (with the possible exception of persons who are active users of alcohol and illegal drugs). Many communities persist in denying accommodation through exclusionary zoning practices and other devices, although well-managed housing for low-income people has proven time after time to be an asset to a neighborhood. The best strategy is simply to exercise one's right to move in and then simply become a good neighbor; any furor usually dies down quickly as fears of problems go unrealized. Shelters can help by establishing in-house programs which prequalify guests for moving to permanent housing.

*Panel 8–7*

## Insurance Companies' Housing Efforts

The insurance industry's Center for Corporate Public Involvement has encouraged member companies to play a significant role in developing housing for the homeless.

Central Life Assurance Company employees formed ACTION, a grassroots volunteer group to assist the homeless, in the summer of 1988. The group, which receives donations of time and services from the parent company, raised significant funds through a walk-a-thon for the Des Moines, Iowa, chapter of Habitat for Humanity and for a city shelter.

The New England (a life insurance company) has set a goal for itself to raise $3 million for the creation of 196 single-room occupancy (SRO) units in Boston, Massachusetts. In cooperation with a real estate investment firm and the local Pine Street Inn shelter, New England Life is devising a housing development plan that will allow private investors to make profits through federal tax credits.

(Panel text reprinted from *Council Communique*, The Interagency Council on the Homeless, August/September 1990.)

*Panel 8–8*

## An "Adopt a Room" Program

A group should follow these steps to Adopt A Room:

1. An adopting group chooses the type of room to adopt, fills out the Adoption Form in this brochure, and mails the form to the Interfaith Assembly on Homelessness and Housing (IAHH).

2. IAHH will place the group on its Adoption Waiting List.

3. IAHH will pair groups on the Waiting List with housing for the homeless built by nonprofit developers.

4. Three to six months' time may elapse between the initial commitment to adopt and the actual furnishing of a room. Adopting groups can use this period to raise funds from their membership or acquire high-quality used furniture.

5. IAHH will send the adopting group a description of the room and the furnishings that need to be acquired. IAHH can arrange a tour of the room. Suggestions on when and how to acquire the furnishings will also be made.

6. When the adoption project is almost complete, IAHH will schedule a day for the adopting groups and other volunteers to deliver the furniture and decorate the rooms.

7. IAHH will also facilitate direct cash contributions in lieu of furniture purchases from individuals, corporations, foundations, and congregations.

8. The room adopters can join with the developers and the new tenants to celebrate the grand opening of the new housing.

(Panel text reprinted from "Adopt-A-Room," Interfaith Assembly on Homelessness and Housing, One Lincoln Plaza, Suite 308, Boston, MA 02111.)

## CONCLUSIONS

In conclusion, shelter workers can do much to recognize that the creation of access to housing is a major part of solutions to the problems of homelessness. Shelters should seek to become so adept at assisting guests to gain access to housing, and to become so effective at generating access to housing, that eventually the shelters will put themselves out of business.

# Responding to Homelessness

Popular conceptions of homeless persons are often vivid, usually poignant, but rarely adequate. An outstretched hand at a subway entrance, an elderly woman pushing an overloaded cart, a bottle gang of disheveled alcoholics, a young family despairing in a motel room—all are images that represent part of the homelessness problem, but none captures fully the experiences or feelings of those who become homeless.

Helping persons who are homeless requires both a broader understanding and a more focused knowledge of intersecting systemic and personal problems and of multiple methods of response. Such understanding develops naturally, but only partially, with experience; but it includes more practical information and a wider sense of vision than purely academic knowledge.

So we have combined our review of academic research with more detailed clinical information and broader policy analysis. When we apply these diverse perspectives, we can better appreciate how difficult the problems of the homeless are and how many avenues are available for response.

## INTRODUCTION

The equation introduced in Chapter 1 explained homelessness as a product of variation in four factors: poverty, unaffordable housing, deficient social services and supports, and personal disability. Each chapter has focused on those aspects of these problems that can be ameliorated by service delivery personnel. We have also pointed out how these problems are compounded by their interrelations.

Some of these interrelations can be viewed as a downward spiral of effects: for example, deficiencies in social supports increase the risk of mental and physical illness; severe and persistent illness increases the risk of poverty; inability to afford housing leads to difficulties in maintaining social supports and in securing social services.

Some interrelations among the factors causing homelessness invert otherwise beneficent influences. Social supports may lose much of their positive influence on health and well-being: "Homelessness represents a condition so devastating that personal ties are almost ineffectual" (LaGory et al., 1990:99). Efforts to maintain social supports may lead to self-destructive rather than self-enhancing behavior—"bottle gangs" become a means of sustaining human companionship (Bahr, 1973). Substance abuse and bizarre behavior may become useful street survival strategies (Koegel, 1991; Koegel and Burnam, 1987; Morgan, Geffner, Kiernan, and Cowles, 1985; Shandler and Shipley, 1987; Snow, Baker, Anderson, and Martin, 1986).

Discoveries such as these call into question many popular stereotypes and textbook solutions. The traumatic life histories and current experiences of homeless persons are not so easily understood. But when armed with the insights of multiple disciplines and informed about both individual and system operations, service providers will find new, more effective methods of response.

## METHODS OF RESPONSE

Homelessness can be the object of response at the individual and the system levels. The difficulties experienced by individuals that precipitate their becoming homeless and that shape their experiences while homeless can be ameliorated on a person-by-person basis. But systemic changes are needed to improve the methods of responding to the problems of homelessness as a whole and for reducing the incidence of homelessness throughout society.

### Individual Level

We have reviewed a range of possible responses to the problem of homeless individuals; these responses can be classified as emergency, supportive, therapeutic, and long-term. Each type of response is appropriate to a different type of problem.

#### Emergency Care

Service providers must be ready to respond to health care emergencies and other acute personal crises in a manner that is both sensitive and effective. For example, knowing how to aid a shelter guest who is suffering with delirium tremens is essential, but so is providing aid in a sensitive manner that can begin to build a long-term service relationship.

#### Supportive Relations

Building supportive relationships with homeless persons, and encouraging them to build supportive relations with others, can be the first step in lessening the misery and loneliness they so often experience. For some, the effort to increase supportive relationships should focus on facilitating the renewal or strengthening of ties with family members or friends. For others, the first step must be to develop a relationship with a case manager, nurse, or other shelter staff member or volunteer. Each shelter guest should have someone with whom to share problems in a nonclinical setting.

### Therapeutic Help

But therapeutic relationships are also important for the many homeless persons who experience mental illness, who struggle with substance abuse, or who are depressed about their personal circumstances. One goal of those clinicians who are establishing supportive relationships with shelter guests should be to help those who are in need of therapeutic aid to begin these critical relationships. Clinicians who establish therapeutic relationships must be flexible and understanding about the nature of therapy with homeless clients: until or unless residential stability can be restored, therapeutic gains are likely to be slow in coming and quick to dissipate. Failure to offer therapeutic help, however, is likely to mean even greater misery for many.

### Long-Term Assistance

Long-term service provision to individuals should proceed from a developmental perspective: the goal should be to increase community involvement and to decrease those health problems and resource insufficiencies that impede regular community living. In some cases, long-term plans should include regular participation in Alcoholics Anonymous or similar self-help organizations, compliance with prescriptions for psychotropic medications, or regular therapy sessions; in other cases, long-term plans may focus entirely on strategies to maintain sufficient economic resources and supportive friendships in the community.

Even when responding to the immediate problems of individuals who are homeless, a broader vision is required. Homeless individuals may be chronically without shelter; they may cycle back and forth between regular residences and street living; or they may be homeless for only a brief time. Too many individuals live on the verge of becoming homeless. Action at the individual level should recognize both the importance of lessening the likelihood of a return to homelessness and also the value of simply decreasing the time that individuals spend on the street.

## System Level

The destructive process by which persons first become homeless and then are increasingly unable to reestablish a settled existence cannot be arrested without making available the array of economic, social, and institutional resources that are required to respond to the plight of each type of homeless individual. Many of those who work with homeless persons have been in the forefront of efforts to improve the operation of service organizations, to increase resources available to homeless persons, and to change social service policies.

*Improving Efficiency*

Improving efficiency in service delivery means using available resources in a more focused fashion so that responses to the problems of each homeless person are appropriate to that person's needs and capacities. Our guidelines for assessing and referring shelter guests can improve service efficiency. Establishing a relationship with local university faculty can provide additional resources for developing an adequate assessment process. Participating in local associations or coordinating groups involving other shelters and agencies will result in more successful referral practices.

Maintaining a cordial and supportive shelter atmosphere provides a foundation for successful assessment and referral practices. A chaotic shelter environment will impair the effectiveness of service delivery personnel and give guests the message that their personal feelings are of little concern. Providing clean facilities, some personal space, basic privacy, and at least a few social opportunities should be seen as minimal requirements.

*Increasing Resources*

Insufficient resources to preserve both health and residential stability are at the heart of the homelessness problem; generating economic prosperity is the primary solution. Even during economic contractions, however, advocacy can draw greater attention to the homelessness problem and elicit greater funding for partial solutions.

Efforts to increase resources for the homeless can take many forms (Garrett and Schutt, 1990):

1. Encourage local newspapers and television stations to increase their focus on the problems of the homeless. Write letters to the editor or draft an article for the "Op Ed" section of the paper. Invite media to the shelter or agency; call the hosts of talk shows.

2. Call or write elected representatives in Congress, the state legislature, or local governance organizations. Engage politicians in dialogue about homelessness and discuss experiences with effective and ineffective policies. Get involved in election campaigns and invite candidates and elected officials to visit local shelters or agencies.

3. Put interested homeless persons to work by organizing a group to contact elected officials or the local media.

4. Be informed! Find out about funding opportunities, pending bills and legislation, technical assistance programs, and results from demonstration projects. Register with national and professional organizations that distribute material about homelessness.

5. Get in touch with a coalition for the homeless—virtually every state and many cities have them.

6. Try to stimulate the interest and active involvement of local civic organizations, social clubs, and church groups. Distribute lists of ways they can help, such as fundraising efforts, meals programs, and volunteer work.

7. Attend professional meetings and network with other service providers and administrators. Share ideas about service programs and proposals for new policies.

8. Help out when those who seek to provide low-income housing encounter community resistance. The intimate knowledge of homeless people resulting from direct service work can help to reassure and persuade those who might otherwise cry, "Not in My Back Yard!"

## Changing Social Service Policies

The phenomenon of homelessness in the late twentieth century has been shaped by three major social policies: deinstitutionalization of public psychiatric patients, destruction of low-cost housing, and decreased income supports to the poor. Without reexamination and refinement or change of these policies, large numbers of individuals will continue to be homeless.

Social policies that result in more housing and supports, less poverty and disability are the most straightforward solution. Numerous specific comprehensive proposals have been made (e.g., Bassuk, 1986b; Hope and Young, 1986; Institute of Medicine, 1988; Lamb, 1984; Torrey, 1988) and some programs have demonstrated the effectiveness of a multipronged approach (Garrett and Schutt, 1989; Levine, Lezak, and Goldman, 1986).

But fiscal and political constraints as well as historical experience suggest that comprehensive efforts will not become the norm. Historically, American welfare policy has vacillated between a preference for indoor and for outdoor relief, between reliance on the public and the private sectors, between rehabilitation through and deterrence of welfare dependence (Katz, 1986). In some respects, the increase in homelessness in the 1980s represented another swing in the policy pendulum—away from a greater preference for public indoor relief, with some rehabilitative aspects; but homelessness itself indicates the problems with the alternative approach of private outdoor relief.

In spite of repeated policy failures and confusions, it is clear that the prevalence and course of homelessness is shaped in part by explicit social policies. The research evidence seems consistent with several general policy principles (Schutt, 1990):

1. Prevention of the experience of homelessness is likely to be far less costly than responding only to the needs of those who already are homeless. Even in strictly economic terms, the costs associated with maintaining homeless persons or families often far exceed what would have been required to maintain regular residences (Kozol, 1988).

2. Homelessness refers not to one particular residential state, but to forms of residential instability, ranging from brief episodes of doubling up or shelter living to long-term street survival. It is unlikely that any set of policies can prevent all individuals and families from ever experiencing an episode of homelessness. A more realistic policy goal would be to arrest the progression of residential instability by making support services readily available when loss of a regular residence is imminent.

3. The past is not a prescription for the future. Those who are aware of the depth of the current homelessness problem may find appealing the prior era of

*Panel 9–1*

**Resources for Agencies Serving Homeless People**

Enacted on July 22, 1987, the Stewart B. McKinney Homeless Assistance Act created more than 20 different grant programs that offer assistance to protect and improve the lives and safety of homeless people. These include:

- Adult Education for the Homeless Program, which provides assistance to state educational agencies for literacy training and basic skills for homeless adults (U.S. Department of Education).
- Community Demonstration Projects for Alcohol and Drug Abuse Treatment, administered by the National Institute on Alcohol Abuse and Alcoholism.
- Community Mental Health Services Demonstration Projects (National Institute on Mental Health).
- Emergency Food and Shelter National Board Program, administered by the Federal Emergency Management Agency.
- Homeless Veterans Reintegration Projects and the Job Training for the Homeless Demonstration Program, both administered by the U.S. Department of Labor.

The McKinney Act also established the Interagency Council for the Homeless, which gives it omnibus responsibilities, such as reviewing and evaluating all federal programs assisting homeless people, recommending improvements in programs conducted by federal, state, and local agencies, providing technical assistance to eligible agencies, and disseminating information about homelessness.

Here is a partial list of McKinney Act programs and private organizations that will be useful to a shelter or agency:

National Coalition for the Homeless
105 East 22nd Street
New York, NY 10010

The National Coalition, a network of agencies dedicated to serving the homeless, is especially oriented to housing and shelter issues. Monthly newsletter: *Safety Network*.

Interagency Council for the Homeless
451 Seventh Street, S.W., Suite 10158
Washington, DC 20410-0000

The Council reviews, monitors and recommends improvements in federal assistance programs. The Council maintains regional offices and publishes a bimonthly bulletin: *Interagency Communique*.

Health Resources and Services
    Administration (HRSA)
5600 Fishers Lane, Parklawn Building,
    Room 7A-22
Rockville, MD 20857

The HRSA administers grants under the McKinney Act to public and private nonprofit agencies to support health service delivery programs, including alcohol and drug abuse, mental illness, and primary health services.

National Institute on Alcohol Abuse and
    Alcoholism
Homeless Demonstration and Evaluation
    Branch
5600 Fishers Lane, Parklawn Building
Rockville, MD 20857

The NIAAA sponsors Community Demonstration Projects focusing on alco-

*Panel 9–1*   (Continued)

hol and other drug problems among the homeless. Through the National Clearinghouse (listed below), it also disseminates information and research results from the Demonstration Projects.

National Clearinghouse for Alcohol and
Drug Information
P.O. Box 2345
Rockville, MD 20852

The Clearinghouse provides information and literature services on alcohol and other drug problems.

National Institute of Mental Health
Office of Programs for the Homeless
   Mentally Ill
5600 Fishers Lane, Parklawn Building,
   Room 11C-23
Rockville, MD 20857

The NIMH sponsors research and service demonstration projects and disseminates research findings focusing on mental illness among homeless people through:

The National Resource Center on
   Homelessness and Mental Illness
Policy Research Associates, Inc.
262 Delaware Avenue
Delmar, NY 12054

The National Resource Center offers comprehensive information and technical assistance on services and programs serving mentally ill homeless people. It publishes a quarterly newsletter: *Access.*

HUD User
U.S. Department of Housing and Urban
   Development (HUD)
P.O. Box 6091
Rockville, MD 20850

HUD administers five programs under the McKinney Act to serve the housing needs of homeless people, including the elderly, the mentally ill, the handicapped, and families with children.

Housing Assistance Council, Inc.
1025 Vermont Avenue, N.W., Suite 606
Washington, DC 20005

The Council is a nonprofit corporation dedicated to increasing the housing supply for rural, low-income populations. It offers technical assistance and seed money for eligible rural housing programs, as well as training, research, and information services.

U.S. Department of Labor
200 Constitution Avenue, N.W.
Washington, DC 20210

Under Title VII, Section 731, of the McKinney Act, the Department of Labor administers funds for job-training demonstration programs for the homeless. Grants can be applied to basic skills and literacy, job-search and counseling activities, and to job training.

Veterans Administration
810 Vermont Avenue, N.W.
Washington, DC 20420

Programs for homeless veterans are operated out of 56 VA medical centers nationwide. In 1987, the VA created two new programs: Homeless Chronically Mentally Ill Veterans Program and the Domiciliary Care for Homeless Veterans Program.

More information about McKinney and non-McKinney Act programs is available from the Interagency Council. See also Garrett and Schutt (1990) for an expanded list of organizational resources.

contained skid row neighborhoods, cubicle and SRO hotels; several prominent psychiatrists have urged a reinvigorated role for psychiatric hospitals (Lamb, 1990; Torrey, 1988; cf. Lamb, 1984). Yet the social problems generated by these earlier practices were legion; to return to them is to ignore the insights of previous generations of researchers and the problems that stimulated new policies.

4. In order to increase the returns to efforts to make improvements in any one term in the homelessness equation, efforts are needed with respect to the other terms. Effective treatment of alcoholism, for example, requires a stable residential setting that supports sober living habits (Garrett, 1989).

5. Disciplinary paradigms can limit as well as expand analytic vision; policy advice, therefore, should be sought from a variety of perspectives. For example, psychiatrists who treat chronic mental illness as a discrete state rooted in medical dysfunction (Torrey, 1988), or sociologists who view mental illness as a segment of an arbitrarily dichotomized continuum of mental health (Mirowsky and Ross, 1989), or even as a consequence of societal labeling (Goffman, 1961), see only a portion of the complex reality of mental illness.

6. Shelter staff and directors often are uncomfortable with their mission and fearful of contributing to a new "shelter industry." As a result, shelters may resist the provision of more than strictly emergency help (Schutt, 1987). Yet in addition to developing new housing, the most important step shelters can take to return their clients to housing is to make available to shelter users as broad an array of services as possible.

7. No one approach will be effective for everyone. Some research indicates that schizophrenics tend to manage better in group housing with support services. Homeless alcoholics often need substantial recovery assistance before they are ready for independent living.

8. Homelessness is a manifestation of a larger complex of interrelated social problems. Homelessness will decline in tandem with reductions in drug abuse, child abuse and neglect, and alcoholism, and with improvements in education, familial and community-based social supports, jobs, and health care. An adequate supply of affordable housing is a prerequisite for the effectiveness of any new service policies.

9. Inaction has consequences. Overrepresented among today's homeless are yesterday's abused children, untreated patients, AIDS victims, and high school dropouts.

10. Ongoing research is a necessity, not a luxury. Future policies as well as current decisions must rest on careful evaluation of the effects of every social program. Although research to date provides guidance for social policy, homelessness is far too complex a social phenomenon to presume that all the important questions have been answered.

## CONCLUSIONS

It has been more than 10 years since the upsurge of homelessness in America in the 1980s. During this time, hundreds of research projects and thousands of service providers have identified the nature of the homelessness problem and have tested the means of responding effectively to it. It has become clear that homelessness is both cause and consequence of multiple systemic and personal difficulties; but another message also emerges from these years of experience: through the creative application of effective policies and programs, the difficulties of homeless persons can be lessened and the prevalence of homelessness itself reduced.

# Appendix

## Long Island Shelter Intake

---

| Last Name | First Name | Middle Initial |
|---|---|---|

### INTRODUCTORY STATEMENT

Hello. I would like to ask you some questions about your situation, your health, and your current needs. The information you provide will be used by staff to help you; it may also be used in statistical reports on the people who come here. You will not be linked to any information that leaves the shelter. None of the identifying information you provide will be released to any person other than those responsible for the provision of shelter services. You have a right to refuse to provide this information as well as a right to refuse to answer any particular questions. Can I proceed with the questions?

In case of an emergency, may we share this information with other health care providers?

Yes: _____
                Signature

No: _____
                Signature

*Families only*

| Children's Names | Date of Birth | School |
|---|---|---|

_____

_____

_____

And can you tell me who referred you to the Long Island Shelter?

_____

**1.** What is your Social Security Number? _____ - _____ - _____

## Contact Information

**2.** Last known address _____

**3.** Person to contact in emergency

Name _____

Address _____

Phone _____

**4.** Relationship _____

**5.** Last Contact _____ / _____ / _____
                   Month               Day             Year

Comments:

## Background

**6.** Date form completed _____ / _____ / _____
                                Month             Day             Year

**7.** _____
     Last name                  First name             Middle initial

**8.** Are you a U.S. citizen? 1. Yes    2. No

**9.** How old are you? _____

**10.** Birth date _____ / _____ / _____

**11.** Birth place (state, nation) _____ (city) _____

**12.** Sex
    1. Male
    2. Female

**13.** What is your racial or ethnic background?
    1. White
    2. Black
    3. Hispanic
    4. Asian, Pacific
    5. Am. Indian, Alaskan
    6. Other (specify) _____

**14.** What is your religion?
    1. Protestant
    2. Catholic
    3. Jewish
    4. None, no preference
    _____
    5. Other (specify) _____
    6. Don't know

**15.** Do you read and write English?
    1. Speaks only
    2. Reads/Writes
    3. Neither

**16.** How many years of formal schooling have you had? _____

**17.** Any other education?
    1. GED
    2. Vocational
    3. Special school
    4. Other _____
    5. None

Comments:

## Social Support

**18.** Marital status
    1. Married _____
    2. Single _____
    3. Divorced _____
    4. Widowed _____
    5. Separated _____
    6. Living together _____

**19.** Do you have any children? 1. Yes   2. No
    1. At shelter     2. Boston     3. Elsewhere
       (Circle all that apply)

**20.** Relatives in Boston area? 1. Yes   2. No

**21.** Friends in Boston area? 1. Yes   2. No

**22.** Is there any one special person you feel you can depend on in times of special need?

    1. Yes _____

    2. No _____

Comments:

## Veteran Status

**23.** Are you a veteran?
1. Yes
2. No (go to Q30)

**24.** Years served? _____ to _____

**25.** Where discharged _____

**26.** Branch
1. Army
2. Navy
3. Air Force
4. Marines
5. Coast Guard
6. National Guard
7. Other

**27.** Discharge
1. Honorable
2. General
3. Dishonorable, bad conduct

**28.** Service disability
1. Yes \_\_\_\_\_ ?
2. No

**29.** Any veterans benefits?
1. Yes $\_\_\_\_\_ per month
2. Have applied
3. No

Comments:

## Benefits

**30.** Thinking back over the past year, how often has it been difficult for you to afford things such as food, clothing, or medical care?
1. Never or hardly ever
2. Once in a while
3. Sometimes
4. Pretty often
5. Always or almost always

**31.** Have you received any financial benefits in the past month?

| 1. Yes | *Type* | *Source* | *Office/Worker** | *Amount* |
|---|---|---|---|---|
| | \_\_\_\_\_ | _____ | _____ | _____ |
| | \_\_\_\_\_ | _____ | _____ | _____ |
| | \_\_\_\_\_ | _____ | _____ | _____ |

Write "No" if no contact

2. No

**32.** Would you like to talk to someone about benefits?
1. Yes
2. No
3. Not sure

Comments:

# Work

**33.** Are you employed now?
   1. Full-time    $ _____ per
   2. Part-time    week
   3. No          (go to Q36)

**34.** Have you worked in the past?
   1. Yes
   2. No (go to Q38)

**35.** Last date worked
   _____ / _____ / _____
     Month      Day       Year

**36.** Longest job (in last 5 years)
   _____ days
   _____ months
   _____ years

**37.** What kind of work do you usually do?
   1. Professional, technical (advanced education required)
   2. Clerical, secretarial
   3. Craftsman (skilled)
   4. Semiskilled (machine operation)
   5. Unskilled, permanent (e.g., guard)
   6. Unskilled, temporary (day labor)
   7. Migrant labor
   8. Other _____

**38.** Do you have any special job-related skills?
   1. Yes _____
                 (specify)
   2. No

**39.** Are you looking for work?
   1. Yes
   2. No

**40.** Would you like to see someone about job possibilities?
   1. Yes
   2. No
   3. Not sure

Comments:

## Residential History

**41.** Where have you usually slept in the last 6 months?
1. Own apartment/house
2. Family
3. Friend
4. Rooming house, hotel
5. Hospital
6. Jail
7. Subway, streets
8. Shelter
9. Other (specify) _____

**42.** Was that in Boston or elsewhere?
1. Boston
2. Other Massachusetts
3. Other New England
4. New York
5. Other U.S.
6. Non-U.S.

**43.** In what community was your last fixed residence? _____

**44.** When did you first use any shelter? _____ (month) _____ (year)

**45.** How long have you been without a regular place to stay?

_____ years  _____ months  _____ weeks  _____ days

**46.** How did you become homeless? (Circle all that apply.)
1. Substance abuse
2. Financial
3. Fire
4. Eviction
5. Transience (relocation)
6. Family problems
7. Emotional or nervous problems
8. Job problems
9. Other (specify) _____

**47.** Have you been physically assaulted or robbed since you have not had a place to stay?
1. Assaulted
2. Robbed
3. Both assaulted and robbed
4. No

**48.** Would you like to see someone about housing possibilities?
1. Yes
2. No
3. Not sure

Comments:

## Health Assessment

**49.** Do you have any health problems?
1. Yes
2. No (go to Q53)
3. Not sure (go to Q53)

**50.** What are those health problems? _____

_____

_____

_____

_____

**51.** Are you taking any prescribed medications?
   1. Yes          Medication          Date last taken     Need prescription filled?

   _____          _____     1. Yes   2. No

   _____          _____     1. Yes   2. No

   _____          _____     1. Yes   2. No

   2. No

**52.** Has a nurse or doctor said that you should be taking medication?
1. Yes
2. No

**53.** Have you been hospitalized for for a physical problem this year?
1. Yes—emergency only
2. Yes—emergency and overnight
3. Yes—inpatient—one day or more number of days ____
4. No (go to Q56)

**54.** When discharged (most recent)

_____ / _____ / _____
Month        Day        Year

**55.** Name of last hospital _____

**56.** Have you been seen in a health clinic this year?
1. Yes
2. No

**57.** What is the last problem you were hospitalized or seen in a clinic for?

_____

**58.** Do you have health insurance, Medicaid, or Medicare?
1. Yes
2. No
3. Not sure

**59.** Do you have a doctor?
1. Yes
2. No
3. Not sure

60. Would you like to speak to a nurse about any physical health problems?
    1. Yes
    2. No
    3. Not sure

61. Would you like to speak to a dentist about dental problems?
    1. Yes
    2. No
    3. Not sure

62. Have you ever been hospitalized for     63. When discharged? (most recent)
    an emotional or nervous problem?
    1. Yes                                     _____ / _____ / _____
    2. No (go to Q65)                            Month        Day         Year

64. Where was that? _____ (last location)

65. Have you ever received treatment at a mental health center or other facility as
    an outpatient?
    1. Yes
    2. No (go to Q68)

66. Where was that?    5. Solomon-Carter-Fuller    67. When discharged? (most
    1. Bay Cove        6. Mass Mental Health           recent)
    2. West Ros Pk     7. Hospital
    3. Dorchester      8. Other (specify)           _____ / _____ / _____
    4. Lindemann          _____             Month       Day        Year

    Therapist's name: _____

68. Would you like to speak to someone about a mental or nervous condition?
    1. Yes
    2. No
    3. Not sure

69. Do you feel you can manage all right tonight, or are you worried about hurting
    yourself or someone else?
    1. Can manage
    2. Worried about hurting
    3. Not sure

Comments:

## Substance Abuse

**70.** About how often do you drink?
   1. Daily
   2. Few times a week
   3. About once a month
   4. Less often
   5. Never (go to 74)

**71.** When did you have your last drink?

_____ / _____ / _____
   Month        Day        Year

**72.** How much did you drink then?

_____

**73.** How much do you usually drink when you drink? _____

**74.** Were you ever treated for drinking?
   1. Yes
   2. No (go to Q76)

**75** When were you last treated? _____ / _____ / _____
                                      Month      Day      Year

**76.** Do you feel you have a problem with drinking?
   1. Yes
   2. No
   3. Not sure

**77.** Would you like to see someone about an alcohol problem now?
   1. Yes
   2. No
   3. Not sure

**78.** About how often, if ever, do you use street drugs?
   1. Daily
   2. Few times a week
   3. About once a week
   4. Less often
   5. Never (go to Q82)

**79.** Which drugs are those? _____

**80.** When did you last use street drugs? _____ / _____ / _____
                                              Month      Day      Year

**81.** What were they? _____

**82.** Were you ever treated for drug use?
   1. Yes
   2. No

**83.** Would you like to see someone about a drug problem now?
   1. Yes
   2. No
   3. Not sure

Comments:

## Legal History

**84.** Do you have any legal problems at present?
1. Probation
2. Parole
3. Pending arraignment
4. Other (specify) _____
5. None

**85.** Were you ever jailed or imprisoned?
1. Jail
2. Prison
3. No

**86.** Would you like to see someone about a legal problem?
1. Yes
2. No

Comments:

## Services

**87.** What social service agencies have you dealt with recently? (Circle all that apply.)
1. Mass. Rehabilitation Commission
2. Department of Public Welfare
3. Department of Social Services
4. Social Security Administration
5. Other homeless shelters
6. Vocational rehabilitation agency
7. Veteran's Administration
8. Commission for the Blind
9. Agency for Elderly Assistance
10. Boston Housing Authority
11. Bridge
12. St. Francis House
13. Travelers' Aid
14. Salvation Army
15. BCH Social Services
16. Department of Immigration
17. Other (specify) _____
18. None

**88.** Are you still in contact with any of these agencies?
1. Yes (List and give caseworker names.)
2. No

Comments:

**89.** How have you felt about not having a regular place to stay?
 1. Distressed
 2. So-so
 3. OK

## Referrals

| *Agency* | *Office* | *Contact* | *Date of Referral* |
|---|---|---|---|
| | | | |
| | | | |
| | | | |
| | | | |
| | | | |

## Final Assessment
(Answer all questions)

| *Observations* | *Yes* | *No* |
|---|---|---|
| Extremely withdrawn | 1 | 2 |
| Depressed | 1 | 2 |
| Excessively drowsy | 1 | 2 |
| Slurred speech | 1 | 2 |
| Rambling, incoherent talking | 1 | 2 |
| Hand tremors | 1 | 2 |
| Muscle twitching/jerking | 1 | 2 |
| Irritabilitity | 1 | 2 |
| Unable to sit still | 1 | 2 |
| Under influence of alcohol | 1 | 2 |

*Impressions*                          1 = Completely    5 = Not at all

| | | | | | |
|---|---|---|---|---|---|
| A. Physical appearance | | | | | |
| Groomed | 1 | 2 | 3 | 4 | 5 |
| Clean | 1 | 2 | 3 | 4 | 5 |
| B. Mental functioning | | | | | |
| Alert | 1 | 2 | 3 | 4 | 5 |
| Oriented | 1 | 2 | 3 | 4 | 5 |
| Able to remember | 1 | 2 | 3 | 4 | 5 |

1 = Completely   5 = Not at all

C. Emotional state
    Relaxed                                 1     2     3     4     5
    Happy                                      1     2     3     4     5
    Cooperative                         1     2     3     4     5

D. Validity of respondent's answers        1     2     3     4     5

# References

Agar, M. (1973): *Ripping and Ruggin: A Formal Ethnography of Urban Heroin Addicts.* New York: Seminar Press.

Alcoholics Anonymous. (1991): *Twelve Steps and Twelve Traditions* (45th ed.). New York: AA World Services.

American Psychiatric Association (1987): *Diagnostic and Statistical Manual of Mental Disorders* (3rd ed. revised). Washington, DC: American Psychiatric Association.

Anderson, N. (1923): *The Hobo: The Sociology of the Homeless Man.* Chicago: University of Chicago Press.

Anderson, N. (1934): *Homeless in New York City.* New York: Board of Charity.

Anderson, N. (1940): *Men on the Move.* Chicago: University of Chicago Press.

Appleby, L., and Desai, P. D. (1985): Documenting the relationship between homelessness and psychiatric hospitalization. *Hospital and Community Psychiatry* 36:732–737.

Appleby, L., Slagg, N., and Desai, P. N. (1982): The urban nomad: A psychiatric problem? In *Current Psychiatric Therapies*, vol. 21, pp. 253–262. J. H. Masserman, ed. New York: Grune & Stratton.

Arce, A. A., and Vergare, M. J. (1984): Identifying and characterizing the mentally ill among the homeless. In *The Homeless Mentally Ill*, pp. 75–89, H. R. Lamb, ed. Washington, DC: American Psychiatric Association.

Arce, A. A., Tadlock, M., Vergare, M. J., and Shapiro, S. H. (1983): A psychiatric profile of street people admitted to an emergency shelter. *Hospital and Community Psychiatry* 34:812–817.

Argeriou, M., McCarty, D., and MacDonald, B. (1989): *Do-It-Yourself Sober Housing.* Paper prepared for the Stabilization Services Project, Division of Substance Abuse Services, Massachusetts Department of Public Health. Boston: Stabilization Services Project.

Atencio, A. R. (1982): *Emergency Housing in the City and County of Denver.* Denver, CO: Department of Social Services.

Bachrach, L. L. (1982): Young adult chronic patients: An analytic review of the literature. *Hospital and Community Psychiatry* 33:189–197.

Bachrach, L. L. (1984a): Asylum and chronically ill psychiatric patients. *American Journal of Psychiatry* 142:975–978.

Bachrach, L. L. (1984b): The homeless mentally ill and mental health services: An analytical review of the literature. In *The Homeless Mentally Ill*, ed. H. R. Lamb, pp. 11–53. Washington, DC: American Psychiatric Association.

Bachrach, L. L. (1986): Dimensions of disability in the chronic mentally ill. *Hospital and Community Psychiatry* 37:981–982.

Bahr, H. M. (1965): *The Homeless Man.* New York: Bureau of Applied Social Research, Columbia University.

Bahr, H. M. (1968): *Homelessness and Disaffiliation.* New York: Columbia University, Bureau of Applied Social Research.

Bahr, H. M. (1970): *Disaffiliated Man: Essays and Annotated Bibliography on Homelessness.* Toronto: University of Toronto Press.

Bahr, H. M. (1973): *Skid Row: An Introduction to Disaffiliation.* New York: Oxford University Press.

Bahr, H. M., and Caplow, T. (1968): *Old Men, Drunk and Sober*. New York: New York University Press.

Bahr, H. M., and Garrett, G. R. (1971): *Disaffiliation among Urban Women*. New York: Columbia University, Bureau of Applied Social Research.

Bahr, H. M., and Garrett, G. R. (1976): *Women Alone*. Lexington, MA: Lexington Books.

Ball, F. J., and Havassy, B. E. (1984): A survey of the problems and needs of homeless consumers of acute psychiatric services. *Hospital and Community Psychiatry* 35:917–921.

Barbieri, R., and Fricke, D. (1989): The crisis in affordable housing. *GAO Journal* 5:28–33.

Barrow, S., and Lovell, A. (1982): *Evaluation of Project Reach Out, 1981–1982*. New York: New York State Psychiatric Institute.

Barrow, S., and Lovell, A. (1983): *The Referral of Outreach Clients to Mental Health Services: Progress Report for 1982–1983*. New York: New York State Psychiatric Institute.

Barrow, S. M., Hellman, F., Lovell, A. M., Plapinger, J. D., and Struening, E. L. (1989): *Effectiveness of Programs for the Mentally Ill Homeless: Final Report*. New York: Community Support Systems Evaluation Program, New York State Psychiatric Institute.

Bassuk, E. L. (1984): The homelessness problem. *Scientific American* 251:40–45.

Bassuk, E. L., ed. (1986a): *The Mental Health Needs of Homeless Persons*. San Francisco: Jossey-Bass.

Bassuk, E. L. (1986b): Characteristics of sheltered homeless families. *American Journal of Public Health* 76:1–5.

Bassuk, E. L., and Gerson, S. (1978): Deinstitutionalization and mental health services. *Scientific American* 238:46–53.

Bassuk, E. L., and Rosenberg, L. (1988): Why does family homelessness occur? A case-control study. *American Journal of Public Health* 78:783–788.

Bassuk, E. L., Rubin, L., and Lauriat, A. (1984): Is homelessness a mental health problem? *American Journal of Psychiatry* 141:1546–1550.

Bassuk, E. L., Rubin, L., and Lauriat, A. (1988): Characteristics of sheltered homeless families. *American Journal of Public Health* 76:1097–1101.

Bassuk, E. L. (1990): Identifying and managing psychiatric disorders in homeless families. In *Community Care for Homeless Families: A Program Design Manual*, ed. Bassuk, E. L., Carman, R. W., and Weinreb, L. F. with Herzig, M. M. pp. 147–157. Washington, DC: Interagency Council on the Homeless.

Bauman, J. F. (1987): *Public Housing, Race, and Renewal*. Philadelphia: Temple University Press.

Baxter, E., and Hopper, K. (1981): *Private Lives/Public Spaces: Homeless Adults on the Streets of New York City*. New York: Community Service Society.

Baxter, E., and Hopper, K. (1984): Shelter and housing for the homeless mentally ill. In *The Homeless Mentally Ill*, ed. H. R. Lamb, pp. 109–139. Washington, DC: American Psychiatric Association.

Beier, A. L. (1985): *Masterless Men: The Vagrancy Problem in England 1560–1640*. New York: Methuen.

Bennett, T., Bock, B., Clark, T., Curran, R., Johansen, B., Mansfield, C., McInnis, B., and Provan, A. (1990): *AIDS and HIV: A Manual for Shelter and Residential Program Providers*. Boston: Massachusetts Department of Public Health and Massachusetts Shelter Providers Association.

Blumberg, L., Shipley, T., and Shandler, I. (1973): *Skid Row and its Alternatives: Research and Recommendations from Philadelphia*. Philadelphia: Temple University Press.

Blumberg, M. (1990): *AIDS: The Impact on the Criminal Justice System*. Columbus, OH: Merrill Publishing.

Bogue, D. J. (1963): *Skid Row in American Cities*. Chicago: Community and Family Study Center, University of Chicago.

Boland, K. A. (1986): *To Have a Home. . . . A Report on Maine's Homeless and At-Risk Population*. Augusta: Maine Task Force to Study Homelessness.

Breakey, W. R. (1987): Treating the homeless. *Alcohol, Health and Research World* 11:42–46, 90.

Breton, M. (1984): A drop-in program for transient women: Promoting competence through the environment. *Social Work* 29:542–546.

Brickner, P. W., and Scanlan, B. C. (1990): Health care for homeless persons: Creation and implementation of a program. In *Under the Safety Net: The Health and Social Welfare of the Homeless in the United States*. ed. P. W. Brickner, L. K. Scharer, B. A. Concanan, M. Savarese, and B. C. Scanlan, pp. 15–31. New York: Norton.

Brickner, P. W., Filardo, T., Iseman, M., Green, R., Concanan, B., and Elvey, A. (1984): Medical aspects of homelessness. In *The Homeless Mentally Ill*, ed. H. R. Lamb, pp. 243–259. Washington, DC: American Psychiatric Association.

Brickner, P. W., Scharer, L. K., Concanan, B., Elvy, A., and Savarese, M. eds. (1985): *Health Care of Homeless People*. New York: Springer Publishing.

Brickner, P. W., Scharer, L. K., Concanan, B. A., Savarese, M., and Scanlan, B. C., eds. (1990): *Under the Safety Net: The Health and Social Welfare of the Homeless in the United States*. New York: Norton.

Brown, C., MacFarlane, S., Paredes, R., and Stark, L. (1982): *The Homeless in Phoenix: Who Are They and*

*What Should Be Done?* Phoenix, AZ: South Community Mental Health Center for the Consortium for the Homeless.

Burt, M. R., and Cohen, B. (1988): *State Activities and Programs for the Homeless: A Review of Six States.* Washington, DC: The Urban Institute.

Burt, M. R., and Cohen, B. (1989): *America's Homeless: Numbers, Characteristics and Programs That Serve Them.* Washington, DC: Urban Institute Press.

Cahalan, D., Cisin, I., and Crossley, H. M. (1970): *American Drinking Practices: A National Study of Drinking Behavior and Attitudes.* New Brunswick, NJ: Rutgers Center of Alcohol Studies.

Carliner, M. S. (1987): Homelessness: A housing problem? In *The Homeless in Contemporary Society*, R. D. Bingham, R. E. Green, and S. B. White, eds. pp. 119–128. Newbury Park, CA: Sage.

Carter, W. W. (1985): *Beyond Summers Street: Homelessness in Charleston, West Virginia.* Charleston, WV: City of Charleston.

Caton, C. L. M. (1990): *Homeless in America.* New York: Oxford University Press.

Chicago Committee on Alcoholism (1955): Survey on alcoholism. *Quarterly Journal of Studies on Alcoholism* 16:619.

Church, W., Galbreath, S., and Raubeson, A. (1985): *Single Room Occupancy Development Handbook.* Los Angeles, CA: Community Redevelopment Agency.

Coalition for the Homeless. (1985): *Single Room Occupancy Hotels: Standing in the Way of the Gentry.* New York: Coalition for the Homeless.

Comfort, M., Shipley, T. E., White, K., Griffith, E. M., and Shandler, I. W. (1990): Family treatment for homeless alcohol/drug-addicted women and their preschool children. *Alcoholism Treatment Quarterly* 7(1):129–148.

Cook, H. (1910): *Report to the Social Secretary of the Municipal Lodging House for October, 1910.* New York: New York Charity Organization Society.

Cooper, M. A. (1987): The role of religious and nonprofit organizations in combating homelessness. In *The Homeless in Contemporary Society*, ed. R. D. Bingham, R. E. Green, and S. B. White. pp. 130–149. Beverly Hills: Sage.

Corrigan, E., and Anderson, S. (1984): Homeless alcoholic women on Skid Row. *American Journal of Psychiatry* 10:393–408.

Crystal, S. (1985): Health care and the homeless: Access to benefits. In *Health Care of Homeless People*, ed. P. W. Brickner, L. K. Scharer, B. Concanan, A. Elvy, and M. Savarese, pp. 279–287. New York: Springer Publishing.

Crystal, S., Ladner, S., and Towber, R. (1986): Multiple impairment patterns in the mentally ill homeless. *International Journal of Mental Health* 14:61–73.

Culver, B. F. (1933): Transient unemployed men. *Sociology and Social Research* 17:519–535.

Curtiss, J., Garrett, C., Geffner, E. I., Hughes, L., Lubran, B., Murray, P., O'Neill, J. V., Power, R., Schwartz, R., Shandler, R., White, K., and Wittman, F. (1991): *A Guide to Housing for Low-Income People Recovering from Alcohol and Other Drug Problems*, ed. F. Wittman. Rockville, MD: U.S. Department of Health and Human Services, National Institute on Alcohol Abuse and Alcoholism.

Danziger, S., and Gottschalk, P. (1985): The impact of budget cuts and economic conditions on poverty. *Journal of Policy Analysis and Management* 8:587–593.

Dennis, D. L., Gounis, K., Morrissey, J. P., and Holz, B. (1986): *The Early Development and Utilization of the Builders for Family and Youth Residential Care Center for Adults.* Albany: Bureau of Planning and Evaluation Research, New York State Office of Mental Health.

Division of Substance Abuse (1983): *Drug Use among Tenants of Single Room Occupancy (SRO) Hotels in New York City.* Albany: New York State Division of Substance Abuse.

Dockett, K. H. (1986): *Homeless Mentally Ill People: An Analysis of the Referral Network.* Washington, DC: Center for Applied Research and Urban Policy, University of the District of Columbia.

Dockett, K. H. (1989): *Street Homeless People in the District of Columbia.* Washington, DC: U.S. Department of Agriculture.

Dolbeare, C. (1983): The low income housing crisis. In *America's Housing Crisis: What Is To Be Done?*, ed. C. Hartman, pp. 29–75. Boston: Routledge & Kegan Paul.

Drake, R. E., and Adler, D. A. (1984): Shelter is not enough: Clinical work with the homeless mentally ill. In *The Homeless Mentally Ill*, ed. H. R. Lamb, pp. 141–151. Washington, DC: American Psychiatric Association.

Erickson, J., and Wilhelm, C., eds. (1986): *Housing the Homeless.* New Brunswick, NJ: Center for Urban Policy Research, Rutgers—The State University.

Fagan, R. W., and Mauss, A. (1978): Padding the revolving door: An initial assessment of the uniform alcoholism and intoxication treatment act in practice. *Social Problems* 46:232–247.

Farr, R. K., Koegel, P., and Burnam, A. (1986): *A Study of Homelessness and Mental Illness in the Skid Row Area of Los Angeles.* Los Angeles: Los Angeles County, Department of Mental Health.

Filardo, T. (1985): Chronic disease management in the homeless. In *Health Care of Homeless People*, ed. P. W. Brickner, L. K. Scharer, B. Concanan, A. Elvy, and M. Savarese, pp. 19–31. New York: Springer Publishing.

Finn, P. E. (1985): The health care system's response to the decriminalization of public drunkenness. *Journal of Studies on Alcoholism* 46:7–23.

Finn, P. E., and Sullivan, M. (1988): *Police Response to Special Populations: Handling the Mentally Ill, Public Inebriate, and the Homeless*. Washington, DC: National Institute of Justice Research in Action Series.

Fischer, P. J. (1989): Estimating the prevalence of alcohol, drug and mental health problems in the contemporary homeless population: A review of the literature. *Contemporary Drug Problems* 16: 333–390.

Fischer, P. J., and Breakey, W. R. (1987): Profile of the Baltimore homeless with alcohol problems. *Alcohol, Health and Research World* 11:36–37, 61.

Fischer, P. J., Shapiro, S., Breakey, W. R., Anthony, J. C., and Kramer, M. (1986): Mental health and social characteristics of the homeless: A survey of mission users. *American Journal of Public Health* 76: 519–524.

Fischer, P. J. Breakey, W. R., Shapiro, S., and Kramer, M. (1986): Baltimore mission users: Social networks, morbidity, and employment. *Psychosocial Rehabilitation Journal* 9:31–63.

Flynn, K. (1985): The toll of deinstitutionalization. In *Health Care of Homeless People*, ed. P. W. Brickner, L. K. Scharer, B. Concanan, A. Elvy, and M. Savarese, pp. 189–203. New York: Springer Publishing.

Flynn, R. L. (1986): *Making Room: Comprehensive Policy for the Homeless*. Boston: City of Boston.

Fodor, T. (1985): *Toward Housing the Homeless: The Single Occupancy Alternative*. Cambridge, MA: Interactive Development Planning Associates.

Fried, M. (1963): Grieving for a lost home: Psychological costs of relocation. In *The Urban Condition: People and Policy in the Metropolis*, ed. L. Duhl, pp. 151–171. New York: Basic Books.

Garrett, G. R. (1965): The migrant laborer: A sociological study. Paper presented at the annual United Good Neighbors conference, Seattle, March.

Garrett, G. R. (1970): *Drinking Behavior of Homeless Women*. New York: Columbia University, Bureau of Applied Social Research.

Garrett, G. R. (1973): Drinking on skid row: The case of the homeless woman. Paper presented at the annual meeting of the American Sociological Association, New York City, August.

Garrett, G. R. (1987): *The Homeless Alcoholic*. Paper presented at the NIAAA invited conference on the homeless with alcohol problems, Rockville, MD, April.

Garrett, G. R. (1989): Alcohol problems and homelessness: History and research. *Contemporary Drug Problems* Fall:301–332.

Garrett, G. R., and Bahr, H. M. (1973): Women on skid row. *Quarterly Journal of Studies on Alcohol* 34:1228–1243.

Garrett, G. R., and Bahr, H. M. (1974): A comparison of self-report and quantity-frequency classifications of drinking. *Quarterly Journal of Studies on Alcohol* 35:1294–1306.

Garrett, G. R., and Bahr, H. M. (1976): Family backgrounds of skid row women. *Signs: A Journal of Women in Culture and Society* 2:369–381.

Garrett, G. R., and Schutt, R. K. (1986): Homeless in the 1980s: Social services for a changing population. Paper presented at the annual meeting of the Eastern Sociological Society, New York City, April.

Garrett, G. R., and Schutt, R. K. (1987a): The homeless alcoholic: Past and present. In *Homelessness: Critical Issues for Policy and Practice*, ed. Kneerim, J., pp. 29–32. Boston: Boston Foundation.

Garrett, G. R., and Schutt, R. K. (1987b): Social services for homeless alcoholics: Assessment and response. *Alcohol, Health and Research World* 11:50–53.

Garrett, G. R., and Schutt, R. K. (1987c): Networking by the homeless alcoholic. *Alcohol, Health and Research World* 11:58–59.

Garrett, G. R., and Schutt, R. K. (1989): Homelessness in Massachusetts: Prescription and analysis. In *Homelessness in the United States: State Surveys*, ed. Jamshid A. Momeni, pp. 73–89. New York: Praeger.

Garrett, G. R., and Schutt, R. K. (1990): *Working with the Homeless* (3rd ed.). Boston: Center for Communications Media, University of Massachusetts at Boston.

Gelb, A. (1991): Measuring the drug problem. *The Atlanta Journal-The Atlanta Constitution*. February 3, C2–C3.

General Accounting Office. (1987): *Homelessness: Implementation of Food and Shelter Programs Under the McKinney Act*. U.S. General Accounting Office/RCED-88-63.

Giffen, P. (1963): *Sentencing in a Magistrate's Court*. Toronto, Ontario: Alcoholism and Drug Addiction Research Foundation.

Goetcheus, J., Gleason, M. A., Sarson, D., Bennett, T., and Wolfe, P. B. (1990): Convalescence: For those without a home—Developing respite services in protected environments. In *Under the Safety Net: The Health and Social Welfare of the Homeless in the United States*, ed. P. W. Brickner, L. K. Scharer, B. A. Concanan, M. A. Savarese, and B. C. Scanlan, pp. 169–183. New York: Norton.

Goffman, E. (1961): *Asylums: Essays on the Social Situation of Mental Patients and Other Inmates*. New York: Doubleday.

Goldfinger, S. M. (1990): Introduction: Perspectives on the homeless mentally ill. *Community Mental Health Journal* 26:387–390.

Goldfinger, S. M., and Chafetz, L. (1984): Developing a better service delivery system for the homeless mentally ill. In *The Homeless Mentally Ill*, ed. H. R. Lamb, pp. 91–108. Washington, DC: American Psychiatric Association.

Goode, E. (1989): *Drugs in American Society*, 3rd ed. New York: Knopf.

Gronfein, W. (1985): Psychotropic drugs and the origins of deinstitutionalization. *Social Problems* 32: 437–454.

Gunston, S. (1988): *The Road Back: Alcoholism and Your Health*. Boston: Positive Lifestyles.

Hammett, T. M. (1986): *AIDS in Correctional Facilities: Issues and Options*, 3rd ed. Washington, DC: National Institute of Justice, U.S. Department of Justice.

Hartman, C. W. (1986): The housing part of the homelessness problem. In *The Mental Health Needs of Homeless Persons*, ed. E. L. Bassuk, pp. 71–85. San Francisco: Jossey-Bass.

Hartman, C. W. (1967): The politics of housing. *Dissent*. November-December.

Hartman, C. W., ed. (1983): *America's Housing Crisis: What Is to Be Done?* Boston: Routledge & Kegan Paul.

Hatfield, A. B., Farrell, E., and Starr, S. (1984): The family's perspective on the homeless. In *The Homeless Mentally Ill*, ed. H. R. Lamb, pp. 279–300. Washington, DC: American Psychiatric Association.

Health and Welfare Council of Central Maryland (1985): *Where Do You Go from Nowhere*. Baltimore: Maryland Department of Human Resources.

Heckler, M. M. (1984): *Helping the Homeless: A Resource Guide*. Washington, DC: U.S. Department of Health and Human Services.

Henshaw, S. (1968): *Camp LaGuardia: A Voluntary Total Institution for Homeless Men*. New York: Columbia University, Bureau of Applied Social Research.

Heskin, A. D. (1987): Los Angeles: Innovative local approaches. In *The Homeless in Contemporary Society*, ed. R. D. Bingham, R. E. Green, and S. B. White, pp. 170–183. Beverly Hills: Sage.

Hirsch, K. (1989): *Songs from the Alley*. New York: Anchor.

Homelessness Information Exchange (HIE) (1988): *City Assistance Packet*. Washington, DC: Homelessness Information Exchange.

Hope, M., and Young, J. (1984): From back wards to back alleys: Deinstitutionalization and the homeless. *Urban and Social Change Review* 17:7–11.

Hope, M., and Young, J. (1986): *The Faces of Homelessness*. Lexington, MA: Lexington Books.

Hopper, K., and Hamberg, J. (1984): *The Making of America's Homeless: From Skid Row to New Poor, 1945–1984*. New York: Community Service Society.

Horn, J., Skinner, H. A., Wanberg, K., and Foster, F. M. (1984): *Alcohol Dependence Scales (ADS)*. Toronto: Addiction Research Foundation of Ontario.

Ille, M., Lynn, B., and Wetzel, M. (1991): *Creating Drug-Free and Alcohol-Safe Public Housing*. Paper presented at the conference on *Housing Initiatives for Homeless People with Alcohol and Other Drug Problems*, sponsored by the National Institute on Alcohol Abuse and Alcoholism, National Institute on Drug Abuse, and Interagency Council on the Homeless, in cooperation with the University of California, San Diego. San Diego: Bahia Hotel, February 28–March 2.

Institute of Medicine, Committee on Health Care for Homeless People (1988): *Homelessness, Health, and Human Needs*. Washington, DC: National Academy Press.

Jacobs, J. (1961): *Death and Life of Great American Cities*. New York: Vintage Press.

Jellinek, E. M. (1946): Phases in the drinking history of alcoholics. *Quarterly Journal of Studies on Alcohol* 7:1–88.

Jellinek, E. M. (1968): *The Disease Concept of Alcoholism*. New York: National Council on Alcoholism.

Johnson, A. K. (1988): *Homeless Shelters as a System: Community Coordination and Budgets*. Paper presented to the Homelessness Study Group, Committee for Health Services Research, Medical Care Section, American Public Health Association, Boston.

Jones, B. E., ed. (1986): *Treating the Homeless: Urban Psychiatry's Challenge*. Washington, DC: American Psychiatric Press.

Kasinitz, P. (1984): Gentrification and homelessness: The single room occupant and the inner city revival. *Urban and Social Change Review* 17:9–14.

Katz, M. B. (1986): *In the Shadow of the Poorhouse: A Social History of Welfare in America*. New York: Basic Books.

Kellermann, S. L., Halper, R. S., Hopkins, M., and Nayowith, G. B. (1985): Psychiatry and homeless-ness: Problems and programs. In *Health Care of Homeless People*, ed. P. W. Brickner, L. K. Scharer, B. Concanan, A. Elvy, and M. Savarese, pp. 179–188. New York: Springer Publishing.

Kessler, R. C., and McLeod, J. D. (1985): Social support and mental health in community samples. In *Social Support and Health*, ed. S. Cohen and S. L. Syme, pp. 219–240. New York: Academic Press.

Kinney, J., and Leaton, G. (1987): *Loosening the Grip: A Handbook of Alcohol Information*. St. Louis: Times Mirror Mosby.

Koegel, P. (1987): *Ethnographic Perspectives on Homeless and Homeless Mentally Ill Women*. Washington, DC: Public Health Service.

Koegel, P., and Burnam, M. A. (1987): Traditional and nontraditional homeless alcoholics. *Alcohol, Health and Research World* 11:28–34.

Koegel, P., and Burnam, M. A. (1992): Problems in the assessment of mental illness among the homeless: An empirical approach. In *Homelessness: The National Perspective*, ed. M. J. Robertson and M. Greenblatt, pp. 77–99. New York: Plenum Press.

Korenbaum, S. (1984): *Helping the Homeless: A Resource Guide*. Washington, DC: Department of Health and Human Services [cited as HHS].

Korenbaum, S. and Burney, G. (1987): Program planning for alcohol-free living centers. *Alcohol, Health and Research World* 11:68–73.

Kozol, J. (1988): *Rachel and Her Children: Homeless Families in America*. New York: Crown.

Ladner, S., Crystal, S., Towber, R., Callender, B., and Calhoun, J. (1986): *Project Future: Focusing, Understanding, Targeting, and Utilizing Resources for the Homeless Mentally Ill, Elderly, Youth, Substance Abusers and Employables*. New York: Human Resources Administration.

LaGory, M., Ritchey, F. J., and Mullis, J. (1990): Depression among the homeless. *Journal of Health and Social Behavior* 31:87–101.

Lamb, H. R. (1982): Young adult chronic patients: The new drifters. *Hospital and Community Psychiatry* 33:465–468.

Lamb, H. R., ed. (1984): *The Homeless Mentally Ill*. Washington, DC: American Psychiatric Association.

Lamb, H. R. (1990): Will we save the homeless mentally ill? *American Journal of Psychiatry* 147:649–651.

Lamb, H. R., and Talbott, J. A. (1986): The homeless mentally ill: The perspective of the American Psychiatric Association. *Journal of the American Medical Association* 256:498–501.

Laubach, R. (1916): Why They Are Vagrants: A Study Based Upon an Examination of One-Hundred Men. Unpublished doctoral dissertation, Columbia University.

Lettieri, D. J., Nelson, J. E., and Sayers, M. A. (eds.). (1985): *Alcoholism Treatment Assessment Research Instruments*. Rockville, MD: National Institute on Alcohol Abuse and Alcoholism.

Levine, I. S. (1984): Homelessness: Its implications for mental health policy and practice. *Psychosocial Rehabilitation Journal* 8:6–16.

Levine, I. S., and Fleming, M. (1987): *Human Resource Development: Issues in Case Management*. Washington, D.C.: Center for State Human Resource Development and Community Support and Rehabilitation Branch, National Institute of Mental Health.

Levine, I. S., Lezak, A. D., and Goldman, H. H. (1986): Community support systems for the homeless mentally ill. In *The Mental Health Needs of Homeless Persons*, ed. E. L. Bassuk, pp. 27–41. San Francisco: Jossey-Bass.

Levy, L. T., and Henley, B. (1985): Psychiatric care for the homeless: Human beings or cases. In *Health Care of Homeless People*, ed. P. W. Brickner, L. K. Scharer, B. Concanan, A. Elvy, and M. Savarese, pp. 205–219. New York: Springer Publishing.

Lipton, F. R., and Sabatini, A. (1984): Constructing support systems for homeless chronic patients. In *The Homeless Mentally Ill*, ed. H. R. Lamb, pp. 153–172. Washington, DC: American Psychiatric Association.

Lipton, F. R., Sabatini, A., and Katz, S. E. (1983): Down and out in the city: The homeless mentally ill. *Hospital and Community Psychiatry* 34:817–821.

Lipton, F. R.., Nutt, S., and Sabatini, A. (1988): Housing the homeless mentally ill: A longitudinal study of a treatment approach. *Hospital and Community Psychiatry* 39:40–45.

Long, L. A., and Jacobs, E. L. (1986): *A Curriculum for Working with the Homeless Mentally Ill*. Long Island City: LaGuardia Community College.

Mair, A. (1986): The homeless and the post-industrial city. *Political Geography Quarterly* 5:351–368.

Mandell, B. and Schram, B. (1985): *Human Services: Introduction and Intervention*. New York: Macmillan.

Mapes, L. V. (1985): Faulty food and shelter programs draw charge that nobody's home to homeless. *National Journal* 9:474–476.

Maxwell, M. A. (1984): *The Alcoholics Anonymous Experience: A Close-Up View for Professionals*. New York: McGraw-Hill.

McAdam, J. M., Brickner, P. W., Scharer, L. K., Groth, J. L., Benton, D., Kiyasu, S., and Wlodarczyk, D.

(1990): Tuberculosis in the homeless: A national perspective. In *Under the Safety Net: The Health and Social Welfare of the Homeless in the United States*, ed. P. W. Brickner, L. K. Scharer, B. A. Concanan, M. Savarese, and B. C. Scanlan, pp. 234–249. New York: Norton.

McCarty, D., Argeriou, M., Krakow, M., and Mulvey, K. (1990): Stabilization services for homeless alcoholics and drug addicts. *Alcoholism Treatment Quarterly* 7:31–46.

McCook, J. (1893): A tramp census and its revelations. *Forum* 15:753–766.

McKusick, L. (1990): *Important Information for All People About HIV Disease, Testing for HIV, Stages of HIV Disease, Therapies*. San Francisco: Center for AIDS Prevention Studies.

McLellan, A. T., Luborsky, L., Woody, G. E., and O'Brien, C. P. (1980): An improved diagnostic evaluation instrument for substance abuse patients: The Addiction Severity Index. *Journal of Nervous and Mental Disease* 168:26–33.

Mechanic, D., and Aiken, L. H. (1987): Improving the care of patients with chronic mental illness. *New England Journal of Medicine* 317:1634–1638.

Mendelson, J. H., and Mello, N. K. (1985): *Alcohol: Use and Abuse in America*. Boston: Little, Brown.

Milburn, N. (1990): Drug abuse among homeless people. In *Homelessness in the United States*, ed. J. Momeni, pp. 61–79. Westport, CT: Greenwood Press.

Milburn, N., and Booth, J. (1988): *Drug Abuse among Sheltered Homeless People*. Paper presented at the 116th annual meeting of the American Public Health Association, Boston, November.

Mirowsky, J., and Ross, C. E. (1989): *Social Causes of Psychological Distress*. New York: Aldine de Gruyter.

Morgan, R., Geffner, E. I., Kiernan, E., and Cowles, S. (1985): Alcoholism and the homeless. In *Health Care of Homeless People*, ed. P. W. Brickner, L. K. Scharer, B. Concanan, A. Elvy, and M. Savarese, pp. 131–150. New York: Springer Publishing.

Morrissey, J. P., Dennis, D. L., Gounis, K., and Barrow, S. (1985): *The Development and Utilization of the Queens Men's Shelter*. Albany: Bureau of Evaluation Research, New York State Office of Mental Health.

Morrissey, J. P., Gounis, K., Barrow, S., Struening, E. L., and Katz, S. F. (1986): Organizational barriers to serving the mentally ill homeless. In *Treating the Homeless: Urban Psychiatry's Challenge*, ed. Jones, B. E. Washington, DC: American Psychiatric Press.

Morse, G., Shields, N. M., Honneke, C., Calsyn, R. J., Burger, G. K., and Nelsen, B. (1985): *Homeless People in St. Louis: A Mental Health Program Evaluation, Field Study, and Follow-Up Investigation*. Jefferson City, MO: Minnesota Department of Mental Health.

Morse, G., Calsyn, R. J., Volker, M., Muether, R. O., and Harmann, L. (1988): *Community Services for the Homeless: Preliminary Experimental Results*. Paper presented in the symposium, *Mental Health Services for the Homeless*, 141st annual meeting of the American Psychiatric Association, May 7–13, Montreal.

Mulkern, V., and Bradley, V. J. (1986): Service utilization and service preferences of homeless persons. *Psychosocial Rehabilitation Journal* 10:23–29.

Mulkern, V., and Spence, R. (1984): *Illicit Drug Use among Homeless Persons: A Review of the Literature*. Rockville, MD: National Institute on Drug Abuse.

Multnomah County Social Services Division (1984): *The Homeless Poor*. Portland, OR: Department of Social Services.

National Institute on Alcohol Abuse and Alcoholism (NIAAA) (1983): *National Drug and Alcoholism Treatment Utilization Survey*. Rockville, MD: National Institute on Alcohol Abuse and Alcoholism.

National Institute on Drug Abuse (1990): *National Household Survey on Drug Abuse*. Rockville, MD: National Institute on Drug Abuse.

National Institute on Alcohol Abuse and Alcoholism (NIAAA) (1988): *Synopses of Community Demonstration Grant Projects for Alcohol and Drug Abuse Treatment of Homeless Individuals*. Washington, DC: National Institute on Alcohol Abuse and Alcoholism, U.S. Department of Health and Human Services.

Neuner, R., and Schultz, D. (1986): *Borrow Me a Quarter*. Anoka, MN: Minnesota Institute of Public Health.

Newton, S. P., and Duffy, C. P. (1987): Old town Portland and an oldtime problem. *Alcohol, Health and Research World* 11:62–65.

Oxford House Service Board (1988): *Oxford House Manual*. Silver Spring, MD: Oxford House Publishing.

Pahl, J. (1979): Refuges for battered women: Social provision or social movement? *Journal of Voluntary Action Research* 8:25–35.

Peele, R., Gross, B., Arons, B., and Jafri, M. (1984): The legal system and the homeless. In *The Homeless Mentally Ill*, ed. H. R. Lamb, pp. 261–278. Washington, DC: American Psychiatric Association.

Peterson, W. J. (1955): *The Culture of the Skid Road Wino*. Unpublished Master's thesis, State College of Washington.

Philadelphia Health Management Corporation (1985): *Homelessness in Philadelphia: People, Needs, Services*. Philadelphia: Philadelphia Health Management Corporation.

Phillips, M. H., Kronenfeld, D., and Jeter, V. (1986): A model of services to homeless families in shelters. In *Housing the Homeless*, ed. J. Erickson and C. Wilhelm, pp. 322–334. New Brunswick, NJ: Center for Urban Policy Research, Rutgers University.

Phoenix South Community Mental Health Center (1983): *The Homeless of Phoenix: Who Are They? And What Should be Done?* Phoenix: Phoenix South Community Mental Health Center.

Pine Street Inn (1985): *Lobby Volunteer Handbook*. Boston: Pine Street Inn.

Pittman, D. J., and Gordon, C. W. (1958): *Revolving Door: A Study of the Chronic Police Case Inebriate*. New Brunswick, NJ: Rutgers Center of Alcohol Studies Monograph Series.

President's Commission on Law Enforcement and Administration of Justice. (1967): *Task Force Report: Drunkenness*. Washington, DC: U.S. Government Printing Office.

Preston, S. H. (1984): Children and the elderly in the U.S. *Scientific American* 251:44–49.

Raba, J. M., Joseph, H., Avery, R., Torres, R. A., Kiyasu, S., Prentice, R., Staats, J. A., and Brickner, P. W. (1990): Homelessness and AIDS. In *Under the Safety Net: The Health and Social Welfare of the Homeless in the United States*, ed. P. W. Brickner, L. K. Scharer, B. A. Concanan, M. Savarese, and B. C. Scanlan, pp. 215–233. New York: Norton.

Rapp, C. (1992): The strengths model of social work: Power in the people. In *The Strengths Perspective of Case Management with Persons Suffering from Severe Mental Illness*, ed. Saleebey, D. White Plains, NY: Longman. In press.

Rainwater, L. (1967): The lessons of Pruitt-Igoe. *Public Interest*, pp. 116–126.

Redburn, F. S., and Buss, T. F. (1986): *Responding to America's Homeless: Public Policy Alternatives*. New York: Praeger.

Reyes, L. M. (1987): *Local Responses to the Needs of Homeless Mentally Ill Persons*. Washington, DC: United States Conference of Mayors.

Rice, S. A. (1918): The homeless. *The Annals of the American Academy of Political and Social Science* 77: 140–153.

Richmond, M. R. (1917): *Social Diagnosis*. New York: Russell Sage.

Ridgely, S., Goldman, H., and Talbott, J. (1986): *Young Adult Chronics*. Washington, DC: National Institute of Mental Health.

Ridgway, P. (1986): *Case Management Services for Persons Who Are Homeless and Mentally Ill: Report from an NIMH Workshop*. Boston: The Center for Psychiatric Rehabilitation, Sargent College of Allied Health Professions, Boston University.

Ridlen, S., Asamoah, Y., Edwards, H. G., and Zimmer, R. (1990): Outreach and engagement for homeless women at risk of alcoholism. *Alcoholism Treatment Quarterly* 7:99–110.

Robbins, T. (1986): New York's homeless families. In *Housing the Homeless*, ed. J. Erickson and C. Wilhelm, pp. 26–36. New Brunswick, NJ: Center for Urban Policy Research, Rutgers—The State University.

Robertson, M. J., Koegel, P., and Ferguson, L. (1989): Alcohol use and abuse among homeless adolescents in Hollywood. *Contemporary Drug Problems* 16:415–452.

Robinson, P. (1984): Personal communication, June 22, 1984. Cited in Mulkern, V. and Spence, R. (1984): *Alcohol Abuse/Alcoholism Among Homeless Persons: A Review of the Literature. Final Report*. Rockville, MD: National Institute on Alcohol Abuse and Alcoholism.

Rog, D. J. (1988): *Engaging Homeless Persons with Mental Illness into Treatment*. Alexandria, VA: National Mental Health Association.

Rog, D. J., Andranovich, G. D., and Rosenblum, S. (1987): *Intensive Case Management for Persons Who are Homeless and Mentally Ill: A Review of Community Support Program and Human Resource Development Program Efforts*. Washington, DC: Cosmos Corp.

Rooney, J. (1961): Group processes among skid row winos. *Quarterly Journal of Studies on Alcohol* 22: 444–460.

Ropers, R. H., and Boyer, R. (1987a): Homelessness as a health risk. *Alcohol, Health and Research World* 11:38–41, 89–90.

Ropers, R. H., and Boyer, R. (1987b): Perceived health status among the new urban homeless. *Alcohol, Health and Research World* 11:38–41.

Ropers, R. and Robertson, M. J. (1984): *The Inner-city Homeless of Los Angeles: An Empirical Assessment*. Los Angeles: Los Angeles Basic Shelter Project.

Rosecan, J., Spitz, H., and Gross, B. (1987): Contemporary issues in the treatment of cocaine abuse. In *Cocaine Abuse: New Directions in Treatment and Research*, ed. H. Spitz and J. Rosecan, pp. 299–323. New York: Brunner/Mazel.

Rosenheck, R., Gallup, P., Leda, C., Gorchov, L., and Errera, P. (1989): *Reaching Out across America: The Third Progress Report on the Department of Veterans Affairs Homeless Chronically Mentally Ill Veterans Program*. West Haven, CT: Northeast Program Evaluation Center, Department of Veterans Affairs Medical Center.

Rosnow, M., Shaw, T., Concord, C. S., Tucker, P., and Palmer, J. (1985): *Listening to the Homeless: A Study of Homeless Mentally Ill Persons in Milwaukee*. Milwaukee: Human Resources Triangle, Inc.

Rossi, P. H. (1988): *First out: Last in: Homelessness in America*. The 1988 Jensen American Sociological Association Lecture, annual meeting of the American Sociological Association, Atlanta.

Rossi, P. H. (1988): *Down and Out in America: The Origins of Homelessness*. Chicago: University of Chicago Press.

Rossi, P. H., and Wright, J. D. (1987): The determinants of homelessness. *Health Affairs* 6:19–32.

Rossi, P. H., Fisher, G. A., and Willis, G. (1986): *The Condition of the Homeless of Chicago*. Amherst and Chicago: Social and Demographic Research Institute, University of Massachusetts; NORC, A Social Science Research Center.

Roth, D., and Bean, G. J. (1986): New perspectives on homelessness: Findings from a statewide epidemiological study. *Hospital and Community Psychiatry* 37:712–719.

Roth, D., and Bean, J. (1987): Alcohol problems and homelessness. *Alcohol, Health and Research World* 10:14–15.

Rubington, E. (1958): The chronic drunkenness offender. *Annals of the American Academy of Political and Social Science* 315:65–72.

Rubington, E. (1968): The bottle gang. *Quarterly Journal of Studies on Alcohol* 29:943–955.

Rubington, E. (1973): *Alcohol Problems and Social Control*. Columbus, OH: Merrill Publishing.

Runck, B. (1986): *Coping with AIDS*. Rockville, MD: National Institute of Mental Health.

Sadd, S. (1985): The revolving door revisited: Public inebriates' use of medical and nonmedical detoxification services in New York City. In *The Homeless with Alcohol-Related Problems*, ed. F. D. Wittman, pp. 12–16. Rockville, MD: National Institute of Alcohol Abuse and Alcoholism.

Sadd, S., and Young, D. W. (1987): Nonmedical treatment of indigent alcoholics: A review of recent research findings. *Alcohol, Health and Research World* 11:48–49.

Saltonstall, M. B. (1984): *Bridge over Troubled Waters/Runaways and Youth on the Streets of Boston: One Agency's Response*. Boston: The Bridge Inc.

Schutt, R. K. (1986): *Organization in a Changing Environment: Unionization of Welfare Employees*. Albany: State University of New York Press.

Schutt, R. K. (1987): Shelters as organizations: Full-fledged programs or just a place to stay? In *Homelessness: Critical Issues for Policy and Practice*, ed. J. Kneerim, pp. 43–47. Boston: The Boston Foundation.

Schutt, R. K. (1988): *Homeless in Boston, 1986–1987: Change and Continuity*. Report to the Long Island Shelter, Boston.

Schutt, R. K. (1989): Objectivity and outrage. *Society* 26:14–16.

Schutt, R. K. (1990): The quantity and quality of homelessness: Research results and policy implications. *Sociological Practice Review* 1:77–87.

Schutt, R. K. (1991): Service interests of homeless persons: An assessment of three perspectives. *Journal of Sociology and Social Welfare* 18. In press.

Schutt, R. K., and Garrett, G. R. (1985): *The Long Island Shelter Interview Study: Validating Intake Procedures*. Report to City of Boston, Department of Health and Hospitals.

Schutt, R. K., and Garrett, G. R. (1986): *Homeless in Boston in 1985: The View from Long Island*. Boston: University of Massachusetts at Boston.

Schutt, R. K., and Garrett, G. R. (1987): Homelessness in three dimensions: Professors, practitioners, and politicians. *ASA Footnotes* 15 (January):8.

Schutt, R. K., and Garrett, G. R. (1988): Social background, residential experiences and health problems of the homeless. *Psychosocial Rehabilitation Journal* 12:67–70.

Schwartz, S. R. and Goldfinger, S. M. (1981): The new chronic patient: Clinical characteristics of an emerging subgroup. *Hospital and Community Psychiatry* 32:470–474.

Sebastian, J. G. (1985): Homelessness: A state of vulnerability. *Family and Community Health* 8:11–24.

Segal, S. P., and Baumohl, J. (1980): Engaging the disengaged: Proposals on madness and vagrancy. *Social Work* 25:358–365.

Segal, S. P., and Baumohl, J. (1985): News and views: The community living room. *Social Casework: The Journal of Contemporary Social Work* 66:111–116.

Selzer, M. L. (1971): The Michigan Alcoholism Screening Test: The question for a new diagnostic instrument. *American Journal of Psychiatry* 127:1653–1658.

Shandler, I. W., and Shipley, T. E., Jr. (1987): New focus for an old problem: Philadelphia's response to homelessness. *Alcohol, Health and Research World* 11:54–56.

Shelton v. Tucker, 364 U.S. 449 (1960).

Shipley, T. E., Moor, J. O., and Shandler, I. W. (1987): *Homeless Alcoholics in Philadelphia: An Update*. Unpublished manuscript, Department of Psychology, Temple University.

Snow, D. A., Baker, S. G., Anderson, L., and Martin, M. (1986): The myth of pervasive mental illness among the homeless. *Social Problems* 33:407–423.

Solarz, A. L. (1985): *An Examination of Criminal Behavior among the Homeless*. Paper presented at the annual meeting of the American Society of Criminology, San Diego.

Solarz, A. L. (1986): *Criminal Victimization among the Homeless*. Paper presented at the annual meeting of the American Society of Criminology, Atlanta.

Solenberger, A. (1911): *One Thousand Homeless Men*. New York: Russell Sage.

Solomon, C. D. (1985): *Aid to Families with Dependent Children (AFDC): Needs Standard, Payment Standards, and Maximum Benefits*. Congressional Research Service, Report No., 85–224, December 11, Table 5.

Somers, S. A., Rimel, R. W., Shmavonian, N., Waxman, C. D., Reyes, L. M., Wobido, S. L., and Brickner, P. W. (1990): Creation and evolution of a national health care for the homeless program. In *Under the Safety Net: The Health and Social Welfare of the Homeless in the United States*, ed. P. W. Brickner, L. K. Scharer, B. A. Concanan, M. Savarese, and B. C. Scanlan, pp. 56–66. New York: Norton.

Sosin, M. R., Colson, P., and Grossman, S. (1988): *Homelessness in Chicago: Poverty and Pathology, Social Institutions and Social Change*. Chicago: The Chicago Community Trust.

Spradley, J. P. (1970): *You Owe Yourself a Drunk: An Ethnography of Urban Nomads*. Boston: Little, Brown.

Stark, L. (1985): Strangers in a strange land: The chronically mentally ill homeless. *International Journal of Mental Health* 14:95–111.

Stark, L. (1987): A century of alcohol and homelessness: Demographics and stereotypes. *Alcohol, Health and Research World* 11:8–13.

Statewide Task Force on the Homeless (1985): *Final Report: Florida's Homeless, A Plan for Action*. Tallahassee: Department of Health and Rehabilitative Services, State of Florida.

Steiner, G. Y . (1966): *Social Insecurity: The Politics of Welfare*. Chicago: Rand McNally.

Stoil, M. (1987): Salvation and sobriety. *Alcohol, Health and Research World* 11:14–17.

Stoner, M. R. (1983): The plight of homeless women. *Social Service Review* 57:565–581.

Stoner, M. R. (1984): An analysis of public and private sector provisions for homeless people. *Urban and Social Change Review* 17:3–8.

Straus, R. (1946): Alcohol and the homeless man. *Quarterly Journal of Studies on Alcoholism* 7:360–404.

Sullivan, R. (1986): A consumer perspective on Saint Francis House. In *Case Management for Persons Who are Homeless and Mentally Ill: Report from an NIMH Workshop*, Ridgway, P., pp. 14–17. Boston: The Center for Psychiatric Rehabilitation, Sargent College of Allied Health Professions, Boston University.

Surber, R. W., Dwyer, E., Ryan, K. J., Goldfinger, S. M., and Kelly, J. T. (1988): Medical and psychiatric needs of the homeless: A preliminary response. *Social Work* 33:116–119.

Susser, E., Goldfinger, S. M., and White, A. (1990): Some clinical approaches to the homeless mentally ill. *Community Mental Health Journal* 26:459–476.

Sutherland, E. H., and Locke, H. J. (1936): *Twenty Thousand Homeless Men: A Study of Unemployed Men in Chicago Shelters*. Chicago: Lippincott.

Terry, R. (1986): *Journal Notes*. Boston: University of Massachusetts at Boston, unpublished manuscript.

Tessler, R. C., and Dennis, D. L. (1989): *A Synthesis of NIMH-Funded Research Concerning Persons Who Are Homeless and Mentally Ill*. Washington, DC: Program for the Homeless Mentally Ill, Division of Education and Service Systems Liaison, National Institute of Mental Health.

Toff, G. E. (1988): *Results from a Survey on State Initiatives on Behalf of Persons Who are Homeless*. Washington, DC: Intergovernmental Health Policy Project, George Washington University.

Torrey, E. F. (1988): *Nowhere to Go: The Tragic Odyssey of the Homeless Mentally Ill*. New York: Harper & Row.

Tucker, W. (1990): *The Excluded Americans: Homelessness and Housing Policies*. Washington, DC: Regnery Gateway.

Turner, J. C., and Shifren, I. (1979): Community support systems: How comprehensive? In *New Directions for Mental Health*, ed. H. R. Lamb, vol. 2, pp. 1–13. San Francisco: Jossey-Bass.

U.S. Conference of Mayors (1987): *Local Responses to the Needs of Homeless Mentally Ill Persons*. Bethesda, MD: National Institute of Mental Health, May, 1987.

U.S. Department of Housing and Urban Development (HUD) (1984): *A Report to the Secretary on the Homeless and Emergency Shelters*. Washington, DC: Office of Policy Development and Research, U.S. Department of Housing and Urban Development.

U.S. Department of Housing and Urban Development (HUD) (1989): *A Report on the 1988 National Survey of Shelters for the Homeless*. Washington, DC: Office of Policy Development and Research, U.S. Department of Housing and Urban Development.

Vaillant, G. E. (1983): *The Natural History of Alcoholism*. Cambridge: Harvard University Press.

Vernez, G., Burnam, A., McGlynn, E. A., Trude, S., and Mittman, B. S. (1988): *Review of California's Program for the Homeless Mentally Disabled*. Santa Monica: RAND.

White, A. (1988): Triple-trouble: Homelessness, substance abuse and mental illness. *Community Psychiatrist* 3:7–8.

Winters, W., and Venturelli, P. (1987): *Drugs and Society*. Boston: Jones and Bartlett.

Wiseman, J. (1970): *Stations of the Lost: The Treatment of Skid Row Alcoholics*. Englewood Cliffs, NJ: Prentice Hall.

Wittman, F. D., and Madden, P. (1988): *Alcohol Recovery Programs for Homeless People: A Survey of Current Programs in the U.S.* (Report prepared for the NIAAA.) Berkeley: Prevention Research Center, Pacific Institute for Research and Evaluation.

Wittman, F. D. (1987): Alcohol, architecture, and homelessness. *Alcohol, Health and Research World* 11: 74–79.

Wobido, S. L., Frank, T., Merritt, M., Orlin, S., Prisco, L., Rosnow, M., and Sonde, D. (1990): Outreach. In *Under the Safety Net: The Health and Social Welfare of the Homeless in the United States*, ed. P. W. Brickner, L. K. Scharer, B. A. Concanan, M. Savarese, and B. C. Scanlan, pp. 328–339. New York: Norton.

Wolch, J., Dear, M., and Akita, A. (1988): Explaining homelessness. *Journal of the American Planning Association* 54:443–453.

Wright, J. D. (1989): *Address Unknown: The Homeless in America*. New York: Aldine de Gruyter.

Wright, J. D., and Weber, E. (1987): *Homelessness and Health*. New York: McGraw-Hill.

Wright, J. D., and Weber, E. (1988): *Homelessness and Health: A Special Report*. New York: McGraw-Hill.

Wright, J. D., Knight, J. W., Weber-Burdin, E., and Lam, J. (1987): Ailments and Alcohol: Health status among the drinking homeless. *Alcohol, Health and Research World* 11:22–27.

Wright, J. D., Weber-Burdin, E., Knight, J. W., and Lam, J. A. (1987): *The National Health Care for the Homeless Program: The First Year*. Amherst: Social and Demographic Research Institute, University of Massachusetts.

Wynne, J. (1984): *Women in San Diego: A New Perspective on Poverty and Despair in America's Finest City*. San Diego: County of San Diego Department of Health Services Alcohol Program.

# Index